Global Bioethics and Human Rights

Global Bioethics and Human Rights

Contemporary Issues

Edited by
Wanda Teays,
John-Stewart Gordon,
and Alison Dundes Renteln

ROWMAN & LITTLEFIELD
Lanham • Boulder • New York • Toronto • Plymouth, UK

Published by Rowman & Littlefield
4501 Forbes Boulevard, Suite 200, Lanham, Maryland 20706
www.rowman.com

10 Thornbury Road, Plymouth PL6 7PP, United Kingdom

British Library Cataloguing in Publication Information Available

Library of Congress Cataloging-in-Publication Data

Global bioethics and human rights : contemporary issues / edited by Wanda Teays, John-Stewart Gordon, and Alison Dundes Renteln.
     pages cm
  Includes bibliographical references and index.
  ISBN 978-1-4422-3213-6 (cloth : alk. paper) — ISBN 978-1-4422-3214-3 (pbk. : alk. paper) — ISBN 978-1-4422-3215-0 (electronic) 1. Bioethics. 2. Human rights. I. Teays, Wanda, editor of compilation.
  QH332.G5626 2014
  174.2—dc23

                                                                2013049315

∞™ The paper used in this publication meets the minimum requirements of American National Standard for Information Sciences—Permanence of Paper for Printed Library Materials, ANSI/NISO Z39.48-1992.

Printed in the United States of America

We Dedicate This Book

To Ibrahim—*Wanda*
To my family—*John*
To Paul, David, and Michael—*Alison*

Contents

Contents

Acknowledgments

We would like to thank the two reviewers whose constructive comments and suggestions helped us polish this book.

Thanks also to both philosophy editor Jon Sisk and assistant editor Benjamin Verdi for their support and encouragement, and to Elaine McGarraugh and Rowman & Littlefield's production team.

We are grateful to our contributors, whose insightful essays make this book such a valuable collection. We deeply regret the death of Bernard Gert, whose important essay on a global framework for bioethics opens this book. Thanks to his daughter and philosopher Heather Gert for adding the polishing touches at the end.

Thanks also to librarian Willow Bunu for her generous help with electronic and other resources. Her research skills made all the difference in the supplementary materials for the text.

Finally, we want to thank all of you who have come to this text. Together we can affirm the importance of a global bioethics—and one that puts human rights and justice at its core.

Introduction to the Text

Wanda Teays, John-Stewart Gordon, and Alison Dundes Renteln

The exciting field of global bioethics encompasses numerous issues of international concern. For those interested in bioethics, contemporary moral problems, and international health ethics, this book will be a welcome addition. In the twenty-first century scholars must address new challenges in moral reasoning and ethical decision making with respect to medicine, research, and health care.

This volume provides an overview of global bioethics with contributions from leading thinkers. It also offers a set of original chapters that grapple with key questions, such as: What does global bioethics mean? What should be the role of human rights and human dignity in debates about bioethics? What is the best way to approach cultural and moral conflicts related to health care and matters of life and death? And what sorts of concerns arise in relation to public health? These four sets of concerns provide the organizational structure of this volume.

This book is not meant to provide a comprehensive treatment of every topic nor complete coverage of all worldviews on the subject. The general idea, rather, is to bring together a cross section of thinkers who look at bioethics in terms of a broader context—crossing the traditional views of bioethics in the United States and continental Europe by also paying attention to the new and illuminating perspectives, such as those of Asian and African bioethics.

The range of topics along with the interdisciplinary and cross-cultural aspects of the chapters give us a window on bioethics as an international field with global concerns and transnational conflicts that need to be articulated and discussed. Bioethics is in transition to a more inclusive and global field. Its issues are not just theoretical but need also to be studied with respect to applications, particular cases, cultural considerations, and alternative frameworks that reach global expression from one country to the next.

The Western approach—previously so dominant in bioethics—can no longer be seen as inviolable—as the only way of doing bioethics (see, for example, Ryan 2004, Callahan 2009).[1] The contributions show us how to assess bioethical issues in a more global and interdisciplinary way not easily evaluated with the earlier models and presuppositions. Thanks to their insights, we gain a clearer focus on contemporary bioethical problems and tools of analysis that can be taken to a wider variety of cases and ethical issues in general. This allows us to listen to different voices and understand competing points of view. This also allows us to observe how factors such as culture, religion, social context, and politics can, or should, shape the cross-cultural dialogue. Against this new background, we are better able to examine issues, incorporate diverse points of view, and solve global problems.

Our contributors raise important questions for us to consider: Do we need a global language? Is there a way to construct a global bioethics? Do ethnic, religious, or cultural differences create a set of obstacles for an international dialogue on bioethics? The range of perspectives expressed in the chapters deepens our understanding and provides a framework to rethink moral conflicts, public policies, and professional obligations. We are then better equipped to deal with cases and decision making as bioethics finds its footing on the world stage.

WHY GLOBAL BIOETHICS?

Bioethics has become global because of four main reasons. First, globalization influences how we perceive the world. In traveling, moving, and interacting with people of other cultures, we encounter new ways of life, different worldviews, and pluralism in ethical reasoning and decision making. National boundaries aren't what they used to be. Actions taken in one area reverberate and may even transform individuals, groups, and entire societies.

Second, globalization changes decision making in both ethical and nonethical matters by highlighting interdisciplinary, intercultural, and interreligious issues. The rise of the new biotechnologies dealing with such issues as human enhancement, cloning, xenotransplants, and prolonging the human life span has far-reaching consequences. For example, human enhancement could irreversibly alter the genetics of humankind if globally applied. Some say it may undermine the very sense of being human and our understanding of human dignity. Others say there could be potentially devastating harm because we do not fully know and understand what we are doing when genetic enhancement is used to improve the human condition.

Third, the existence of contagious diseases that may lead to pandemics should make us cautious, and it warrants international cooperation in problem solving. That is why we need to develop a global action plan for emergency cases in public health. In addition, research on human subjects in the developing world and on indigenous populations is a matter of global concern. For example, there are serious questions regarding the exploitation of vulnerable groups by Western pharmaceutical companies and others undertaking clinical trials and stretching the notion of "informed" consent.

Last, we need to examine unequal treatment in the access to health care medical personnel and to other resources—and to address injustices due to violations of individual health. In addition, we cannot ignore concerns about moral status and the value placed on different cultures and traditions with regard to health care. For example, the widespread use of sex selection and the resulting "gendercide" have raised important bioethical concerns.

Respecting the various cultural traditions of other countries does not mean that a particular social practice is morally permissible. It only means that we should be sensitive to different values and, at the same time, apply a global approach—that is, human rights in bioethics—to protect individuals, minority groups, and other vulnerable populations.

One of the goals of this book is to give us tools to help analyze these tensions and help us resolve the problems we face. The selection of cases presented in the four parts of this book help us better see the range of issues that come into play in a global bioethics—making the volume a timely and valuable resource.

Among the topics our authors tackle are such pressing dilemmas as foreign health workers, HIV/AIDS, disability rights, the assessment of risk in public health settings, and the importance of systemic change to bring about change in global health inequalities. Others look at the moral conflicts when doctors and nurses participate in lethal injections and harvesting organs in capital punishment cases or when medical personnel are torn between conflicting loyalties in the ongoing war on terror.

The authors also look at the patients—such as the thousands of illegal immigrants held in detention centers struggling with inadequate health care, or the vulnerable human subjects asked to give informed consent for medical experimentation, or those coming to terms with dire prognoses in which no option looks good. Institutions and political and cultural contexts are also scrutinized, as with chapters on cultural conflicts inherent in different types of surgery, Aboriginal research protocols, and global perspectives on long-term care for the elderly.

The chapters provide a thought-provoking overview of ethical issues facing doctors and patients, researchers and practitioners, as well as individuals, families, and communities. They bring in bioethical concerns raised by human rights groups and watchdog agencies around the world. They offer insight into different ways of assessing and resolving ethical dilemmas and set out frameworks for addressing global health. In addition, the chapters show that the worldview and assumptions of one society may not easily translate to another. They also show us that our own values and assumptions may not be universally shared or applied across cultures and continents.

Consequently, we may need to reexamine our conceptual frameworks and reassess policies and methodologies (Durante 2009). In recognizing the need for an open mind in doing global bioethics, we must appreciate the differences as well as acknowledge the commonalities. Many concepts, theoretical frameworks, and concerns of bioethics are shared across different cultures, religions, and societies. In spite of shared values, however, our authors question whether there is a unified view or universal set of values that can be applied from one society to the next. That is one of the concerns debated here.

The world has become both smaller and larger. It is smaller in the sense that what occurs in places around the world can have international consequences, as the environmental disasters in Bhopal, Chernobyl, and Fukushima demonstrate—thus the need for globalization. And it is larger in the sense that cultures and religions once considered marginally important to the field of bioethics bring challenges that require new ways of thinking—thus the need for pluralism.

The chapters by Ilhan Ilkiliç on Muslim views on truth-telling in patient-doctor relations, Godfrey B. Tangwa on human rights and sexual/reproductive health in Africa, Cecilia Wee on Confucianism and killing versus letting die, and Vibhuti Patel on sex selection in India all illustrate this point. The diverse points of view included here will provide readers with a deeper and richer understanding of the new developments in the field. This book stands out as an interdisciplinary contribution ranging across ethics, philosophy, medicine, law, international relations, political science, religion, anthropology, and the history of science.

Global bioethics includes concerns once relegated to the sidelines—such as research bias; vulnerable populations; public health care; the role of race, class, disability, and gender in access to medical resources; and international collaboration on global health, incarceration, detention, and torture. These new perspectives bring important ideas that broaden our understanding of the field. Global perspectives are integral to the future of bioethics. We also need, as Lawrence O. Gostin and Ames Dhai point out, international collaboration on the pressing problems and injustices that we face.

Bioethicists recognize the importance of clarifying rights and duties in dealing with patients and policies. For example, competing interests must be balanced, such as those focused on human rights. We must also assess the role of culture and determine how concepts such as nonmaleficence, informed consent, competence, and personal autonomy should figure into our decision making. Differing interpretations may directly influence theories and policies. And long-term implications of our decisions may also warrant consideration.

Bioethics is not just a compilation of the points of view of theorists, experts, or professional organizations. Actions, decisions, regulations, and codes can have wide-ranging repercussions and spark dialogues across national and cultural boundaries. The chapters in part 2 show how human rights merit further discussion—and inclusion—as we take a wider view of the discipline. The integration of human rights into bioethics has been a key change in the field and warrants our attention (as noted, e.g., by Thomasma 1997).

Cultural considerations also have a role to play in the analysis of bioethical issues, as noted by Patricia A. Marshall's (2005) work on human rights and international health research. In the past few decades there has been a growing recognition of the impact of culture in legal proceedings and on societal norms, as shown in part 3. It is of utmost importance that we recognize the relevance of culture for bioethics and that we examine how cultural and religious factors shape the ways problems are articulated and addressed.

The diversity of ideas and perspectives in the chapters show that there is less homogeneity than previously presumed. This is evident with respect to patient rights, individual autonomy, allocation of resources, access to medical treatment, and participation in medical decision making. Where the decisions are made (home, hospital, prison, battlefield, and so on) and by whom can also merit our analysis.

Doctors and patients from different cultures or societies often have quite different interpretations of concepts that are fundamental to the discipline. There is no uniform worldview, so we must stand guard against unwarranted assumptions that result in distorted interpretations and lead to indefensible actions. This book uncovers how perceptions can differ with respect to rights and responsibilities, moral obligations, institutional structures, limits on self-determination, allocating resources, and assessing the fiduciary duties of medical caregivers.

Not all problems can be looked at abstractly and separate from the world around us. Not all concepts can be extracted from the time and place in which they arose. Many cases are shaped by the social context, and many problems are embedded in relationships, while others can be approached with a degree of detachment. Furthermore, not all theoretical models apply equally to the range of problems that we face.

We must reexamine how theories and concepts apply—or need to be modified—when the cases and contexts put the differing worldviews to the test. The task is personal, in the sense that the decisions we make may influence, even transform, a single life. The task is global, in the sense that decisions could be precedent setting and have long-term universal consequences. Finally, ethical theories play a role by laying a foundation, or groundwork, for the discussion that follows.

The terms of the inquiry, the parameters of the problem, and the criteria of assessment are shaped by the framework we use. For that reason, we have to keep the theoretical models and ethical systems in mind as we undertake a global bioethics. Having a sense of the theoretical frameworks helps guide our thinking as we examine the different cases in the four sections of this book.

THE FUTURE CHALLENGES OF GLOBAL BIOETHICS

Contemporary bioethics has become global. No longer is one country or one way of thinking such as the Western worldview setting the path for the field of bioethics. The playing field has expanded, and the players come from a much wider population than the old days when physicians and philosophy professors were at the helm. Bioethical decision making has also undergone a transformation.

In some areas of the world, paternalism still holds sway, and doctors' opinions and recommendations carry the day. In some areas, patients' rights have been strengthened or expanded to include family members or surrogate decision makers. The medical team has also evolved to include nurses, medics, psychologists, psychiatrists, or other once-peripheral medical personnel. These changes are not incidental. The boundaries of the discipline will likely expand as well, with nurses, psychologists, patients and family members, and other caregivers playing a greater role in bioethical decision making.

Here, the great challenge will be to reconcile the diverse worldviews and the different religious beliefs, values, cultures, and traditions. At first sight, it seems that global diversity makes it almost impossible to solve global bioethical problems. However, the idea of a common language in bioethics—a *lingua franca*—might help provide an international standard for conflict resolution. Many believe that a human rights approach—which provides a yardstick in fields such as international law and policy—might serve the same function for bioethics. It remains to be seen, however, if this can bridge the cultural gaps so more sensitivity is shown to bioethics issues that are international in scope.

Finally, all this is being played out on the world stage and not just within national boundaries. As a result, a global approach is essential. These new challenges obligate us to draw from a wider range of scholarship and points of view. Scholars from many disciplines have contributed valuable insights to cases, theoretical debates, and issues of policy. Bioethics has benefited from the diverse range of voices, and the global approach we recommend will continue to reshape the field.

THE STRUCTURE OF THIS BOOK

The text is divided into four parts, each starting with theoretical frameworks and then moving to a selection of contemporary issues expressed in real-world case studies. The parts are:

Part 1: Theoretical Perspectives
Part 2: Human Rights
Part 3: Culture
Part 4: Public Health

The chapters in these four sections offer sufficient depth and breadth to serve as a main text or supplementary volume for courses in bioethics, contemporary moral problems, public health ethics, medicine, medical anthropology, and related areas. It could also serve as a valuable supplementary/secondary or reference text, particularly given the diverse perspectives and range of cases included here.

The four sections work together to offer both an overview and specific applications that show how the different worldviews and values shape the practice of bioethics. They start with a consideration of theory and the framing of issues, and then show how particular applications, including specific cases, are used to see different ways the theoretical concerns reach expression or are challenged when we expand the territory on a global scale.

Part 1: The first section looks at ways the same ultimate concerns become manifest and how those concerns undergird the topics. The unit moves from theoretical discussions to explorations of the way those concepts and theories reach expression in real-world cases and how they are rethought and restructured. What will it mean to have bioethics be seen as a dialogue—an interaction—from a range of cultures that, up until now, have been marginal in bioethics? Bringing them into bioethics means it has become different from what it was in the past.

Part 2: The second section starts with the interface of global bioethics, human dignity, and human rights and proceeds to a historical overview of the issues we would confront on an international scale and the work by the United Nations on disability rights. These beginning chapters provide a useful historical background on global bioethics and human rights. The remaining chapters illustrate how human rights and human dignity undergird a range of contemporary issues—such as torture, immigration detention, lethal injection in capital punishment, and human rights and reproduction. All bring up ethical concerns on pressing international concerns.

Part 3: The third section looks at culture, bringing in global perspectives. It starts with theoretical issues, such as (1) the question of truth-telling, (2) the changing notion of "family" and "parenting," and (3) diverse worldviews with respect to surgery. We then go to concrete examples alluded to in part 1, with different topics introduced by new voices. These chapters also show how different values and worldviews are often crucial when evaluating key concepts and conflicts. Case studies range over sex selection in India, Confucian versus Western views of euthanasia, human experimentation in Nigeria, and medical research of Aboriginal peoples.

What comes to the fore is the need to examine different claims asserted in the context of global decision making. What are the different interests that should be served—or curtailed/limited? And how do we see the particular aspects of moral and cultural conflicts evolving from one time or place to the next?

Part 4: The last section focuses on public health. What sorts of injustices need our attention? And where in that do we have choices—and what values weigh into our decision making? The authors in this section explore the theoretical underpinnings of the issues and different ways of approaching moral conflicts that arise. The section starts with the ethical challenges in international health and the need to address current health inequities. Some of those are systemic and, thus, call for close scrutiny. The second chapter continues the discussion on global health and recommends a framework for international collaboration to bring about systemic change. The next chapter shifts the spotlight to the United States and the very timely question of health equity in the Affordable Care Act.

There are three cases centering on global bioethics and public health examined in part 4—all on vital concerns. Their focus is on the international phenomenon of aging and long-term care, safety and acceptable risk in public health, and in the last chapter, the intersection of bioethics and environmental catastrophes. Each one pinpoints public health concerns and raises important issues for us to examine and find ways to address.

Bringing the issues of bioethics into the world we inhabit is shown throughout the four sections of this volume. The authors show the importance of concepts and theories on both conceptual and practical levels. As a result, we note that many phenomena influence decision making: values and traditions, individual and collective worldviews, social norms, and political contexts factor into ethical decision making from one country to the next.

This volume brings in voices previously missing or marginalized in bioethics. Some raise issues that mainstream and/or Western societies have not had to face. Some call upon us to reexamine our assumptions, values, biases, and prejudices. And still others help us better see that, whereas some bioethics issues are shaped by culture, others are cross-cultural and international in scope. This global dimension leads to a greater appreciation of the importance of bioethics and the complexity of the issues that it deals with.

RESOURCES AND FURTHER READING

Resources in the field of global bioethics and human rights strengthened this text. This includes references for further reading, electronic resources, and a guide to bioethics films and documentaries ("Global Bioethics on the Screen"). An additional resource is an appendix on human rights and disability to accompany the chapter by Akiko Ito, Chief, Secretariat for the Convention on the Rights of Persons with Disabilities, DESA, United Nations. Ito provided this appendix so the reader would have access to the relevant documents on the subject.

Together these resources supplement the readings. And by highlighting ethical issues in print and on the screen, they provide other avenues for learning about global bioethics. As future references, they should be useful for faculty, students, scholars, and general readers who wish to expand the scope of what is covered in this book.

While national borders are arbitrary, most issues and concerns of bioethics are not limited to any particular region. They extend across political, religious, and other boundaries. The world has changed, as has the field of bioethics. It is our hope that this collection will encourage colleagues and students to see the extent to which bioethics has become *global* bioethics.

NOTE

1. Some contend that American scholars dominated the field at the outset (see, for example, Callahan 2009 and Campbell 1999).

REFERENCES

Callahan, D. 2009. "The Contested Terrain of American Bioethics." *Journal International de Bioéthique* 20 (4): 25–33.

Campbell, A. V. 1999. "Presidential Address: Global Bioethics—Dream or Nightmare?" *Bioethics* 13 (3–4): 183–90.

Durante, C. 2009. "Bioethics in a Pluralistic Society: Bioethical Methodology in Lieu of Moral Diversity." *Medical Health Care and Philosophy* 12:35–47.

Dwyer, J. 2003. "Teaching Global Bioethics." *Bioethics* 17 (5–6): 432–46.

Hellsten, S. K. 2008. "Global Bioethics: Utopia or Reality?" *Developing World Bioethics* 8 (2): 70–81.

Marshall, P. A. 2005. "Human Rights, Cultural Pluralism, and International Health Research." *Theoretical Medicine and Bioethics* 26 (6): 529–57.

Ryan, M. A. 2004. "Beyond a Western Bioethics?" *Theological Studies* 65:158–77.

Thomasma, D. C. 1997. "Bioethics and International Human Rights." *Journal of Law, Medicine & Ethics* 25 (4): 295–306.

I

THEORETICAL PERSPECTIVES

Introduction to Part I: Theoretical Perspectives

John-Stewart Gordon

This opening section contains original articles contributing to some major and pertinent issues of global bioethics ranging from more general topics such as global ethical frameworks and universality versus particular moralities to more specific issues such as public health concerns and different approaches to bioethics from one country to the next. The last decades have unmistakably shown that bioethics has become global by virtue of a variety of, at least, the following different reasons:

1. **Biotechnological development and problems:** Genetic engineering and enhancement (e.g., "designer babies," sex selection), gene therapy, cloning, life-prolonging interventions (e.g., end-of-life care, palliative care), and human-animal hybrids.
2. **Global bioethical problems:** Pandemic diseases (e.g., HIV), environmental issues (e.g., oil and nuclear catastrophes, climate change and global warming, biodiversity), poverty and public health inequities (e.g., access to health care and health care resources), expensive health care systems, organ transplantations ("medical tourism"), multiculturalism, female genital circumcision, different concepts of autonomy and physician-patient relationship, global research ethics (e.g., research experiments and clinical trials on human subjects, particularly, in poorer countries), and the rise of the importance of human rights in bioethics.

This situation has led to a growing global awareness in the discipline of bioethics by acknowledging the fact that different traditions, religions, and cultures give rise to diverse value systems. These can create problems for the applicability of universal norms. The global dimension and hazards of some bioethical issues such as pandemic diseases and nuclear pollution call for a common strategy in order to avoid serious harm for human beings, animals, and the environment. This, however, presupposes a so-called common standard for ethical reasoning and decision making by providing a global solution for the particular bioethical problem.

Global bioethical problems call for a global solution. The chapters in this section contribute in a meaningful way to the general purpose of the book to provide some vital insights on important perspectives on global bioethics.

The first half of the chapters in this section are concerned with more general issues on the application of universal norms and its various problems. For example, Bernard Gert and Tom L. Beauchamp both claim that there is a common morality that provides a sufficient ethical guidance in the context of differences regarding culture, religion, and tradition. However, both authors adhere to two completely distinct ethical theories, such as the ten moral rules approach (Gert) and principlism (Beauchamp).

Søren Holm, instead, argues that there is no unproblematic common language such as human rights or a set of core principles that can sufficiently solve concrete bioethical issues. This he does in the third chapter. Each of these chapters brings out key concerns when we try to reconfigure bioethics on a global scale.

Gert and Beauchamp apply their well-known ethical theories and thereby provide a superb insight of how approaches in global bioethics might look like and what vital issues are at stake. The opposite position is defended by Holm, who claims that there are irresolvable moral differences on the theoretical and practical level that undermine an easy application of universal norms.

We then turn to the ways in which bioethical concerns and conflicts reach expression—and extend across national boundaries. Scott Stonington and Pinit Ratanakul have powerfully questioned the idea that cultural differences are not adequately addressed by global bioethics that is particularly shaped by the Western perspective. They claim that the so-called Western universal values such as autonomy, beneficence, nonmaleficence, truth-telling, and justice are inadequate to solve bioethical problems—such as the case of the end-of-life decision making in Thailand—in non-Western societies.

1

A Global Ethical Framework for Bioethics

Bernard Gert[1]

ABSTRACT

Although morality is universal, it allows for some significant variations because of cultural differences. Bioethics is morality applied to medicine and medical research, so a global bioethics should be thought of as an application of the common moral system to medicine and medical research that allows for significant variations in different cultures or societies. Common morality has rules that prohibit killing, causing pain or disability, and deceiving and breaking promises, but there is some variation in the interpretation of these rules as well as in what counts as an adequate justification for violating them. Different societies also have some significant differences in their laws and in the duties that they regard physicians as having. There are also differences in whom they hold to be fully protected by the moral rules. These societal variations have significant effects on what morality encourages, prohibits, and requires physicians to do.

INTRODUCTION

Different cultures give different answers to some of the questions with which bioethics is concerned. This much seems obvious, and it has led many to conclude that there is no universal morality while leading others to conclude that where there is disagreement one of the disagreeing cultures must be mistaken. In this chapter I describe what I believe is the universal moral system and explain how its universality is consistent with limited but true moral disagreement.

To begin, I distinguish the claim that morality is universal both from the claim that it always provides a unique correct solution and from the claim that it is explicitly recognized by every (or any) culture. As with grammatical rules, the moral system is normally followed without conscious reflection.

I next present the ten moral rules that I believe constitute the core of the universal moral system. One source of moral disagreement arises from different interpretations of these rules themselves. For instance, although the rule prohibiting killing is universal, and cultures normally agree on when an action is a killing, certain actions (removing from a ventilator) may constitute killings in some cultures but not in others.

In every culture violations of the moral rules require moral justification, thus universal morality includes not only rules but also a procedure for justifying violations of these rules. I next introduce a two-step procedure for justifying violations of moral rules and consider how, using the identical procedure, members of different cultures can come to different conclusions about whether a particular violation is morally permissible.

In the last section I discuss moral disagreements arising from differences of opinion regarding who or what is fully protected by this moral system, an issue the system itself cannot resolve. In all cultures moral agents must be treated morally, but some cultures include others within morality's sphere of protection as well. And, finally, I note that, although a certain amount of disagreement is consistent with our universal morality, that morality itself puts substantial limits on the permissible ways of resolving the disagreements it sanctions.

MORALITY OR THE MORAL SYSTEM

Morality is a public system that is known by all those who are held responsible for their actions—that is, all moral agents. A public system is a system that has the following two characteristics. In normal circumstances, (1) all persons to whom it applies—that is, those whose behavior is to be guided and judged by that system, understand it—they know what behavior the system prohibits, requires, discourages, encourages, and allows; (2) it is not irrational for any of these persons to accept being guided and judged by that system.

The clearest example of a public system is a game, such as bridge or football. A game has an inherent goal and a set of rules that form a system that is understood by all of the players—they all know what kind of behavior is prohibited, required, discouraged, encouraged, and allowed by the game, and it is not irrational for all players to use the goal and the rules of the game to guide their own behavior and to judge the behavior of other players by them. Although a game is a public system, it applies only to those playing the game, and if one does not want to abide by the rules, one can quit playing the game. No one can quit being governed by morality. Morality is a public system that applies to all people that understand it and can guide their behavior accordingly. Moral agents are subject to moral judgments simply by virtue of being rational persons who are responsible for their actions.

Although there is general agreement about who is subject to moral judgment, there is considerable disagreement about who is protected by morality. Some, for example, Kant, hold that only moral agents are fully protected, whereas others, for example, Bentham, hold that all beings that can suffer pain are protected. Morality has the inherent goal of lessening the amount of harm suffered by those included in the protected group, either all moral agents or a more inclusive group.

It contains rules that prohibit some kinds of actions, for example, killing, and require other kinds, for example, keeping promises; and moral ideals that encourage certain kinds of actions, that is, relieving pain. It also contains a procedure for determining when it is justified to violate a moral rule—when a moral rule and a moral ideal conflict. Morality does not provide unique answers to every question, rather, it sets the limits to legitimate moral disagreement. It is important to realize that unresolvable moral disagreement on some important issues, for example, abortion, is compatible with total agreement in the overwhelming number of situations in which moral judgments are made.

A useful analogy to morality or the moral system is the grammar or grammatical system used by all competent speakers of a language. Almost no competent speaker can explicitly describe the grammatical system that she uses, yet all competent speakers know the grammar of their language in the sense that they use it when speaking and in interpreting the speech of others. If presented with an explicit account of the grammatical system, competent speakers have the final word on its accuracy.

They should not accept any description of the grammatical system if it rules out speaking in a way that they regard as acceptable or allows speaking in a way that they regard as completely unacceptable. Morality or the moral system requires consistency in a way that grammar does not, so moral agents should not accept any description of morality if it conflicts with the overwhelming set of their considered moral decisions or judgments that are consistent.

There is such overwhelming agreement in most moral matters that we do not even make conscious moral judgments about them, for example, causing pain to someone simply because one feels like doing it. But morality involves one's emotions and interests far more than grammar, so people sometimes make moral decisions and judgments that are inconsistent with the vast majority of their considered moral judgments because they are distorted by their emotions or interests. This has the result that sometimes even competent moral agents can be shown that some of their moral decisions or judgments are mistaken.

COMMON MORALITY[2]

When some people claim that there is a common morality, they sometimes mean that there is a universal moral system that provides a unique, correct answer to every moral question. Those who deny that there is a common morality sometimes mean that there is not a unique correct answer to any moral problem.

Not surprisingly, both of these extreme views are mistaken. To claim that there is a common morality is to claim that there is a universal moral system that provides a global framework for all acceptable moral decisions and judgments, but it does not mean that there is a unique, correct solution to every moral problem.

There are, of course, unique, correct answers to many moral questions, but these are usually moral questions than no one ever asks, for example, "Is it morally acceptable to torture someone because I enjoy seeing someone in pain?" Even in most situations in which one might be tempted to do an immoral action, no one consciously deliberates about what is the morally right thing to do, for example, keeping an important promise that it is inconvenient for one to keep. Similarly, in most situations no one consciously makes a judgment about someone who does not do a morally wrong action, say, refrains from cheating in a game.

Bioethics is a field in which people often do consciously deliberate about what is the morally right thing to do, for example, whether to perform an abortion. Physicians also sometimes consciously make judgments about someone who does not give in to the temptation to do the morally wrong action, for instance, does not give an unnecessary antibiotic to a patient who requests it. In what follows I shall provide a brief description of the common morality that provides a global framework for bioethics, but I shall also show that, even when there is complete agreement on the facts, including probabilities of future harms and benefits, there can be unresolvable differences in the decisions and judgments that people make.[3]

MORAL RULES

There is universal agreement that actions such as killing, causing pain or disability, and depriving of freedom or pleasure are immoral unless one has an adequate justification. Similarly, there is universal agreement that deceiving, breaking a promise, cheating, violating the law, and neglecting one's duties would also need justification in order not to be immoral.

When I say that all societies have moral rules that prohibit such actions, all I mean is that doing these kinds of actions are immoral unless one has an adequate justification for doing them. Although there are alternative ways of formulating the moral rules, the following is a list of moral rules that includes all of the kinds of action that need justification. Although these rules are subject to some variation in interpretation, they can be understood by all those held responsible for their actions.

1. Do not kill.
2. Do not deceive.
3. Do not cause pain.
4. Keep your promises.
5. Do not disable.
6. Do not cheat.

7. Do not deprive of freedom.
8. Obey the law.
9. Do not deprive of pleasure.
10. Do your duty.

The rule prohibiting causing pain prohibits causing not only physical pain but also mental pain; the rule prohibiting causing disabilities prohibits causing not only physical disabilities but also mental and volitional disabilities; the rule prohibiting depriving of freedom includes prohibiting depriving of opportunities and resources, and the rule prohibiting depriving of pleasure includes prohibiting depriving of future pleasure as well as present pleasure. The rule prohibiting deceiving can be broken by withholding information as well as by lying, and the rule requiring one to keep one's promises requires keeping informal agreements as well as formal contracts.

Finally, "duty," in the rule requiring one to do one's duty, is meant in its everyday sense, where duties are determined by one's social role, job or profession, or by special circumstances. Someone who takes a job is often told what duties are involved. "Duty" is not used as philosophers customarily misuse it, to mean whatever one morally ought to do. We are morally required to obey all of the moral rules unless we have an adequate justification for not doing so, but in the everyday sense of "duty" it is a misuse to say we have a duty to obey these rules—not to kill, or to do our duties.

Duties in this everyday sense are not derived from our common morality, but in each society duties develop from social roles and from the history and practice of the professions in that society. Knowing about social roles and about the practices of a field or profession in a particular society is not only necessary for understanding what duties people have in that society but it is sometimes also necessary for understanding the interpretation of the moral rules in that society.

In many societies these rules are understood to prohibit not only actual violations but also attempts to violate them, even if the attempt is unsuccessful. They are also often understood to prohibit not only intentional violations but also violations done knowingly but not intentionally. They can even be understood to prohibit some unknowing violations, if the person should have known that his action was a violation of a moral rule or that he was likely to cause harm to someone. But what it means "to cause harm to someone" is not as simple and straightforward as it initially seems. Although one can take "do not kill" to mean "do not cause death," causing death, like causing pain or disability, does not mean simply doing an intentional act that you know will result in a person's death, pain, or disability.

Consider a physician who is deciding whether to comply with a competent ventilator-dependent patient's refusal to stay on the ventilator. If the physician does decide to disconnect the patient from the ventilator, does that count as killing him or even as assisting his suicide? For most people in American society, complying with a competent patient's refusal to stay on the ventilator when one knows that disconnecting the patient from the ventilator will result in the patient's death does not count as either killing the patient or even as assisting his suicide.

This is also the legal view in this society. In every state of the United States, physicians are legally required to take a competent patient off the respirator if the patient refuses to be on it any longer, yet in every state physicians are prohibited from killing patients, even competent patients that have requested to be killed. Further, although all states require complying with a competent patient's refusal to continue on a ventilator, almost all states do not even allow physician-assisted suicide.

However, some religious people in the United States regard taking a competent patient off a respirator even if the patient refuses to be on it any longer as interfering with the will of God and hence as killing the patient, and they do not sanction it. This may also be the view of those societies in which religion has a greater influence on the interpretation of the moral rules than is the case in the United States.

Although no society denies that when physicians comply with a terminal patient's request to be given a lethal injection they are killing that patient, some more secular societies such as the Netherlands consider it morally justified for a physician to kill a patient in these circumstances. Thus, societies can differ from one another not only in their interpretation of the rule prohibiting killing, they can also differ from each other in what they consider to be morally justified cases of killing. These differences do not conflict with all societies accepting that violating the moral rule that prohibits killing needs moral justification.

Like "cause," "deprive" is also not as simple as it initially seems. "Do not deprive of freedom" does not mean simply "do not intentionally do any act that you know will have the result that someone does not have the freedom or opportunity to do something he would have had if you had not done that act." For example, in every country with automobiles and parking lots, if, in the normal course of affairs, you arrive at a parking lot before another person, you do not deprive him of the opportunity to park in that lot if you take the last parking place. You do not even need to justify parking in the last space. Further, no one in any country holds that someone who wins a race fairly has deprived the other runners of the pleasure of winning the race.

However, there may be societal differences concerning whether a teacher who grades a student's exam fairly and gives it a very bad grade has broken the rule prohibiting causing pain. Some might say that she has broken the rule but that she is justified in doing so because it is her duty to grade exams fairly, but others might say that she has not broken the rule at all. Similarly, some might claim that a physician, who tells a patient about his very poor prognosis, even if it is done in a compassionate manner, is still violating the rule against causing pain.

However, similar to what some would say about the teacher, some might claim that the physician is justified in violating the rule because it is her duty to tell her patient the truth about his prognosis, while others might claim that telling the patient the truth does not even violate the rules against causing pain and so does not need to be justified at all. But in some societies, doctors do not regard it as necessary to tell a patient the unpleasant truth in order to proceed with treatment. If the physician only has a duty to tell a member of the patient's family, she is not justified in causing pain to the patient.

Deciding whether to tell a patient bad news can also be influenced by a society's interpretation of the rule prohibiting deceiving. Although every society regards a physician lying to a patient as deceiving, one society may also regard a physician as deceiving a patient if she withholds unpleasant information about the patient's medical condition because doctors have a duty to tell their competent patients about their diagnosis and prognosis.

However, another society, which does not regard a doctor as having a duty to tell patients bad news, for example, Russia, may not regard withholding unpleasant information as deceiving at all. Given this wide variation in the interpretation of the rules, some based on the differences in the duties doctors have in that society, it may seem as if talking about a common morality, or a global framework for bioethics, is a sham. That is because we are discussing interesting cases, where there are legitimate differences in the interpretation of a moral rule. However, most cases are not interesting. In the overwhelming majority of cases, all societies agree when a given moral rule has been violated and also agree on whether the violation is justified.

DISAGREEMENTS BASED ON DIFFERENT INTERPRETATIONS OF A MORAL RULE

Different interpretations of a moral rule can lead to unresolvable moral disagreement, not only between different societies but also within a given society. I include in the category of disagreements based on different interpretations of the rules only those different interpretations that do not involve deciding who is impartially protected by the moral rules.

Even when there is no doubt that all involved are impartially protected by the moral rules, there is sometimes disagreement on what counts as breaking the rule, that is, what counts as killing or deceiving. Even people who agree that complying with a competent patient's refusal to continue on the respirator is not killing sometimes disagree on whether discontinuing food and fluids counts as killing. In addition to the disagreement about whether withholding information counts as deceiving, there is also disagreement about whether dying one's hair counts as breaking that rule.

Some of these disagreements can be resolved, but some cannot, and often some institution will have to make a decision that settles the matter for the people governed by that institution. Hospitals may adopt rules determining when it is allowed to discontinue life-sustaining treatments, and those physicians that follow those rules are not regarded as having killed their patients but only as having allowed them to die.

Because different societies have different legal systems and impose different duties on physicians, the moral rules prohibiting violating the law and neglecting one's duties will differ in the actions that they prohibit and require. For example, in the United States doctors have a duty to tell their competent patients about their diagnosis and prognosis, but in many countries in South America, Israel, and Russia, doctors may tell family members rather than the patient. A universal morality allows for significant cultural or societal variation.

Although there is overwhelming agreement on the moral status of the vast majority of actions, these kinds of actions are those about which no one consciously makes moral decisions and judgments. Normally we consciously make moral decisions and judgments only on actions about which there is some controversy. With regard to these kinds of situations, morality often does not provide a unique solution to every moral problem, even within a particular society.

Moreover, because their legal systems differ and different duties are assigned, societies may differ in the judgments that are made about particular actions even when these judgments are uncontroversial within each society. But the differences in laws and duties does not affect the universality of morality any more than the fact that people make different promises affects the universality of morality. And just as promises can sometimes be justifiably broken, so laws can sometimes be justifiably violated and duties can be justifiably not performed. Morality places significant limits on legitimate moral variation between societies as well as within societies.

MORALLY RELEVANT FEATURES AND THE TWO-STEP PROCEDURE FOR JUSTIFYING VIOLATIONS

In addition to the agreement about the kinds of actions that need moral justification, there is general agreement about the way in which violations of moral rules can be justified. There is overwhelming agreement that what counts as an adequate justification for one person must be an adequate justification for anyone else in the same situation. However, since no two situations are exactly alike in all respects, each society must have some way of determining what counts as the same situation.

When it is said that morality requires impartiality, what should be meant is that the same situation does not change simply because the identity of the persons involved in that situation changes. This does not mean that everyone must agree about whether a violation of a moral rule is justified. Impartiality does not require uniformity; impartiality is compatible with disagreement about what counts as an adequate moral justification for any particular violation, that is, killing or deceiving.

For the same reason, the judges on the Supreme Court of the United States can agree completely on the facts, be impartial, and yet still come to different conclusions. It is also important to realize that morality only requires impartiality when one is concerned with the violation of a moral rule; morality does not require impartiality when following a moral ideal, say, doing something morally good, that is, aiding the needy or relieving pain. Morality allows people to give to whatever charity they prefer; morality does not require impartiality when giving to charities.

One of the most important differences between moral rules and moral ideals is that it is possible for moral rules to be impartially obeyed all of the time. That is why, unless they have an adequate justification for not doing so, people can be required to obey the moral rules all of the time. People are only encouraged, not required, to follow the moral ideals, and no one can even favor following moral ideals all of the time because it is humanly impossible to do so. The moral rules set constraints on one's behavior regardless of what one's goals are, and it is possible for these constraints to be obeyed all of the time. The moral ideals provide goals for one's behavior, but there is a limit on how much time it is possible to spend trying to achieve these goals. Nonetheless, moral ideals express the point of morality more clearly than moral rules, for following them is directly acting to achieve the goal of morality, which is the lessening of suffering harm by all those protected by morality.

Although obeying the moral rules is required and following the moral ideals is only encouraged, when following a moral ideal conflicts with obeying a moral rule, it is sometimes justified to violate the moral rule in order to follow the moral ideal. When there is a conflict between two moral rules, or between obeying a moral rule and following a moral ideal, there is a two-step procedure for deciding what one morally ought to do.

This two-step procedure is used in all societies, though usually not consciously, to determine whether a violation of a moral rule is justified. As stated above, when we are talking about impartiality, everyone agrees that what counts as an adequate justification for one person must be an adequate justification for anyone else in the same situation. But for this statement to serve any purpose or have any force, there must be a specification of what counts as the same situation.

For the purposes of justifying a violation of a moral rule, two situations count as the same situation when all of their morally relevant features are the same. A morally relevant feature is a feature such that if it changes, it can change whether a rational person would regard that violation of a moral rule as justified. In ordinary circumstances, the day of the week, the time of the day, and the season of the year are not morally relevant features. Unless the day, time, or season is related to some other feature, a change in any of them cannot change whether a violation of a moral rule is justified.

I have compiled a list of ten questions, the answers to which are morally relevant features. I do not claim that any change in any of these features would lead a rational person to change his position concerning whether a particular violation is justified. I do claim that for a rational person who does not use any idiosyncratic beliefs, that is, beliefs that are not shared by all rational persons, only a change in these features can change whether that person regards the violation as justified.

Two violations count as being in the same circumstances, or as the same kind of violation, if all of the following questions have the same answers. The answers to these questions are the morally relevant features of the violation.

1. What kind of act is it, that is, what moral rule is it a violation of?
2. What harms are caused, avoided (not caused), and prevented?
3. What are the relevant beliefs and desires of the person harmed?
4. What is the relationship between the parties?
5. What goods are being gained?
6. Is a violation of a moral rule being prevented?

7. Is a violation of a moral rule being punished?
8. Are there alternative actions that will not violate a moral rule or cause less harm?
9. Is the action being done intentionally, or only knowingly?
10. Is the situation an emergency?

When serving on the ethics committee of a hospital, I found that if one did not recognize all of these morally relevant features, one was quite likely to make a moral judgment that no one, including oneself, would accept. For example, an unacceptable moral judgment could result from a failure to recognize that it is a morally relevant feature that two situations differ, in that in one situation there is an alternative action that would result in less harm. Similarly, a seriously mistaken moral judgment may result from a failure to recognize that it is a morally relevant feature if two situations differ in that one situation is an emergency situation. I cannot show that all of the morally relevant features are answers to just these ten questions.

Perhaps in some other society, or even in my society, some other morally relevant features may be discovered. But in each society there must be some way of identifying what counts as the same situation, or the same kind of violation. Describing a situation in terms of its morally relevant features is the first step in the two-step procedure that all people in all societies must use to guarantee that what counts as an adequate justification for one person counts as an adequate justification for anyone else in the same situation.

The second step in the two-step procedure is estimating the results of everyone knowing that they are allowed to violate the rule in these circumstances. If one estimates that *less* harm would result from everyone knowing that they are allowed to violate the rule in these circumstances than from everyone knowing that they are *not* allowed to violate the rule in these circumstances, then one is acting impartially in violating that rule. If everyone would make the same estimate, then the violation is strongly justified; if not everyone would make the same estimate, then the violation is only weakly justified. Weakly justified violations involve serious moral disagreement.

If everyone would estimate that *more* harm would result from everyone knowing that they are allowed to violate the rule in these circumstances than everyone knowing that they are *not* allowed to violate the rule in these circumstances, then the violation is unjustified. What one estimates about the harms and benefits of everyone knowing that violating a rule in the specified situation is allowed is shown by whether one would favor everyone knowing that they are allowed to violate the rule in these circumstances. This has a superficial resemblance to Kant's Categorical Imperative, but both its foundation and its results are significantly different.

DISAGREEMENTS BASED ON DIFFERENCES ABOUT WHEN A VIOLATION OF A MORAL RULE IS JUSTIFIED

In addition to the unresolvable disagreements that arise from differences in the interpretation of the moral rules, there are two other kinds of differences that can lead to unresolvable disagreements between different societies, or even between persons in the same society, about whether a violation of a moral rule is justified. The first is a difference in the ranking of the harms and benefits, although not in what count as harms. Everyone agrees on what the harms are—death, pain, disability, and loss of freedom and loss of pleasure. All rational persons try to avoid these harms unless they have an adequate reason for not avoiding them, to avoid what they take to be a greater harm or to gain a compensating benefit for themselves or someone else.

This may not be obvious, because sometimes one may not appreciate the benefit involved, that is, some cultures require suffering pain in order to gain the status necessary for being a full member of the society, a practice not unlike fraternity hazing. Also, for some religious people, the harm they will avoid is based on religious belief. For example, a Jehovah's Witness may refuse a blood transfusion that will save his life because he believes that having a blood transfusion violates the biblical prohibition against eating blood and so will result in the loss of eternal bliss.

Although there is universal agreement on what counts as harms, people do not all agree on the ranking of these harms. Further, pain, disability, loss of freedom, and loss of pleasure have degrees, and even death occurs at very different ages, so that there is no agreement that one of these harms is always worse than the others. Some people rank dying several months earlier as worse than a specified amount of pain and suffering, while other people rank that same amount of pain and suffering as worse. Thus, for most terminally ill patients, it is rationally allowed either to refuse death-delaying treatments or to consent to them.

Most actual moral disagreements, that is, whether or not to discontinue treatment of a terminally ill incompetent patient, are based on disagreements about the facts of the case—how painful is the disease, how painful is the treatment, and how long would the treatment prolong the patient's life? Differences in the rankings of the harms account for much of the rest of the moral disagreements—how much pain and suffering is it worth to prolong life for three months?

Often the factual disagreements about prognoses are so closely combined with different rankings of the harms involved that they cannot be distinguished. Further complicating the matter, the probability of suffering any of the harms can vary from very low to almost certain, and people can differ in the way that they rank a given probability of one harm against a different probability of another harm. Disagreement about the involuntary commitment of people with mental disorders that make them dangerous to themselves involves a disagreement about both what percent of these people would die if not committed and whether a significant probability of death within one week, say, 2 percent, compensates for a 100 percent probability of three to five days of a very serious loss of freedom and a 30 percent probability of long-term mental suffering.

Actual cases usually involve much more uncertainty about outcomes as well as the rankings of many more harms. Thus, complete agreement on what counts as a harm or evil is compatible with considerable disagreement on what counts as the lesser evil or greater harm in any particular case. It should be apparent that there is also considerable disagreement concerning the rankings of the benefits or goods—consciousness, abilities, freedom, and pleasure—but the rankings of the benefits play a much smaller role in justifying violations of moral rules than the rankings of harms.

Obviously, if people rank the harms differently, even when they agree on all of the facts, they will disagree in their estimates of whether more harm would result from everyone knowing that they are allowed to violate the rule in these circumstances than from everyone knowing that they are not allowed to violate the rule. Hence, they will differ in whether they favor everyone knowing that they are allowed to violate the rule in these circumstances.

Suppose that two people agree that legalizing active euthanasia will result in the same reduction in the amount of pain and suffering of terminally ill patients, and that they also agree that, due to mistakes and pressure, it will result in the same increase in people dying somewhat earlier than they might want to die. If they rank pain and death differently, they may disagree about whether one should legalize active euthanasia. One may hold that death is such a serious evil that avoiding quite a large amount of pain and suffering does not justify any significant increase in the number of earlier deaths, wanted or unwanted; whereas another may hold that death for a terminally ill patient is not as serious as the pain and suffering that results from living longer. Different societies may differ in the rankings that most of their members hold, and many different rankings seem acceptable.

But even if they rank the reduction of pain and suffering and the increase in somewhat earlier deaths exactly the same, they may still disagree because of their differing views of human nature. This difference may be most marked when one is considering people in different societies. People in a relatively homogeneous society may have a different estimate concerning what would be the result of everyone knowing that they can violate the rule against killing terminally ill patients in clearly specified circumstances than people living in a quite heterogeneous society like the United States. People in a homogeneous society may believe that there will be relatively few cases of unwanted earlier deaths due to mistakes and pressure, whereas those in a heterogeneous society may believe that there will be far more unwanted earlier deaths due to mistakes and pressure.

But even within a particular society, people can have different views about what would happen if everyone knows that they are allowed to break a moral rule in the same circumstances. For example, some people hold that when asked about how you like someone's clothes or hair, it is justifiable to deceive them in order to avoid hurting their feelings. They would favor allowing deception in this kind of situation because they believe that everyone knowing that this kind of violation is allowed would result in significant harm being avoided with only a minimal loss of trust. Others would not favor allowing deception in this kind of situation because they believe that the loss of trust would be significant and would outweigh the amount of harm avoided.

This ideological difference concerning human nature may also involve a different ranking of the harms involved, and there may be no way to decide which of these estimates is correct. It may be that one estimate is shared by most in one society and another by most in another society, but there may be no way to decide which of these estimates is correct even in a particular society.

DISAGREEMENTS BASED ON DIFFERENCES ABOUT WHO IS IMPARTIALLY PROTECTED BY THE MORAL RULES

The debates about abortion and animal rights are best understood as debates about who is included in the group that is impartially protected by the moral rules. However, there is no way to resolve this issue, for it makes sense to talk of impartiality only when the group toward which one is supposed to be impartial has been specified. Fully informed rational persons who hold that animals are not protected as strongly as moral agents can disagree about how much they should be protected; that is, they can disagree about how strong a reason has to be to be an adequate reason to justify killing or causing pain to an animal.

People can also disagree about whether fetuses are protected as strongly as moral agents, and if they are not, how much they are protected. They may even disagree about whether a fetus is protected to the same degree at all stages, or whether the fetus deserves more protection as it develops. Some societies do not even hold that neonates are protected as strongly as moral agents, and so allow infanticide with no justification or much less than is needed to justify killing a moral agent.

That there is no unique, correct answer to the question about who is protected as strongly as moral agents is why discussions of abortion and animal rights are so emotionally charged and often involve violence. Morality, however, does set limits to the morally allowable ways of settling unresolvable moral disagreements. These ways cannot involve violence or other unjustified violations of the moral rules, but they must be settled peacefully. Indeed, one of the proper functions of a democratic government is to settle unresolvable moral disagreements by peaceful means.

As mentioned at the beginning of this chapter, some maintain that morality is only, or primarily, concerned with the suffering of harm by moral agents, while others maintain that the harms—death, pain, and loss of freedom—suffered by those who are not moral agents is as important, or almost so, as the harms suffered by moral agents. But even if one regards animals as not included in the group impartially protected by the moral rules, this does not mean that one must hold that they should receive no protection. There is a wide range of morally acceptable options concerning the amount of protection that should be provided to those that are not included in the group toward which morality requires impartiality.

Many hold that although the reasons that are adequate to justify killing or causing pain to animals do not have to be as strong as the reasons that are adequate to justify killing or causing pain to moral agents, some reasons are needed. Few hold that it is morally justifiable to cause pain to animals just because one feels like doing so. Many states have laws prohibiting cruelty to animals to enforce this moral position.

Yet many hold that it is justifiable to use animals in painful medical experiments that will help provide treatments for important human maladies. Many also hold that it is justifiable to kill animals for food, even when alternative vegetarian alternatives are available. Many also hold that it is justifiable to deprive animals of their freedom so that people can enjoy seeing them in zoos, but many now feel that they should be put in larger, more comfortable surroundings than the small cages that were commonly used.

Regardless of the cultural variations in morality, the similarity in the content of morality is sufficiently great that there is general agreement that the world would be a better place if everyone acted morally, and that it gets worse as more people act immorally more often. This explains why we teach children to act morally and why every society has laws that prohibit serious immoral actions. A complete account of morality would discuss the moral virtues, but simply from the account of morality presented, it is obvious why the moral virtues connected with the second five rules—truthfulness, trustworthiness, fairness, honesty, and dependability—are those traits of character that all rational people want others to have and at least pretend to have themselves.

Rational persons favor others acquiring the moral virtues in order to lessen their own risk of suffering harm, and since they know that other rational persons also want them to act morally, they must, at least, pretend to cultivate these virtues in themselves. This explains the truth of La Rochefoucauld's saying, "Hypocrisy is the homage that vice pays to virtue."

CONCLUSION

In conclusion, the fact of disagreement between cultures over issues in bioethics does not force us to choose between the idea that one party to any disagreement must always be acting immorally, and the idea that there is no universal morality. For the reasons I have given, a universal moral system does not mean universal agreement. But it does limit legitimate disagreement.

Where a culture allows the violation of moral rules in such a way that, even by its own lights, it would not do to have everyone know that actions with the same morally relevant features are permissible, that culture permits actions that are immoral. Thus, for instance, no culture could allow everyone to know that actions with the same morally relevant features as Nazi medical experiments were permissible. No one in any culture could want everyone to know that it was generally permissible to cause death, terrible pain, and disability to many persons to satisfy the curiosity and sadistic impulses of a few. Nor, I expect, could any society accept the consequences of everyone knowing that actions with the same morally relevant features as assisting in involuntary female circumcision were permissible.

Nonetheless, as in some of the examples discussed above, there are times when each party to a disagreement can present a sound moral argument for its own moral position. Recognition and careful application of this distinction between morally defensible disagreement and indefensible disagreement certainly has implications for how practitioners should engage with those with whom they disagree. When the other side advocates what is clearly in conflict with morality, sanctioning their customs may be inappropriate.

In other cases, however, cases in which we must admit that morality itself makes no distinction between our own position and the position of those with whom we disagree, nothing more forceful than discussion, or perhaps a vote, is an appropriate way of resolving the disagreement. We may also find that an understanding of how legitimate moral disagreement is possible makes it easier, in appropriate circumstances, to truly respect moral positions that are contrary to our own.

NOTES

1. The editors would like to thank Heather Gert, the author's daughter, for graciously supplying this introduction and conclusion after his untimely death.

2. Tom Beauchamp and James Childress explicitly use the phrase *common morality* in later editions of their text, *Principles of Biomedical Ethics*. In that book, they contrast their understanding of common morality with the one presented in this chapter. However, in a recent paper, Tom Beauchamp acknowledges that the account of common morality presented here is superior to the account provided in *The Theory of Morality* by Alan Donagan that they used to support their four principles.

3. For a full account of this common moral system, see *Morality: Its Nature and Justification*, revised edition (New York: Oxford University Press, 2005). For a shorter account see *Common Morality: Deciding What to Do* (New York: Oxford University Press, 2007). For applications of the common moral system to bioethics, see *Bioethics: A Systematic Approach* by Bernard Gert, Charles M. Culver, and K. Danner Clouser (New York: Oxford University Press, 2006).

2

The Compatibility of Universal Morality, Particular Moralities, and Multiculturalism

Tom L. Beauchamp

ABSTRACT

The topics addressed in this chapter are moral relativism, the objectives of morality, universal morality, particular moralities, multiculturalist theory, and cultural moral imperialism. I argue that cultural relativism is an untenable theory and that a universal common morality transcends all cultural standards. The norms of universal morality are not thick in moral content, but they afford a starting framework that we can use to construct thick, action-guiding norms. The common morality allows for moral disagreement and legitimate differences of opinion about how to best specify universal norms, and thus it supports the development of particular moralities that differ from other particular moralities. However, the common morality does not allow for the so-called multicultural world, which some writers in ethics take to mean a world void of universal moral norms. Their views misrepresent even the commitments of multiculturalist theory. Multiculturalism is the theory that respect is owed to cultural traditions because morality itself demands this form of respect. Multiculturalism asserts that, universally, it is morally wrong to not acknowledge the moral rights of persons merely because their beliefs descend from different cultural histories.

Do all moral beliefs derive from cultural standards, or are there moral standards that transcend cultures and conventions? In one type of theory, morality is relative to cultural arrangements and aspirations. The notion of an objective principle or universal morality has no place in this theory. In another type of theory, universal moral standards such as human rights and basic moral rules are independent of particular cultures, nations, and organizations. I will present a version of the second type of theory. In addressing this problem, I will consider the subjects of moral relativism, the objectives of morality, universal morality, particular moralities, multiculturalism, and cultural moral imperialism. I will argue both in opposition to a relativism of basic moral standards and in support of a universally valid common morality.

THE UNTENABILITY OF CULTURAL RELATIVISMS

Moral relativism is an ancient problem about cultural differences that remains vibrant today. Two types of relativism are examined in this section: descriptive cultural relativism and normative cultural relativism. There are many species of relativism, but these are the two most prominent forms.

Descriptive Cultural Relativism

Defenders of descriptive relativism regard many discoveries in the social sciences as constituting evidence of an extensive diversity of moral practices across cultures. This work has cataloged and described many cultural differences, but these differences do not demonstrate that morally committed people in diverse cultures disagree about universal moral standards that underlie and justify their particular moral beliefs and practices. Simple examples are principles of honesty and truth-telling, virtues of caring and trustworthiness, and ideals of charity and friendliness.

Consider the vast similarity, in virtually every nation, in codes and regulations governing research involving human subjects. There are understandable and justifiable differences from country to country, but the differences pale in comparison to the sea of similarity in the norms governing how this research can and cannot be conducted. A few dozen principles are globally accepted as canonical for research ethics. Here are a few (steeply abridged) examples:

- Disclose all material information to subjects in medical research.
- Obtain individual, voluntary, informed consent for biomedical interventions.
- Maintain secure safeguards for keeping personal information about subjects private and confidential.
- Receive surrogate consent from a legally authorized representative for incompetent subjects.
- Protect subjects in research against excessive risk.
- Ethics review committees must scrutinize and approve research protocols.
- Research cannot be conducted unless its risks and intended benefits are reasonably balanced and risks are minimized.
- Special justification is required if proposed research subjects are vulnerable persons.

Several global organizations and many governments have officially supported these norms in codes and regulations, but the force and authority of the norms themselves is not contingent on any particular form of agreement. As the World Medical

Association says of its "Declaration of Helsinki," and as the U.S. government says of its *Belmont Report*, the "ethical principles" governing research involving human subjects are valid independently of any state of cultural belief or law.[1] Scandals in the history of research involving human subjects have occurred precisely when people in cultures neglected these principles in their laws and practices.

True cultural relativists reject these claims. They subscribe to the thesis that no moral principles of any sort, general or particular, are valid independent of the cultural contexts in which they have arisen and shaped to their present form. Relativists regard the relevant social science data as indicating that moral rightness and wrongness vary from place to place and that there are no absolute or universal moral standards that apply across all societies. Even the concepts of rightness and wrongness themselves are meaningless apart from the specific cultural contexts in which they arise, and patterns of culture can only be understood as unique wholes. In a much quoted statement, anthropologist Ruth Benedict once expressed the thesis as being that the term *morality* means "socially approved habits" and that the expression "It is morally good" is synonymous with "It is habitual."[2]

There is no need to question the anthropological reports on which cultural relativism is erected. Many are informative, solid, scientific studies. However, these studies do not show that there are no basic universal moral principles. More importantly, these descriptive reports of what people in fact believe do not support any normative position about what is right and wrong or about what any person or culture ought to believe. This takes me to the second type of relativism.

Normative Cultural Relativism

Though descriptive cultural relativism contains no normative content about how one ought to behave, the theory can be altered and given normative content. In this theory the statement "What is right at one place or time may be wrong at another" is interpreted to mean that *it is right* in one context to act in a way that *it is wrong* to act in another context. According to cultural normative relativism, one ought to behave in the ways one's culture determines to be correct and not behave in ways one's culture determines to be incorrect.

Cultural normative relativism is usually expressed as a theory based on cultural group beliefs and institutions, not merely on beliefs that appear only within the borders of nation-states. Accordingly, normative relativism does not merely say that when one is in Japan one should act as the Japanese do or when in the United States as the Americans do. It is a cultural, not a geographical, theory about the source of moral correctness.

Normative group relativists hold both that there is no criterion independent of one's culture for making a judgment that a practice is right or wrong or to assess whether the standards of one's social group are the standards one ought to uphold. More generally, normative relativism is the theory that a form of moral conduct is right or wrong for persons if and only if their culture holds that it is right or wrong.

One weakness in this theory is that it is often difficult to determine which group, society, or institution constitutes the culture that should be followed. For example, in pre-Taliban Afghanistan women were often well educated and worked in professions, but under the Taliban-imposed culture they were not allowed to work or to seek an education beyond the age of eight. Should we say that women should be governed by either of these conflicting sets of norms? Can one ever be bound by a coercively imposed culture? What from a moral point of view are one's obligations under these circumstances? Do any of the series of controlling groups in Afghanistan give any of its citizens the normatively correct set of beliefs and action guides? This is not a problem about Afghanistan and its history. Determining how to identify an appropriate cultural group is a serious theoretical problem for normative relativism.

A bigger problem is that, however precisely formulated, normative relativism has no justification for its view that a norm is acceptable merely because the members of a cultural group believe it in a certain way—or because individuals or the members of a religious group believe it in a certain way. This commitment to being morally bound by group norms is at the heart of the theory of normative cultural relativism and cannot be eliminated without abandoning the theory. But the idea that the slave trade, sexual harassment under a severe threat by a superior, excluding women from training as physicians, and denying human rights to "foreigners" ought to be practiced merely because a group believes in the practice has no moral justification or credibility. It is no more than a justification of tradition by appeal to tradition (or of culture by appeal to culture), a clear case of begging the question of moral justification.

Normative relativism has other problems as well. If right and wrong are entirely relative to a culture's standards, no person could ever maintain that his or her culture's standards are wrong or seek any kind of reform. Rejection by individuals of the culture's standards is wrong in this theory, no matter what the standards are. Similarly, if there are no moral norms about exposing research subjects to high risks—coercion and exploitation of nursing home populations, unacceptable occupational risks to health, or unethical billing for health reimbursements—then normative relativism implausibly maintains that the absence of such standards is morally normative in these situations. No reasonable person would accept such a view.

The unacceptability of descriptive cultural relativism and normative cultural relativism does not mean that a multicultural theory is unacceptable. I will later argue that multiculturalism is no relativism at all and is actually an important defense of universal morality and human rights.

THE OBJECTIVE OF MORALITY

I now turn to a thesis about what I will call the objective of morality.[3] This objective is that of promoting human flourishing by counteracting human circumstances in interactions with others that cause the quality of people's lives to worsen. The objective is to prevent or limit problems of indifference, conflict, suffering, hostility, scarce resources, limited information, and the like. This thesis has notable similarities to, though it is broader than, what Bernard Gert, in chapter 1 in this volume, described as the goal of morality: "Morality has the inherent goal of lessening the amount of harm suffered by those included in the protected group."

Following in the path of Thomas Hobbes and David Hume, I accept the following as the background circumstance of morality: From centuries of experience we have learned that the human condition tends to deteriorate into misery, confusion, violence, and distrust unless certain norms are enforced through a public system of norms.[4] When complied with, these norms lessen human misery and foster cooperation. These norms may not be necessary for the *survival* of a society, as some have maintained,[5] but they are necessary to ameliorate or counteract the tendency for the quality of people's lives to worsen and for social relationships to disintegrate. In every well-functioning society norms are in place to prohibit lying, breaking promises, causing bodily harm, stealing, fraud, the taking of life, the neglect of children, and failures to keep contracts. These norms, when socially enforced, achieve the objective of morality.

Many philosophers with different conceptions than the one I just presented nonetheless do not significantly disagree about the general norms that comprise morality. That is, philosophers from many different theoretical standpoints converge on the principles, virtues, rights, and responsibilities that are central to morality, and in doing so they converge on the essential conditions of any system of belief that deserves to be called morality.[6] They also agree on paradigm cases such as the judgment that rules legitimating the slave trade are morally unacceptable, no matter what a culture might think about the legitimacy of these rules.

The universal character of the human experience and of social responses to threatening conditions (by formulating norms that are suitable for the moral life) helps *explain* why there is a common morality, but it does not *justify* the norms.[7] What justifies the norms of the common morality, in the pragmatic theory I accept, is that they are the norms best suited to achieve the objectives of morality. Once the objective(s) of morality have been identified, a set of standards is pragmatically justified if and only if it is the best means to the end identified when all factors—including human limitations, shortcomings, and vulnerabilities—are taken into consideration. If one set of norms will better serve the objective of morality than a set currently in place, then the former should displace the latter.

This account is my own preferred strategy for the justification of moral norms, but I appreciate that others prefer a different justification, such as a contractarian one or the full account and justification of morality found in Gert's *Morality: Its Nature and Justification.*[8] However, I will not further pursue these theoretical matters, because they would make no difference to the arguments I provide hereafter.

THE COMMON MORALITY AS UNIVERSAL MORALITY

What are the principal cross-cultural norms of the common morality?[9] The common morality is comprised of *rules*, *virtues*, *ideals*, and *rights*—each of which I briefly discuss in this section.

Gert and I both understand the common morality as universal morality. It is not relative to cultures or individuals and is to be distinguished from norms that bind only members of particular groups. Gert views the nature and number of the moral rules in the common morality as precisely determinable,[10] whereas I regard these matters as less cleanly demarcated.

I will not address this issue here, but I emphasize that it is of the highest importance in the interpretation of both Gert's theory in chapter 1 of this volume and my account that the focus not be exclusively on moral principles or rules of obligation. "Common morality" references the entire "moral system," to use Gert's preferred language. I will now outline what I see as the main constituent elements in the system (elements that Gert and I catalogue somewhat differently, but not in a way that compromises the core of the common morality).

Universal Rules of Obligation

Here are a few examples (not a complete catalogue) of rules of obligation in the common morality: (1) do not kill; (2) do not cause pain or suffering to others; (3) prevent evil or harm from occurring; (4) rescue persons in danger; (5) tell the truth; (6) nurture the young and dependent; (7) keep your promises; (8) do not steal; (9) do not punish the innocent; and (10) obey the law. These norms have been justified in various ways by various philosophical theories, but I will not treat this problem of justification here. These cross-cultural norms obviously are implemented in different ways in different cultural or group settings, a matter I will later discuss when treating the topic of specification.

Universal Virtues

The common morality also contains standards that are *moral character traits*, or virtues. Here are a few examples: (1) honesty; (2) integrity; (3) nonmalevolence; (4) conscientiousness; (5) trustworthiness; (6) fidelity; (7) gratitude; (8) truthfulness; (9) lovingness; and (10) kindness. These virtues are universally admired traits,[11] and a person is deficient in moral character if he or she lacks these traits. Negative traits amounting to the opposite of the virtues are *vices* (malevolence, dishonesty, lack of integrity, cruelty, etc.). They are substantial moral defects, universally so recognized by persons committed to morality.

Universal Ideals

Moral ideals such as charitable goals, community service, dedication to one's job that exceeds obligatory levels, and service to the poor are also a part of the common morality. These aspirations are not *required* of persons, but they are universally *admired* and *praised* in persons who accept and act on them.[12] Here are four examples that can be interpreted both as ideals of virtuous character and ideals of action: (1) exceptional forgiveness, (2) exceptional generosity, (3) exceptional compassion, and (4) exceptional thoughtfulness.

Universal Rights

In addition to the basic obligations, virtues, and ideals just mentioned, human rights form an important dimension of universal morality. Rights in general are justified claims to something that individuals or groups can legitimately assert against other individuals or groups. Human rights in particular are those that all humans possess.[13]

Many philosophers, political activists, lawyers, and framers of political declarations now regard rights theory as the most important type of theory for expressing a universal moral point of view. Human rights language easily crosses national boundaries and supports international law and policy statements by international agencies and associations. Although human rights are, for this reason, often interpreted as legal rights, this interpretation does not properly capture their status. They are universally valid moral claims, and they have been so understood at least since early modern theories of rights were developed in the seventeenth century.[14]

The point of human rights language is to provide standards that transcend norms and practices in particular cultures that conflict with human rights. However, as James Griffin has rightly pointed out, we are sometimes satisfied that a basic human right exists, yet we are uncertain about what precisely the basic right gives us a right to.[15] This problem should be handled through what I will refer to in the next section as *specification*—the process of reducing the indeterminate character of abstract norms and giving them specific action-guiding content, often in the context of what I will call particular moralities.

PARTICULAR MORALITIES

It might be thought, given my emphasis on universal morality, that I do not allow for any form of pluralism or for local moral viewpoints—as if morality were a monolithic whole that does not permit disagreements and differences of approach. However, this is a misunderstanding of the connection between universal morality and the many moral norms that are particular to cultures, groups, and even individuals. Unlike the common morality, with its notably abstract and therefore content-thin norms, particular moralities present concrete, nonuniversal, and content-rich norms.

Particular moralities include the many responsibilities, ideals, attitudes, and sensitivities found in, for example, cultural, religious, and professional guidelines. Nonetheless—and this is a key matter in understanding why relativism is an unacceptable theory—*all justified particular moralities share the norms of the common morality with all other justified particular moralities.*

In order to have a practical, action-guiding morality, the norms of the common morality must be made specific in content. We cannot erect policies and practices on vague notions such as "respect for persons." All abstract norms must be carefully defined and then carefully fashioned as specific, well-crafted norms that give specific guidance to actions such as truthful disclosure, maintenance of confidentiality, obtaining an informed consent, providing access to medical care, and the like. These more concrete norms often must be made more concrete still for certain contexts. For example, the requirement of obtaining informed consent will be fashioned somewhat differently for contexts of research and for contexts of medical practice.

Consider an example of a rule that sharpens the requirements of a more general norm of avoiding conflicts of interest. The rule to be specified is, "Avoid conflicts of interest in making treatment recommendations" (which itself is a specification of a more general principle of avoiding conflicts of interest). This rule might be specified as follows: "When physicians prescribe pharmaceutical products they must avoid favoring products in which they have a financial relationship if this financial interest influences their judgment." The initial norm of avoiding conflicts endures, even though it is now a more specific rule.

Specification is a process of reducing the indeterminate character of abstract norms and generating more specific norms.[16] Specifying the norms with which one starts, whether those in the common morality or norms from a source such as a professional code, is accomplished by *narrowing the scope* of the norms, not by explaining what the general norms *mean*. As Henry Richardson puts it, specification occurs by "spelling out where, when, why, how, by what means, to whom, or by whom the action is to be done or avoided."[17] All norms are subject to specification, and many already specified rules would need further specification to handle new circumstances of conflict. Progressive specification can continue indefinitely.

To illustrate progressive specification, consider an additional specification that can be made to the rule already specified above, namely, "When physicians prescribe pharmaceutical products they must avoid favoring products in which they have a financial relationship if this financial interest influences their judgment." To this proscription we can add the following words shown in italic type: "When physicians prescribe pharmaceutical products they must avoid favoring products in which they have a financial relationship if this financial interest influences their judgment, *and they must avoid prescribing products if their judgment is influenced by a personal relationship they have with a representative of a company that distributes the product(s).*" These specified rules can be indefinitely specified and turned into a whole policy governing this type of conflict of interest.

Very commonly, more than one line of specification is available when confronting practical problems and moral disagreements, and different persons or groups will offer conflicting specifications. For any moral problem, thoughtful and fair-minded parties may offer several competing specifications, and thereby many different provisions in particular moralities are coherent ways to specify the common morality. This latitude must be permitted in practical moral thinking. We cannot demand more of people than that they faithfully specify norms with an eye to the overall coherence of the resulting particular morality while ensuring that their specifications do not violate the norms of universal morality.

Good examples of particular moralities that contain at least some specifications are *professional moralities* in biomedical research, medical practice, nursing practice, veterinary practice, and the like. These moral codes, declarations, and standards of practice often legitimately vary from other moralities in the ways they handle justice in access to health care, human rights, justified waivers of informed consent, government oversight of research involving human subjects, privacy provisions, and the like.

MULTICULTURALISM AS A UNIVERSALISTIC THEORY

It is an undisputed fact that multiple cultures have constructed unique particular moralities. This fact suggests to several writers in ethics that it is likewise an undisputed fact that morals are relative to cultures—or *pluralistic*, in the word now commonly heard in bioethics. Some writers in bioethics insist that we live in a multicultural world in which many moral cultures can live together peacefully, without need for the outmoded notion of universal, basic norms.

This characterization has matters upside down. In this section I argue that multiculturalism requires and insists on universal norms. Multiculturalism is not a pluralism or relativism. Multiculturalism is a universalistic theory to the effect that particular moralities are owed respect because morality itself demands it. Various writers in bioethics hijacked the term *multicultural world* to suggest the reverse, and especially to suggest that there is no universal morality and no commonly held morality.[18]

THE UNIVERSAL NORMS IN MULTICULTURALISM

The term *multiculturalism* refers to theories that support the moral principle that cultural or group traditions, institutions, perspectives, and practices should be respected and should not be violated or oppressed as long as they do not themselves violate the standards of universal morality. The objective of multiculturalism is to provide a theory of the norms that should guide the protection of vulnerable cultural groups when threatened with marginalization and oppression caused by one or more dominant cultures.

Resistance to forceful dominance and cultural oppression drive multiculturalist theory, which holds that respect is owed to people of dissimilar but peaceful cultural traditions because it is unjust and disrespectful to marginalize, oppress, or dominate persons merely because they are of an unlike culture or subculture. The moral notions at work in this account are universal theses about rights, justice, respect, and nonoppression.[19]

The major demand in multiculturalism is that people of one culture are morally obligated to tolerate and not interfere with the views of those in other cultures (as long as those views are themselves not in violation of universal moral norms). This universally valid demand is independent of any particular culture's values and is not valid *because* a culture accepts it.[20] These are matters of human rights, not of human contracts or cultural arrangements or the current state of national or international law. Without universal norms of toleration, respect, restraint, and the like, a multiculturalist could neither explain nor justify multiculturalism.

In short, the moral obligation to respect the views of people from other cultures is not confined to people in cultures that *recognize* this obligation. By design of multiculturalism as a moral theory, moral obligations of respect and tolerance apply to all cultures whether or not they recognize these norms. Harvey Siegel puts it accurately when he says, "Multiculturalism is itself a culturally transcendent or universal moral, educational, and social ideal in the sense that it is applicable to all cultures . . . and rests upon other equally transcendent, moral imperatives and values."[21]

CULTURAL IMPERIALISM

Some seem to think that my support of transcendent, universal moral standards is merely a disguised form of cultural imperialism. Persons outside of a given culture who press for recognition within that culture of the human rights of women, minorities, children, the ill, the disabled, the oppressed, the marginalized, the economically disadvantaged, and other vulnerable groups have been denounced in some literatures as cultural imperialists who incorporate "Western values" that are uncritically assumed to be universally valid, but that—beneath the veneer of fairness, equity, and respect—simply camouflage the continuance of Western dominance.

These charges of cultural imperialism have understandable roots in hundreds of years of colonial political and economic domination. Despite this perplexing history, threats of "cultural imperialism" today have nothing to do with so-called Western values or with any history of moral imperialism emanating from the Western world or from any history of imperialism from any particular region of the world. Virtually every region of the world has a horrid history of imperialistic control extending from one people to another.

Numerous cultural traditions, past and present, and in all parts of the world, have held that their cultural values are universal values to which everyone should conform. This claim might be correct in the sense that one culture might have understood and insisted on universal norms not recognized by some other culture(s). However, the concern here is the *imposition* of norms by one culture on another.

THE PRACTICAL IMPORTANCE OF CONTROLLING CULTURAL OPPRESSION BY UNIVERSAL NORMS

There is today a convergence of global opinion that cultural differences must not be allowed to obscure the conditions of injustice and oppression that are presented by despotic rulers as nothing more than ways of protecting a culture's traditional values.[22] There are no more important human rights than rights against oppression—a broad category, but today the most consequential form of human rights violation.

Even the governments of many nations that are signatories to the UN Universal Declaration of Human Rights do not protect the basic human rights of women and children, or at least they have an unduly narrow vision of what those rights are. When complaints and resistance movements arise, governments often claim that they are treating women and children in accordance with *their* cultural traditions, but here is a true case in which forms of oppression are being disguised by dominant powers that have no respect for universal values.

Susan Okin has justly argued that conflict between traditional cultural practices and persons subordinated to those practices cannot be resolved by the theory that regional control, based on some tradition, may legitimately be asserted over persons in the local region who do not come from or follow the dominant tradition. She argues that when these conflicts arise, they ought always to be resolved in terms of the rights of the oppressed, never resolved merely in terms of cultural practices or some kind of balancing of competing interests. Neither tradition nor a balancing of interests should be given priority when there are serious human rights violations. The enforcement of human rights that override even long-standing traditional values ought, in this account, to be the primary consideration.[23]

We are often told in writings in ethics that there are important East-West moral differences and that Western values should not be imposed on Eastern nations. However, these alleged differences are virtually never explained in detail and documented. The available empirical literature on the subject often does not support the claims. Amartya Sen points out that the idea of "Asia as a unit" with a set of Asian values different from those of the West makes no sense despite its frequent mention. He notes that about 60 percent of the world lives in Asia, with virtually nothing to solidify it as a uniform moral culture (other than universal morality, which simply solidifies it with the rest of the world): "There are no quintessential values that apply to this immensely large and heterogeneous population, that differentiate Asians as a group from people in the rest of the world."

Sen notes that violations of basic rights of freedom occur routinely in many parts of Asia and that dictatorial heads of state use the excuse that "Asian nations" do not accord the same value to personal autonomy and political freedom as do Western countries and therefore the human rights to freedom extolled in the West are either irrelevant or objectionable.

Sen rightly sees such claims as morally unacceptable, while noting an interesting piece of history: The idea of "Asian values" and "the Orient" were originally the products of a Eurocentric perspective that regarded the whole of the Asian region as united by a body of non-Western standards. Sen briskly criticizes Western governments, including those in the United States and European nations, for indirectly backing this unfounded idea of Eastern values and allowing such a specious conception to serve as an excuse for not giving primacy to human rights.[24]

CONCLUSION

The arguments in this chapter all move to the conclusion that a universal set of moral norms comprises the common morality. Although these norms are thin in their abstract moral content, they are far from empty, and they afford a starting point for the specification of action-guiding norms in particular moralities and practical ethics. They constitute a wall of moral standards that cannot justifiably be violated in any culture or by any group or individual.

NOTES

1. See the 2008 revision of the World Medical Association's "Declaration of Helsinki: Ethical Principles for Medical Research Involving Human Subjects," Part B, "Basic Principles for All Medical Research" (first adopted 1964); *The Belmont Report: Ethical Guidelines for the Protection of Human Subjects of Research* (Washington, DC: DHEW Publication OS 78-0012, 1978). It first appeared in the *Federal Register* on April 18, 1979.

2. Ruth Benedict, "Relativism and Patterns of Culture," in *Value and Obligation*, Richard B. Brandt, ed. (New York: Harcourt Brace and World, 1961), 457.

3. The term and much of my understanding of the issues derive from G. J. Warnock's similar language in *The Object of Morality* (London: Methuen & Co., 1971), esp. 15–26.

4. Cf. Bernard Gert, *Morality: Its Nature and Justification*, revised edition (New York: Oxford University Press, 2005), 11–14.

5. See the sources referenced in Sissela Bok, *Common Values* (Columbia, MO: University of Missouri Press, 1995), 13–23, 50–59 (citing several influential writers on the subject).

6. Cf. Tom L. Beauchamp and James F. Childress, *Principles of Biomedical Ethics*, sixth edition (New York: Oxford University Press, 2009), 260–1, 361–3.

7. John Mackie, *Ethics: Inventing Right and Wrong* (London: Penguin, 1977), 22–23, 107ff.

8. Gert, *Morality: Its Nature and Justification*.

9. Although there is only one universal common morality, there is more than one *theory* of the common morality. For the theories pertinent to this volume, see Bernard Gert, *Common Morality: Deciding What to Do* (New York: Oxford University Press, 2004, paperback edition 2007); and Beauchamp and Childress, *Principles of Biomedical Ethics*, chapters 1, 10.

10. See, in the present volume, Gert's list of ten moral rules. Gert readily acknowledges that there is disagreement among philosophers on the matter and says that there is not even "complete agreement concerning what counts as a moral rule." Gert, *Morality: Its Nature and Justification*, 13.

11. See Martha Nussbaum's assessment that, in Aristotelian philosophy, certain "nonrelative virtues" are objective and universal: "Non-Relative Virtues: An Aristotelian Approach," in *Ethical Theory, Character, and Virtue*, ed. Peter French et al. (Notre Dame, IN: University of Notre Dame Press, 1988), 32–53, especially 33–34, 46–50.

12. See Bernard Gert, *Common Morality: Deciding What to Do*, 20–26, 76–77; Richard B. Brandt, "Morality and Its Critics," in his *Morality, Utilitarianism, and Rights* (Cambridge: Cambridge University Press, 1992), chapter 5.

13. Cf. Joel Feinberg, *Rights, Justice, and the Bounds of Liberty* (Princeton, NJ: Princeton University Press, 1980), esp. 139–41, 149–55, 159–60, 187. See also Alan Gewirth, *The Community of Rights* (Chicago: University of Chicago Press, 1996), 8–9.

14. Pioneering theories of international rights and natural rights—now generally restyled as *human* rights—first prospered in philosophy through the social and political theories of Hugo Grotius, Thomas Hobbes, and John Locke. See Anthony Pagden, "Human Rights, Natural Rights, and Europe's Imperial Legacy," *Political Theory* 31, no. 2 (2003): 171–99.

15. James Griffin, *On Human Rights* (Oxford: Oxford University Press, 2008), 97, 110.

16. Henry S. Richardson, "Specifying Norms as a Way to Resolve Concrete Ethical Problems," *Philosophy and Public Affairs* 19, no. 4 (Fall 1990): 279–310; and "Specifying, Balancing, and Interpreting Bioethical Principles," in *Belmont Revisited: Ethical Principles for Research with Human Subjects*, edited by James F. Childress, Eric M. Meslin, and Harold T. Shapiro (Washington, DC: Georgetown University Press, 2005), 205–27.

17. Richardson, "Specifying, Balancing, and Interpreting Bioethical Principles," 289.

18. Examples are H. Tristram Engelhardt Jr., *The Foundations of Bioethics*, 2nd edition (New York: Oxford University Press, 1996); Robert Baker, "A Theory of International Bioethics: Multiculturalism, Postmodernism, and the Bankruptcy of Fundamentalism," *Kennedy Institute of Ethics Journal* 8, no. 3 (1998): 201–31; Leigh Turner, "Bioethics in a Multicultural World: Medicine and Morality in Pluralistic Settings," *Health Care Analysis* 11, no. 2 (2003): 99–117.

19. Compare the arguments in the essays in Robert K. Fullinwider, ed., *Public Education in a Multicultural Society: Policy, Theory, Critique* (Cambridge: Cambridge University Press, 1996).

20. See the essays by Charles Taylor, Amy Gutmann, Steven C. Rockefeller, Michael Walzer, and Susan Wolf, in *Multiculturalism and "The Politics of Recognition,"* ed. Amy Gutmann (Princeton, NJ: Princeton University Press, 1992).

21. Harvey Siegel, "Multiculturalism and the Possibility of Transcultural Educational and Philosophical Ideals," *Philosophy* 74 (1999): 387–409.

22. See Martha Nussbaum and Jonathan Glover, eds., *Women, Culture, and Development* (Oxford: Oxford University Press, 1995); and Marcia Angell, "The Ethics of Clinical Research in the Third World," *New England Journal of Medicine* 337, no. 12 (1997): 847–49.

23. Susan Moller Okin, "Is Multiculturalism Bad for Women?" in *Is Multiculturalism Bad for Women?*, published as an anthology, edited by Joshua Cohen, Matthew Howard, and Martha C. Nussbaum (Princeton, NJ: Princeton University Press, 1999), 20–24.

24. Amartya Sen, *Human Rights and Asian Values* (New York: Carnegie Council, 1997). The quote is on page 13.

3

Lost in Translation

Can We Have a Global Bioethics without a Global Moral Language?

Søren Holm

ABSTRACT

This chapter will analyze the question of whether a global bioethics can be established if we do not have a prior common moral language. The first part will analyze two different contenders for a global moral language: (1) human rights and (2) a set of core principles (looking closely at Macklin's work). It will argue that neither constitute a shared moral language and will identify the reasons why not. The second part will then discuss whether a hybrid approach involving core human rights interpreted in the light of core moral principles could form the basis for a global bioethics. It will again be argued that such an approach is problematic. The third part will then consider whether we are not better off by accepting that there are irresolvable moral differences at both theoretical and practical levels and accepting that the real moral task is to mediate between these differences in concrete situations.

INTRODUCTION

It is a trite platitude that we live in a connected, global world where the consequences of our actions may spread far and wide, and where perhaps more importantly we are aware that the consequences of our actions may spread far and wide. How are we to deal with the global moral problems that occur in such a world? One suggestion is that because the problems are global they should be analyzed and resolved within an agreed global moral framework. It is this suggestion that will be analyzed critically in this chapter. I will outline the epistemic and social conditions necessary for convergence on a common position and apply this analysis in relation to the convergence on a common set of core or fundamental moral principles. I will also consider the use of human rights as the common minimal framework.

In the analysis I will use the principle of "respect for persons" as the main example of a potentially universal moral principle and the important 1998 book *Against Relativism: Cultural Diversity and the Search for Ethical Universals in Medicine* by Ruth Macklin as the main source of examples. I have chosen to use Macklin's book in this way because I take it to be one of the strongest, best, and clearest defenses of an unabashed universalist position in bioethics.

I furthermore agree with Macklin's universalism at the theoretical level, but I disagree with her concerning the conditions under which theoretical universalism can be converted into concrete ethical judgments. This makes her book and analysis an appropriate touchstone for the more skeptical view I develop here.

The analysis will mainly relate to the possibility of a global ethics, but many of the arguments are also relevant to the possibility of a common ethics within a single multicultural society. But before proceeding further, it is important to briefly make the case for why a common, global ethics might be considered desirable. The world in which we live is not "the best of all worlds." The rights of millions of people are breached without justification, unjustifiable resource inequalities are perpetuated and widened, and the strong are often allowed to prey on the weak with impunity.

There are, thus, many ways in which the world could be made a better place, ethically speaking. Although each of us can do much on our own to make the world a better place, there are also many things that can only be changed if individuals or states work together. The necessary cooperation will plausibly be easier if it is possible to reach agreement on what features of the world we ought to change and why we ought to change them. And this agreement might be believed to require a common set of ethical principles.

If we, for instance, want to identify unjustifiable resource inequalities that ought to be rectified, this seems to presuppose agreement on some account of what justice requires. We may be able to proceed some of the way in the absence of a common global ethics, but getting all the way seems to require one, and it would therefore be a major achievement if we could agree on one.

CONDITIONS FOR CONVERGENCE

Under what general conditions can we reasonably expect convergence on a common moral framework, in a situation in which moral agents 1) start from radically different positions, 2) are able to communicate with each other and engage in moral discourse, and 3) are willing to engage in moral discourse in good faith?[1]

Let us first note that the answer to this question is independent of whether we assume a foundationalist or a coherentist account of moral justification. On either of these accounts the process by which convergence is achieved in discourse between real moral agents is going to be a coherence-seeking process involving all the elements of wide reflective equilibrium as inputs—beliefs/facts about the world, considered moral judgments, and moral theories (Daniels 2008). We will never be in a situation in which we try to agree on our common moral principles without any prior moral commitments. Agreeing on foundationalism or coherentism will be an outcome of the process, not an initial assumption, and it might not even be a necessary outcome.

As a starting point in a convergence-seeking process, the participants will need to try to reach agreement on the ground rules for the process. Here there are major stumbling blocks. The one that is commonly discussed is whether considered moral judgments that are based on (religious) comprehensive worldviews are admissible in the process (Audi and Wolterstorff 1997, Rawls 1996). Robert Audi, for instance, proposes two principles of secular reason and motivation as side constraints on interventions in public political debates:

The Principle of Secular Rationale
"One has a prima facie obligation not to advocate or support any law or public policy that restricts human conduct, unless one has, and is willing to offer, adequate secular reasons for this advocacy or support" (Audi and Wolterstorff 1997: 25).

The Principle of Secular Motivation
"One has a (prima facie) obligation to abstain from advocacy or support of a law or public policy that restricts human conduct, unless one is sufficiently *motivated* by (normatively) adequate secular reason" (Audi and Wolterstorff 1997, 28).

Admitting moral judgments based on religious worldviews will make it more difficult to reach consensus, but not admitting them is also problematic. There are no participants in the process who do not hold a comprehensive worldview that influences their concrete judgments. Only some of these comprehensive worldviews are religious,[2] but a specific nonreligious worldview can be as idiosyncratic, be held as strongly, and can influence concrete judgments as much as a religious one (e.g., a Marxist-Leninist worldview [Luther 1986]).

If nonshared components of comprehensive worldviews are excluded ab initio, it is likely to have one of two effects. It will either mean that those who are strongly committed to their comprehensive worldview will be less interested in engaging with the process, or it will mean that they cannot engage in good faith. They will not be able to state their views in what they see as the strongest possible way, but they will be forced to find ways of stating them that are less satisfactory from their point of view.

Here we seem to be between a rock and a hard place, philosophically speaking. Either we complicate our coherence-building process by letting participants state their initial ethical views clearly and with their own justification, or we run the risk of making it impossible for some participants to engage in the process in good faith. If we choose to exclude nonshared components of comprehensive worldviews, we further have the problem that it becomes unclear how the persons who hold these views should view the outcome of the process.

Let us imagine that wide reflective equilibrium has been obtained around a set of global ethical principles. It then seems possible to claim that participants in the process should accept these principles, because they are a way of making their own moral views more coherent, and thereby presumably more justifiable. But if the input is not "their own moral views," it is difficult to see why they should have any commitment to accepting the outcome.

A slightly different issue that is often confused with the religion issue is the issue of non-negotiable commitments. If any party in the process has non-negotiable commitments, it may block the achievement of coherence, and it may therefore be a necessary component of good faith that everything is up for grabs. But non-negotiable commitments can be held for a variety of reasons, not only religious ones.

The other stumbling block is that real-life coherence-seeking does not take place behind a veil of ignorance. All participants are aware of who they are and of what consequences a given set of common ethical principles will have for them and their descendants. In an ideal world where everyone is motivated by ethical concerns only this would not matter, but it will matter for real-world consensus building.

We can therefore not expect agreement on common, global ethical principles to be reached quickly or without contention. What we can expect is a slow process moving forward in a piecemeal fashion, and maybe not even always moving forward. We may be able to reach agreement that a specific ethical construct is a fundamental ethical principle and part of a common global ethics, whereas other constructs still only have the status of plausible candidates or still have vague scope and content.

What we cannot expect, even if we are committed theoretical universalists, is that agreement on the universal principles is reached quickly or easily.

HOW PRECISE A CONSENSUS CAN WE REACH?

Let us, despite the problems alluded to above, assume that we have reached a consensus that "respect for persons" is a fundamental and universal ethical principle[3] that should guide our global ethics. Are we then in a position to make concrete ethical judgments?

Let us first consider a case in which "respect for persons" is the only moral consideration that is engaged. No other principles are in play, and it is clear that everyone involved falls within the scope of the principle[4]; that is, that they are persons. In such a case we would still need to specify the content of the principle in order to form a judgment. It is a well-known and often repeated criticism of Beauchamp and Childress's principlist approach that whereas we might be able to agree on the importance of the four principles when they are fairly content-less labels, it is much more difficult to agree on their precise content; that is, how much beneficence is required. And the same question must be raised here: What does "respect for persons" actually mean? A brief survey of the literature makes it clear that this is a highly controversial question. John Harris argues that respect for persons has two distinct aspects.

Respect for persons requires us to acknowledge the dignity and value of other persons and to treat them as ends in themselves and not merely instrumentally as means to ends or objectives chosen by others. Respect for persons has two distinct dimensions:

1. Respect for autonomy
2. Concern for welfare

When I suggest that these elements are crucial to any conception of respect for persons I mean simply that no one could claim to respect persons if their attitude to others failed to take account of, and indeed exhibit, these elements (Harris 2003: 10).

But respect for autonomy and concern for welfare seem to be two very different things. Macklin explicates respect for persons primarily as respect for personal autonomy, which avoids many interpretative problems, being primarily a negative condition and therefore a potential candidate for a strict and complete duty.

If, however, Harris is right and respect for persons also encompasses concern for welfare, we are left with the further problem of how to explicate welfare.[5] Is the welfare of a person a purely subjective matter to be decided only from the first-person perspective, or is it (at least partly) an objective matter? To agree on this will be important in order to come to concrete judgment in cases in which a person wants to perform actions that will negatively affect some objective assessment of their welfare or interest. But are we likely to reach consensus on the explication? Or are we likely to reach consensus on what should be incorporated in a list of objective goods conducive to welfare?

This might initially seem not to matter if we take the more restrictive Macklin line equating respect for persons with respect for autonomy and relegating welfare considerations to some other fundamental ethical principle. But thinking that this move will solve the problem is partly an illusion because welfare only ceases to matter if we take respect for autonomy to be absolute in the sense that paternalistic action is never justifiable. If we accept that there are instances where paternalism in respect of a competent person is justified, the question of our account of welfare again raises its head. And given that no philosophical agreement has yet been reached on this issue we would surely expect too much of our consensus process if we believed it would give us a firm answer.

A more complicated problem occurs when we have more than one fundamental moral principle in play and where they are in potential conflict.[6] This is a very old problem, and most moral systems have ways of dealing with it—the processes of specification and balancing in Beauchamp and Childress's work (Beauchamp and Childress 2009).

But in the global context what sometimes happens is that someone brings a moral consideration to the table that is new in the sense that it is outside of the moral system of the other participants in the discourse. This would still happen even if we had an agreed set of global moral principles, because unlike in ideal philosophy, not everyone will have been at the discourse where these principles were agreed.

Let me illustrate this problem with an extended example from Macklin's book. In a chapter on death and birth she discusses organ transplantation in the Philippines and the role of traditional Filipino morality in shaping the practice:

The dead person whose organs are removed is not in a position to make a proper "donation" in an act that stems from the right sort of moral motivation. The relevant concept in the traditional Filipino value system is known as *kusang loob*. For an act to have moral worth it must be done out of *kusang loob*, an idea similar to free will but not exactly the same. If a person needs to be told what to do, or is coerced into performing an action, the act does not come out of *kusang loob*. To have moral worth, an action must also be done without anticipation of reward or personal gain and not purely out of a sense of duty.

The implications for the morality of organ donation are rather straightforward. If a person is not in a position to act from the proper moral motivation, that is, out of *kusang loob*, it is better for the action not to have been done at all. Presumably, then, only if a person had signed an organ donation card, done so in an uncoerced manner and not purely out of a sense of duty, would the donation qualify as being done out of *kusang loob*.

What follows from this picture for ethical relativism? Should we conclude that the medical practice of organ transplantation is ethically wrong in the Philippines because of the value attached to the concept of *kusang loob* but ethically right elsewhere as long as the proper safeguards are followed?

[T]he Filipino concept of *kusang loob* is a feature of a moral system in that culture that does not appear to have an exact counterpart in our own society, at least not with respect to organ donation. *Kusang loob* falls under the category of moral motivation, an aspect of ethical behavior that may legitimately differ from one society to another and is therefore an example of one of the things that turns out to be relative. The application of this concept to organ donation yields the result that organ donation itself is neither morally right nor morally wrong, but its rightness or wrongness depends (among other things) on the moral motivation of the individual whose organs are harvested for transplantation. This marks a cultural and ethical difference from organ donation in other cultures where a donation need not stem from a particular moral motivation. This difference is not at the level of fundamental ethical principles, so it does not confirm the proposition that ethical principles vary from one culture to the next with no deeper underlying principles. (Macklin 1998: 143–44)

I agree with Macklin that nothing in this account of the implications of traditional Filipino values for organ transplantation confirms "the proposition that ethical principles vary from one culture to the next with no deeper underlying principles," but I disagree with the way she justifies this conclusion.

Believing that moral motivation is important in deciding whether an act is morally right or wrong is not a peculiar Filipino concern. The non-Filipino philosopher Immanuel Kant famously argued that motivation in the form of goodwill was the only thing that decided rightness and wrongness:

Nothing can possibly be conceived in the world, or even out of it, which can be called good, without qualification, except a good will.

A good will is good not because of what it performs or effects, not by its aptness for the attainment of some proposed end, but simply by virtue of the volition; that is, it is good in itself, and considered by itself is to be esteemed much higher than all that can be brought about by it in favour of any inclination, nay even of the sum total of all inclinations. (Kant 1985)

The characteristics that make an action problematic in the Filipino case have some overlaps with what makes an action heteronomous and therefore without value in Kantian philosophy. Similar concerns related to motivation or intention can also be found in many other ethical systems. It is therefore impossible to drive a wedge between fundamental ethical principles and concerns with motivation in the way Macklin does. That the right motivation matters in the moral assessment of actions may eventually be one of the fundamental ethical principles that emerges from a consensus process.

There is nothing inherent in the concept of a "fundamental ethical principle" that precludes this. A fundamental ethical principle does not have to be about rights or duties. But if we can't just discount *kusang loob* as a particular Filipino ethical value that can never count as a fundamental ethical principle, how are we to deal with it? If we are really committed to universalism and to moral discourse in good faith, it seems that we will minimally have to consider whether we need to augment our set of fundamental ethical principles with a principle about right, ethical motivation. This will not be necessary if we can plausibly claim that our current set of fundamental ethical principles already contains all the principles that can count as fundamental ethical principles. But it is difficult to see how such a claim can be sustained, at least at the present stage of the discourse where we are still moving forward toward a global, common ethics.

So the introduction of *kusang loob* into the debate as a possible important ethical consideration will, at least temporarily, destabilize our set of fundamental ethical principles. It is only after we have seriously considered whether *kusang loob*, or some suitable modification, can make our set of principles even more coherent that we can make a concrete judgment concerning Filipino as well as non-Filipino organ donation.

This is not a problem if *kusang loob* is an isolated instance of a prima facie, valid, ethical consideration found in a specific culture, but there are of course likely to be many such examples and therefore many circumstances in which concrete judgment might elude us because our set of global common ethics cannot be claimed to be complete.

HUMAN RIGHTS AS THE COMMON FRAMEWORK

But is the analysis above not far too complicated and hair splitting? Could we not simply sidestep the philosophical issues and seek convergence in the area of international human rights law?

The link between public health, medicine, ethics, and human rights was first analyzed in detail by Jonathan Mann, and a turn toward human rights has been prominent in recent developments in "global ethics" (Mann 1997). Most have argued that ethics and human rights are complementary, but at least some commentators foresee a development in which human rights law will eventually subsume bioethics and make bioethics more or less redundant (Faunce 2005).

Roberto Andorno furthermore argues that human rights are best understood as a result of a consensus-seeking process that allows consensus on principles without requiring consensus on justifications. The agreed set of human rights may not be the result of wide reflective equilibrium, but they are nevertheless agreed:

> The global success of the human rights movement in contemporary society is probably due to the fact that a practical agreement about the rights that should be respected is perfectly compatible with theoretical disagreement on their ultimate foundation (14). The Universal Declaration of Human Rights of 1948 is the best example of this phenomenon, because it was drafted by representatives of particularly diverse, even opposed, ideologies. Upon this strong legislative foundation has been built an extensive network of human rights mechanisms designed to develop international standards, monitor their implementation and investigate violations of human rights. (Andorno 2002: 960)

The advantages of moving to a human rights arena are according to proponents of such a move many: 1) states voluntarily agree to be bound by human rights, and such rights therefore have undisputed normative force, 2) that human rights jurisprudence provides an interpretative system for determining the scope and meaning of human rights, and 3) that specific institutions (e.g., the European Court of Human Rights [ECHR]) can provide authoritative interpretations with legal force. If we, therefore, as an example want to know the scope and meaning of the right to private and family life enunciated in Article 8 of the European Convention of Human Rights, we can look at ECHR jurisprudence. Article 8 states that:

1. Everyone has the right to respect for his private and family life, his home and his correspondence.
2. There shall be no interference by a public authority with the exercise of this right except such as is in accordance with the law and is necessary in a democratic society in the interests of national security, public safety, or the economic well-being of the country; for the prevention of disorder or crime; for the protection of health or morals; or for the protection of the rights and freedoms of others.

In relation to sexual matters we would then find that the Article 8 rights in general protect against discrimination because of sexual orientation or activity, but also that not all kinds of sexual activity are protected. In the judgment in *Laskey, Jaggard and Brown v. the United Kingdom* (judgment of February 19, 1997) the ECHR, for instance, found that the organized, consensual, sadomasochistic activities carried out by a group of men were not protected by Article 8.

The human rights framework thus specifies the rights of individuals and provides mechanisms for authoritative interpretation. These rights are furthermore universal in scope and consensually agreed to, at least within the relevant set of jurisdictions (member states of the Council of Europe in the case of the ECHR). It thus seems that human rights give the universalists everything that they could reasonably want, and that they circumvent all of the problems about agreement on precise content discussed above because of the existence of authoritative interpretations.

One possible criticism of this positive picture is that there are problems with our current enumerations of human rights and that we should add some and perhaps also remove some from our lists of binding human rights. I think this a valid criticism (Holm 2009), but not one that I will be pursuing here.

The criticism that I want to pursue here is based on the fact that the precise content of specific human rights is an area of huge contestation. The lawyers for Laskey, Jaggard, and Brown argued that Article 8 protected their activities, and many commentators have agreed with them, but the ECHR disagreed. It is a standard legal fiction that courts interpret laws, they do not make them—or to put it differently, when a court makes a decision on a point of law it simply states what the legal position is, it does not change the legal position. According to this fiction the lawyers for Laskey et al. simply made a legal mistake.[7] Article 8 did not protect these kinds of sexual activities, and it had never done so.

But given recent changes in sexual mores it is quite likely that the Laskey judgment will one day be overturned. This will be of no help to Laskey et al., who have long since served their prison sentences. But it will mean that Article 8 suddenly protects activity that the court had previously denied it protected. Or to put it differently, if Laskey is overturned it will illustrate that the content of human rights is much more fluid and malleable than we might initially believe. It will also illustrate that the initial, voluntary consent of states is almost completely irrelevant to the normative force of their current human rights commitment. The rights that the original signatories signed up to in 1950 when the European Convention on Human Rights and Fundamental Freedoms was signed was a set of rights with very different content than the rights in 2010.

Human rights do give us legal enforceability in some regions of the world, but they do not substitute for a common global ethics. They are a parallel normative system with as many interpretative problems and as much vagueness of content.

THE DISMAL CONCLUSION?

In this chapter I have argued for the conclusion that the likelihood that we will be able to agree on a global moral framework that is sufficiently specific to lead to concrete judgment concerning global moral problems is very small indeed. The justification for this conclusion is not that moral relativism is true. I believe that there are compelling arguments showing moral relativism to be unsustainable as a theoretical position, and I believe that there are good arguments for accepting moral universalism, but that is a matter for another paper.

Alas, the falsity of moral relativism does not guarantee actual convergence on one commonly accepted moral framework. In the chapter I have presented arguments showing that there are very large epistemic and social obstacles standing in the way of actual moral convergence, and that we should not expect overall convergence to happen. And even if we could achieve convergence on principles such as "respect for persons," it is unlikely that we could converge on the precise interpretation of that principle.

This may sound like a dismal conclusion, but one way of seeing it in a more positive light is by realizing that it is essentially the position we have been in since the inception of philosophical ethics among the pre-Socratics. Agreement has rarely been achieved in the theoretical realm, but that has not precluded genuine moral progress and agreement on concrete judgments. We may still not agree on exactly why chattel slavery is wrong, but is it not a sufficient cause for joy that most of us now have an unshakable belief that it is wrong, that laws are in force banning it, and that these laws are almost universally enforced?

In one sense it would be strange indeed if we, at this precise moment in time, achieved what has eluded all our philosophical forerunners—that is, an agreed set of universal, content-full ethical principles.

NOTES

1. The good faith requirement is necessary, but unfortunately it is often absent from real-life moral discourse in which participants often expect other people to change their views, without themselves being willing to change.
2. We will here sidestep the issue of trying to define *religion* or *religious*.
3. Without necessarily assuming foundationalism.
4. In reality we know that reaching agreement on the scope of the person concept at the beginning and end of life is highly contentious.
5. This is, of course, a quite general problem in ethics.
6. I here assume that there is more than one fundamental moral principle, although that is, of course, disputed.
7. As did Laskey et al. themselves, if they thought that their actions were protected.

REFERENCES

Andorno, R. 2002. "Biomedicine and International Human Rights Law: In Search of a Global Consensus." *Bulletin of the World Health Organization* 80 (12): 959–63.

Audi, R., and N. Wolterstorff. 1997. *Religion in the Public Square*. Lanham, MD: Rowman & Littlefield.

Beauchamp, T. L., and J. Childress. 2009. *Principles of Biomedical Ethics*, 6th edition. New York: Oxford University Press.

Daniels, N. 2008. "Reflective Equilibrium." *The Stanford Encyclopedia of Philosophy*, Fall 2008 edition, ed. Edward N. Zalta. http://plato.stanford.edu/archives/fall2008/entries/reflective-equilibrium/.

Faunce, T. A. 2005. "Will International Human Rights Subsume Medical Ethics? Intersections in the UNESCO Universal Bioethics Declaration." *Journal of Medical Ethics* 31:173–78.

Harris, J. 2003. "Consent and End of Life Decisions." *Journal of Medical Ethics* 29:10–15.

Holm, S. 2009. "Global Concerns and Local Arguments: How a Localized Bioethics May Perpetuate Injustice." In *The Philosophy of Public Health*, edited by A. Dawson, 63–72. Farnham: Ashgate.

Kant, I. 1985. *Fundamental Principles of the Metaphysics of Morals*. Translated by Thomas Kingsmill Abbott. http://en.wikisource.org/wiki/Groundwork_of_the_Metaphysics_of_Morals.

Luther, E. 1986. *Ethik in der Medizin*. Halle: Martin Luther Universität.

Macklin, R. 1998. *Against Relativism: Cultural Diversity and the Search for Ethical Universals in Medicine*. New York: Oxford University Press.

Mann, J. M. 1997. "Medicine and Public Health, Ethics and Human Rights." *The Hastings Center Report* 27 (3): 6–13.

Rawls, J. 1996. *Political Liberalism (With a New Introduction and the "Reply to Habermas")*. New York: Columbia University Press.

4

Is There a Global Bioethics?[1]

End of Life in Thailand and the Case for Local Difference

Scott Stonington and Pinit Ratanakul

ABSTRACT

The twenty-first century has seen a debate over whether there should be international standards in medical ethics and human rights. Critics worry that such standards risk overlooking important cultural differences in the way people conceptualize medical decision making. The question for a global bioethics, then, is what bioethical guidelines and framework should guide developing countries that are building allopathic medical systems. This chapter examines the issue—including the presumed universality of Western bioethics values such as autonomy, beneficence, nonmaleficence, truth-telling, and justice. It concludes that Western bioethics is inadequate to solve the problems in non-Western societies.

INTRODUCTION

Over the past decade, several scholars have advocated for international standards in medical ethics and human rights (Benatar 2005, Kim 2000, Farmer 2001). Others have countered that such standards risk ignoring important cultural differences in the way people conceptualize medical decision making (Adams 2002, Butt 2002, Cohen 1999, Pelligrino, Mazzarella, and Corsi 1992, Turner 2005). Within this debate hangs a question for international bioethics: As developing countries build allopathic medical systems, what should their bioethics be? In this chapter, we explore possible answers to this question, ultimately arguing that Western bioethics is insufficient to solve the problems that arise in the practice of allopathic medicine in non-Western contexts.

As an example, we discuss recent conflicts over the use of mechanical ventilators in Thailand. Thailand is a center of cutting-edge allopathic medical care in Asia. It has a universal health care system, which provides many Thais with access to mechanical ventilation. So many Thais are placed on mechanical ventilators at the end of life that it has become one of the largest drains on Thailand's universal health care system (Alpha Research 2005). Furthermore, the use of ventilators has become a source of vehement national debate, mostly as a result of several prominent political figures who received overly aggressive medical care at the end of life (Ratanakul 2000, Jackson 2003). As in Western hospitals, the ascension of mechanical ventilation has introduced a host of difficult ethical dilemmas for doctors, families, and patients (Kaufman 2005, Klessig 1992). How will Thais go about solving these dilemmas? On which principles of bioethics will they rely?

To answer these questions, we start with a case that illustrates a common ethical dilemma about withdrawal of mechanical ventilation in Thai intensive care units. We then explore some concepts from Western bioethics to see if they help resolve this dilemma. Finally, we explain some of the local ethics behind the case and discuss the concept of a Thai bioethics to address the use of ventilators in Thailand.

A CASE SCENARIO

The following fictional case is based on thirty ethnographic interviews and two months of participant-observation fieldwork by Scott Stonington in 2005. The case contains themes that arose frequently during this research.

Gaew, a thirty-nine-year-old Thai construction worker, falls from a scaffold and hits his head on the pavement. He is unconscious by the time he arrives at one of Bangkok's cutting-edge emergency rooms. He is intubated and placed in the intensive care unit. Gaew's physician, Dr. Nok, informs Gaew's brother, Lek, that Gaew has little chance of recovery due to his lack of brain activity.

Lek does not know what to do—he wants to give his brother the best care possible, but he knows his brother is suffering. He would like to remove Gaew's ventilator. Dr. Nok replies that this is impossible because it is unethical to remove ventilators. Very few physicians in Thailand withdraw ventilators from patients (Ratanakul 2000). They have a complex array of reasons for declining to withdraw ventilator support, including their medical training, fear of litigation, and belief in the sanctity of life.

As with most Thai physicians, Dr. Nok's refusal to withdraw the ventilator is explicitly Buddhist. The first precept of Buddhism forbids killing. Other Buddhist doctrines teach that the last part of the body to die is the breath. For a Thai Buddhist physician, pulling out a patient's ventilator may feel like pulling out the patient's soul. If Dr. Nok withdraws Gaew's ventilator, she will necessarily have "ill will" or "repugnance" in her mind (Keown 1998, 2005).

In Buddhist terms, Dr. Nok's own karma is at stake. Karma is a moral law, central to lay Thai Buddhism, which describes chains of cause and effect that result from individual behavior.

Actions generate either merit or demerit, and the balance of these two currencies determines one's spiritual future (Ratanakul 2000, Keown 2005, Keown 1995). If Dr. Nok's mind contains ill will or repugnance, she will accrue demerit, and this will negatively affect her in this and future lifetimes.

Neither Lek nor Dr. Nok asks what Gaew would have wanted in his current situation. They do not ponder this question because in lay Thai Buddhism, the self is seen as different from moment to moment—so Gaew is not the same person now as he was ten days ago. To Dr. Nok and Lek, an advance directive seems ludicrous. How could a person know what he would want years later, in a different state of consciousness (Ratanakul 2000)?

Dr. Nok is ready with a strategy for circumventing their dilemma. She tells Lek that together they must help Gaew "let go." She explains that it is Gaew's mental attachments that are keeping him alive and suffering on the ventilator. When Dr. Nok says "attachments," she uses the Thai word for "knot of problems" (*bpom bpan ha*), implying a gnarled set of worries tangling Gaew's mind and keeping him from achieving mental clarity and letting go of life. She asks Lek what Gaew might be worried about. Lek replies that Gaew wanted to be ordained as a monk before dying. Although they cannot know what is in Gaew's mind in his new state of consciousness, this is a possible element in his "knot."

Dr. Nok suggests that Lek go to Bangkok and ordain as a monk for several days in Gaew's stead, then return to tell Gaew what he has done. She explains that even though Gaew has little brain activity, when all of the senses subside, the spirit may still take in sound (Keown 2005). She hopes that when Gaew hears about his brother's ordination, he may let go and die with the ventilator still attached and running. This way, she and Lek can relieve Gaew's suffering without compromising their karma.

HOW WOULD WESTERN BIOETHICS HANDLE THIS CASE?

There has been a recent fervor of discussion in many Western medical schools about culture and bioethics (Turner 2005). Medical students and physicians are being trained in "cultural competence" to help them handle a culturally diverse society. This training usually focuses on prototypic cases meant to exemplify particular cultural or ethnic groups. In general, it is assumed that the principles of Western bioethics—autonomy, beneficence, nonmaleficence, truth-telling, and justice—are universal. Different cultures are seen as emphasizing these principles differently, rather than as operating on unique principles of their own.

A classic example, taught in many U.S. medical schools, is the story of the "Asian" elder who comes into the hospital, and whose son says, "Please, do not tell my father that he has cancer." Most Western physicians would analyze this situation as follows: The son believes that knowing about the illness will hurt his father; the son values beneficence (doing what is best for the patient) over autonomy (the patient's prerogative to make decisions for himself); and thus he wants to conceal the illness from his father. In this analysis, the principles of bioethics are held to be universal—the son's culture simply makes him value these principles in a unique proportion.

This approach proves unhelpful in understanding Gaew's case. Dr. Nok's refusal to remove the ventilator is not based on Gaew's wishes, it is not based on what is best for Gaew, and it is not about what is most truthful, or what is best for Thais as a whole. None of these fundamental principles of Western bioethics—autonomy, beneficence, nonmaleficence, truth-telling, or justice—sufficiently explain Lek and Dr. Nok's dilemma. Even though the hospital taking care of Gaew is a center of allopathic medicine—a form of medicine grown out of the West—it is nonetheless a zone governed at least partially by non-Western bioethical principles.

A tool central to the practice of bioethics in Western hospitals is delineating between different kinds of dilemmas. The most widely read textbook of bioethics in the West, by Beauchamp and Childress, distinguishes between at least three kinds of dilemmas: (1) ethical dilemmas, in which two ethical principles dictate opposite actions; (2) self-interest dilemmas, in which the decision maker's own self-interest conflicts with a decision dictated by an ethical principle; and (3) practical dilemmas, in which something logistical prevents an ethical decision from being enacted (Beauchamp and Childress 2001). Making these distinctions is often the first task that a physician must complete during an ethics consult. One must separate the entangled needs of doctors and family members from the ethical principles that determine how to treat a patient.

So what kind of dilemmas are Lek and Dr. Nok confronting? Are the principles governing their behavior ethical, practical, or self-interested? Take, for example, Dr. Nok's reason for not withdrawing the ventilator: to do so would be revoking a patient's life. At first, this sounds like an ethical principle, a kind of nonmaleficence. But on closer inspection, the principle beneath her action diverges significantly from nonmaleficence.

In a Buddhist framework, killing is ethically wrong because it defiles the mind of the killer. Even if Dr. Nok thinks that withdrawing the ventilator is the most compassionate thing for Gaew, it would be spiritually disadvantageous for her. As one Thai physician explained, "It may be the best thing for the patient [to withdraw the ventilator], but how could you find someone who would do it?" A Thai physician would not want to take the risk of acquiring spiritual demerit.

It would then be tempting to say that Dr. Nok's situation represents a self-interest dilemma. An ethical decision—compassionately relieving suffering by removing the ventilator—is in conflict with Dr. Nok's concern for her own spiritual fate. But this interpretation also breaks down because the precise thing that would generate demerit for Dr. Nok is ill will toward Gaew.

In a Buddhist ethical framework, it is impossible to withdraw a ventilator with beneficent intent. In Dr. Nok's case, self-interest and ethical duty are so intertwined as to be indistinguishable. The distinction made between self-interest and ethical dilemmas collapses. The first task of a Western ethicist—to determine the type of dilemma at work—proves an impasse in Gaew's case.

The fact that a Western bioethical approach fails in Gaew's case may be a indication of the limitations of the "one-size-fits-all" bioethics used in Western hospitals as much as it is an illustration of local differences in ethical reasoning (Damien Keown, personal correspondence). Western bioethics is a young discipline, and it draws on only a minority of the rich history of Western ethical philosophy (Jonsen 1998). Nonetheless, the conceptual tools of Western bioethics dominate policy, law, bureaucracy, and physician decision making in Western hospitals. These concepts are beginning to have weight in policymaking in Thailand (Lindbeck 1984). Gaew's case makes it clear that one must examine local ethical concepts before uncritically importing Western bioethical tools.

DOES THAILAND NEED A THAI BIOETHICS?

Dr. Nok's solution to Gaew's end-of-life is instructive as an introduction to what a Thai bioethics might look like. Dr. Nok and Lek cannot remove Gaew's ventilator, and yet their compassion and duty demand that they relieve his suffering. They circumvent this dilemma by helping Gaew to let go of his life peacefully. This strategy has a positive effect on the karmic fate of everyone involved. They relieve Gaew's suffering. Lek acquires merit by ordaining as a monk.

These decisions are based on the logic of karmic morality. They also illustrate the Buddhist principle of interdependence. Interdependence means that doctors, patients, and relatives must think about the emotions and interests of all parties involved in a medical decision. This is in contrast to the Western concept of autonomy, which allows a patient to make decisions without consideration of the feelings and responsibilities of other people concerned. Dr. Nok's solution to Gaew's end of life is not just for Gaew, it is also for herself and for Lek. It is an ethics of compassion that must relieve the suffering of all people concerned.

Pinit Ratanakul, as a member of a team of Thai scholars, has worked for the last ten years to develop an applied ethics using principles such as karma, compassion, and interdependence (Ratanakul 1988, 1990, 1999; Boyd, Ratanakul, and Deepudong 1998). In the West, the main purpose of a countrywide policy is to resolve conflicts between individuals over medical decisions. However, because the concept of interdependence is so central for most Thais, Thailand's bioethical policies may differ dramatically from those found in the West.

CONCLUSION

The purpose of this exploration has been to illustrate the need for Thailand and other countries to develop bioethical systems using local concepts. It would be a mistake, however, to leave our analysis of Thai bioethics without considering the term *Thai*. This has long been a problem with writings on "Asian values" or "Asian thinking."

In this article, we have emphasized Buddhism as a major ethical system, but it is one of many such systems engaged in decisions about the end of life in Thailand. Buddhist monasteries, lay Buddhist organizations, advocates of medical technology, public health officials, and lobbyists for the booming medical tourism industry are all engaged in vehement debate over what should guide Thailand in making medical decisions (Ratanakul 2000, Jackson 2003). As with other countries, Thailand is not a place with a single ethics. In the same way that one cannot import concepts from the West to solve dilemmas in Thailand, one cannot haphazardly select a view within Thailand and label it as *Thai*.

Nonetheless, there is an urgent need for solutions to the "ventilator problem"—both to patch the failing universal health care system and to help Thais make difficult decisions about intervention at the end of life. Thailand is just beginning the long process of integrating its multitude of local voices and concepts into nationwide ethical standards. This new Thai ethics promises to be much more effective at solving Thailand's ethical problems than tools imported uncritically from the West.

ACKNOWLEDGMENTS

This research was made possible by the University of California Pacific Rim Research Program and the University of California San Francisco Office of International Programs. I would like to thank Warapong Wongwachara for translation, insight, and comments in all phases of fieldwork. I would like to thank Gay Becker, Vincanne Adams, China Scherz, Olivia Para, Sherry Brenner, and Damien Keown for help with this manuscript.

NOTE

1. Open access article from *PLOS Medicine*, October 2006, Vol. 3, no. 10. Reprinted with the permission of Scott Stonington and Pinit Ratanakul.

REFERENCES

Adams, V. 2002. "Randomized Controlled Crime: Postcolonial Sciences in Alternative Medicine Research." *Social Studies of Science* 32 (5–6): 659–90.

Alpha Research. 2005. "Thailand Public Health, 2005–2006." Nonthaburi (Thailand): Alpha Research.

Beauchamp, T. L., and J. F. Childress. 2001. *Principles of Biomedical Ethics*. New York: Oxford University Press.

Benatar, S. R. 2005. "Achieving Gold Standards in Ethics and Human Rights in Medical Practice." *PLOS Medicine* 2 (8): e260.

Boyd, A., P. Ratanakul, and A. Deepudong. 1998. "Compassion as Common Ground." *Eubios Journal of Asian and International Bioethics* 8:34–37.

Butt, L. 2002. "The Suffering Stranger: Medical Anthropology and International Morality." *Medical Anthropology* 21:1–24; discussion 25–33.

Cohen, L. 1999. "Where It Hurts: Indian Material for an Ethics of Organ Transplantation." *Daedalus* 128 (4): 135–65.

Farmer, P. 2001. *Infections and Inequalities: The Modern Plagues.* Berkeley: University of California Press.

Jackson, P. A. 2003. *Buddhadasa: Theravada Buddhism and Modernist Reform in Thailand.* Chiang Mai (Thailand): Silkworm Books.

Jonsen, A. R. 1998. *The Birth of Bioethics.* New York: Oxford University Press.

Kaufman, S. R. 2005. *And a Time to Die: How American Hospitals Shape the End of Life.* New York: Scribner.

Keown, D. 1995. *Buddhism and Bioethics.* New York: St. Martin's Press.

———. 1998. "Suicide, Assisted Suicide and Euthanasia: A Buddhist Perspective." *Journal of Law and Religion* 13 (2): 385–405.

———. 2005. "End of Life: The Buddhist View." Lancet 366 (9489): 952–5.

Kim, J. Y. 2000. *Dying for Growth: Global Inequality and the Health of the Poor.* Monroe, ME: Common Courage Press.

Klessig, J. 1992. "The Effect of Values and Culture on Life-Support Decisions." *Western Journal of Medicine* 157:316–22.

Lindbeck, V. 1984. "Thailand: Buddhism Meets the Western Model." *Hastings Center Report* 14 (6): 24–26.

Pellegrino, E. D., P. Mazzarella, and P. Corsi. 1992. *Transcultural Dimensions in Medical Ethics.* Frederick, MD: University Publishing Group.

Ratanakul, P. 1988. "Bioethics in Thailand: The Struggle for Buddhist Solutions." *Journal of Medicine and Philosophy* 13 (3): 301–12.

———. 1990. "Thailand: Refining Cultural Values." *Hastings Center Report* 20 (2): 25–27.

———. 1999. "Love in Buddhist Bioethics." *Eubios Journal of Asian and International Bioethics* 9:45–46.

———. 2000. "To Save or Let Go: Thai Buddhist Perspectives on Euthanasia." In *Contemporary Buddhist Ethics*, edited by D. Keown, 169–82. Richmond, Surrey (United Kingdom): Curzon.

Turner, L. 2005. "From the Local to the Global: Bioethics and the Concept of Culture." *Journal of Medicine and Philosophy* 30 (3): 305–20.

Discussion Topics: Part I

Wanda Teays

1. If you think about international and cross-cultural issues in medicine, health care, public health, and biomedical research, what do you think are important to focus upon as we set a direction for global bioethics?
2. How can we bring in the different voices and concerns across different groups and socioeconomic levels so that global bioethics can shape policies and methodologies to address injustice in health care? What kinds of changes should occur in institutions such as hospitals and universities in terms of the training of doctors, nurses, and other caregivers?
3. In his global framework of bioethics, Bernard Gert sets out the following moral rules that he thinks are universal. Share your thoughts on his choices. Would you make any changes? His list is as follows: (1) do not kill, (2) do not deceive, (3) do not cause pain, (4) keep your promises, (5) do not disable, (6) do not cheat, (7) do not deprive of freedom, (8) obey the law, (9) do not deprive of pleasure, and (10) do your duty.
4. Consider what *duty* entails. What importance does duty play when it comes to your own health—or caring for the health of another (such as a family member)?

   Answer the following:
   a. Gert says that, "Duties in [the] everyday sense are not derived from our common morality, but in each society duties develop from social roles and from the history and practice of the professions in that society."
   b. This ties the notion of duty to social roles (which affects us as individuals) and professional roles (which affects doctors, nurses, researchers, etc.). Are there any other things that shape our sense of duty?

5. Gert also looks at harm. He says, "what it means 'to cause harm to someone' is not as simple and straightforward as it initially seems." Why not?
   Answer the following:
   a. Can you think of examples that would support his claim—that causing harm is not as simple/straightforward as we might imagine?
   b. Assuming Gert is right, how can this help us when constructing a global—and more expansive—bioethics?

6. Do you think there is any value or set of values that are universal? If not, should bioethicists work toward creating some common values that we can draw upon in addressing ethical dilemmas that are found in different societies or countries?

7. In his chapter on universal morality and multiculturalism, Tom Beauchamp notes: "True cultural relativists . . . subscribe to the thesis that no moral principles of any sort, general or particular, are valid independent of the cultural contexts in which they have arisen and shaped to their present form."

   This puts considerable emphasis on the cultural context and, thus, requires us to have some familiarity with the cultural context in order to assess the validity of moral principles.
   Answer the following:
   How might a cultural relativist respond to Gert's list (set out above in question #3)?

8. When dealing with patients from different cultures or of different religions, misinterpretations are possible. When there are language barriers, we turn to translators to ensure channels of communication are in place.
   Answer the following:
   Should there be something like *culture* translators to enable better communication in the face of cultural differences (or barriers)? Share your thoughts and three to four recommendations as to how this might be achieved.

9. Tom Beauchamp raises important issues around morality and culture in his chapter. He points out: "It is often difficult to determine which group, society, or institution constitutes the culture that should be followed." For example, in pre-Taliban Afghanistan women were often well educated and worked in professions, but under the Taliban-imposed culture they were not allowed to work or to seek an education beyond the age of eight.

   He then asks: "Should we say that women should be governed by either of these conflicting sets of norms? Can one ever be bound by a coercively imposed culture? What from a moral point of view are one's obligations under these circumstances?"
   Answer the following:
   How would you answer these questions? Share your thoughts on any ONE of them.

10. Is there a way to *mediate* moral disputes around bioethical issues—and, thus, go beyond the traditional debate (or adversarial) model? Not all moral

problems have a clear "winner." Offer two or three ideas for constructing or putting to use a mediation model.

11. Søren Holm asks if we can have a global bioethics without having a prior common moral language. He argues that the main contenders for a global moral language are (1) human rights and (2) a set of core principles (see, e.g., Gert). Set out the strengths and weaknesses of these two contenders, noting which one *you* think would be the better choice for a global moral language.

12. The road to a global moral language is not without complications. One concern that Holm raises is *non-negotiable commitments*—where a person's religions, politics, worldview, and more create a challenge (or obstacle) that can't be brushed aside. He asserts: "A slightly different issue that is often confused with the religion issue is the issue of non-negotiable commitments. If any party in the process has non-negotiable commitments, it may block the achievement of coherence, and it may therefore be a necessary component of good faith that everything is up for grabs. But non-negotiable commitments can be held for a variety of reasons, not only religious ones."
    Answer the following:
    What should medical caregivers do when their patients assert non-negotiable commitments due to religion, tradition, culture, politics, or the like?

13. In laying the groundwork for a global bioethics, diversity is key. Becoming more open-minded seems important as well. What other qualities or dispositions need to be taken into account?

14. In their chapter, Scott Stonington and Pinit Ratanakul suggest that Western bioethics cannot easily—if at all—solve the problems of non-Western societies. The trouble seems to be the "one size fits all" mentality of Western bioethics. They examine a case in which "decisions are based on the logic of karmic morality" and illustrate the Buddhist principle of interdependence. They conclude: "Interdependence means that doctors, patients, and relatives must think about the emotions and interests of all parties involved in a medical decision. This is in contrast to the Western concept of autonomy, which allows a patient to make decisions without consideration of the feelings and responsibilities of other people concerned."
    Answer the following:
    a. What needs to shift for Western doctors, patients, and relatives to think about the emotions and interests of all involved in the decision?
    b. Set out the benefits of Western bioethics moving to an approach that recognizes more interdependence in the participants.

15. How can global bioethics address concerns of ordinary people around the world—and not just privilege the views of doctors and researchers?

16. When looking at theoretical perspectives of global health, we also need to consider the way we define our terms. That is not as easy as we might think, but arriving at some commonality is necessary for both communication

and policymaking. Look, for example, at the controversy over the eighteen-year-old Montreal swimmer Victoria Arlen, a paralympic gold medalist in the 100-meter freestyle. Arlen spent almost two years in a coma and is now confined to a wheelchair. On August 10, 2013, she was disqualified from the Paralympic Swimming World Championships in Montreal due to "insufficient evidence to suggest there was a permanent impairment," according to Craig Spence, the paralympic committee spokesperson (See Rachel Lau, "Swimmer and Olympic Gold-Medalist Disqualified for Not Being 'Disabled' Enough," *Global News*, August 14, 2013).

Answer the following:

Investigate the case and share your thoughts on whether Arlen should be disqualified and then offer a working definition of disability for swimmers in the paralympics.

II

HUMAN RIGHTS

Introduction to Part II: Human Rights

John-Stewart Gordon

This section combines two important bioethical topics that are intertwined. These are global bioethics and human rights. The underlying idea is that a global bioethics necessarily needs to appeal to a common or universal standard, a *lingua franca*, in order to resolve bioethical problems in cross-cultural contexts. This universal standard—as many influential (bio)ethicists argue—can be identified with a human rights approach.

Human rights are first and foremost universal moral rights that bind all human beings in all places and at all times, irrespective of whether they are legally enforced or not. For example, Jonathan Mann convincingly claims that the "human rights framework provides a more useful approach for analysing and responding to modern public health challenges than any framework thus far within the biomedical tradition" (1996: 924–25). The contrary view has been brought to the fore by Holm, who examines the strengths and weaknesses of using human rights in bioethics in the previous section. There are, at least, four main reasons why one should rely on human rights in the context of global bioethics that deals with cross-cultural issues:

1. **Universality:** The universality of human rights provides a good universal framework in order to deal with global issues in bioethics.
2. **Established legal framework:** Human rights are already part of international law and are, therefore, best suited to resolve bioethical conflicts at the international and national level, if one could establish a so-called international "bio-law."
3. **Force of language:** Human beings are by nature vulnerable. Violations of human rights usually cause serious health-related problems that undermine the (good) health of human beings. The language of human rights has an

important rhetorical, moral, and popular force. No one—even human rights violators—wants to be acknowledged as a person who violates human rights.

4. **Relation of rights and health:** The most fundamental human rights such as the right to life, the right to physical integrity, and the rights to health care and health care resources are closely tied to the field of biomedicine.

Historically speaking, the use of human rights in legal documents in the context of bioethics during the last decades has been a success story—the Nuremberg Code (1947), the Declaration of Helsinki (1964) and its revised versions, the proposed International Ethical Guidelines for Biomedical Research Involving Human Subjects (1982), the Declaration concerning the human genome and human rights (1997), the European Conventions of Human Rights and Biomedicine (1997), and the additional protocol of the European Convention regarding the prohibition of cloning human beings (1998).

One must admit, however, that many philosophers and, in particular, bioethicists still hesitate to use the concept of human rights by virtue of its unclear ontological, legal, and moral status. For example, critics argue that the application of human rights in non-Western cultures and traditions is a form of Western ethical imperialism since they originated in the West and should not be used elsewhere (e.g., female genital circumcision); or, people simply deny that there are any universal basic rights that bind all human beings in all places at all times. Despite such reservations, it seems crystal clear that global bioethics and human rights share some features that give rise to a fruitful cooperation in order to deal with complex bioethical issues on a global level.

The chapters of the second part can be seen as a further refinement of the first part concerning global perspectives on bioethics. For example, I thoroughly examine the notion of human dignity against the background of human rights in bioethics by showing that human dignity is a valuable concept that can be used for ethical reasoning and decision making on a global scale once a so-called cognitivist theory of dignity has been established.

In his illuminating chapter, Robert Baker provides some valuable historical insights on the parallel development and accidental divorce of bioethics and human rights in the last century. He eventually argues that one should reconcile both concepts. One could say that Baker's request to reconcile bioethics and human rights has been put into practice on an international level by the UN Convention on the Rights of Persons with Disabilities. In Akito Ito's chapter, she examines the implementation phase of the Convention and particularly pays attention to cultural rights against the background of some pertinent issues for policymaking to support national implementation. Her case is a good example of how bioethics and human rights merge together in order to protect vulnerable human beings.

In her intriguing chapter about torturous actions performed by medical personnel in the context of nontherapeutic medical experimentation and participation in abuse and torture, Wanda Teays examines a vast range of important cases. She concludes that medical professionals should report abuses more often and that medical organizations must address such ethical issues more straightforwardly in order to facilitate a systematic change.

Rita Manning's alarming chapter points into the same direction when she discusses the complex situation of the right to health care of detained immigrants and how the Immigration and Customs Enforcement (ICE) in the United States deals with the situation. The grossly inadequate medical care leads to many cases of medical neglect and abuses, and thereby it causes numerous deaths among the detained immigrants. This abuse must stop—Manning sees a special obligation to the vulnerable people housed by the ICE.

Taking the recent development of the death penalty in China as the starting point, Cher Weixia Chen examines two vital concerns in the context of lethal injection—first, the participation of medical staff in lethal injections and, second, the practice of harvesting organs from executed prisoners. Both challenging issues are deeply concerned with human rights and bioethics. After having discussed these issues, Chen eventually offers some recommendations concerning the need for proper guidelines that should be in order.

The last chapter shows us how global bioethics has had an impact on specific countries, and vice versa. By examining the different approaches and the perspective each offers on bioethics, we get a richer sense of this discipline. Godfrey B. Tangwa argues that, as a derivative of ethics, human rights are a powerful heuristic device for assessing and affecting ethical conduct. He focuses on sexual and reproductive health within the context of a particular culture—that of the Nso' of Cameroon, Africa. His examination highlights the complex nature of the interplay between culture, ethics, and human rights—and its importance in Africa today.

The chapters included in part 2 help us see how the ideas and principles of one group or region can travel to another, thus showing us how bioethics takes shape as a global discipline. The authors' work with the chapters in the first section on theoretical perspectives to give us an overview of global bioethics. In addition, they help us to see how much can be gained by this wider approach to the field.

1

Human Dignity, Human Rights, and Global Bioethics

John-Stewart Gordon[1]

ABSTRACT

This chapter examines the notion of human dignity in bioethics and focuses, in particular, on the potential contribution of human dignity for global bioethics. It is argued that the notion of human dignity in bioethics should be supported by the concept of human rights in order to establish a so-called cognitivist theory of dignity that can be used in global bioethical discourses. All in all, this chapter offers a systematic analysis of the role of human dignity in bioethics and highlights the pros and cons of the debate.

INTRODUCTION

The notion of human dignity is, without a doubt, one of the most controversial and lively discussed concepts in bioethics. The last seventy years are rife with intriguing approaches on how to understand the nature of human dignity and its relation to human rights in bioethics on many different levels. This includes legal documents, ethical guidelines, books, and research articles. The vast range of different views on (human) dignity is divergent and varies from "incoherent and unhelpful" to "illuminating and important" by virtue of the unclear ontological, epistemological, as well as moral and legal status of the notion of human dignity.

The consequence is that many bioethicists attempt to completely avoid "dignity-talk," since they argue that this notion is—simply speaking—too vague, reactionary, and redundant to facilitate and enhance the bioethical debate in general and to solve complex cases in particular (e.g., Kuhse 2000, Macklin 2003, Cochrane 2009,

Pacholczyk and Schüklenk 2010). Furthermore, physicians and researchers occasionally claim that the appeal to human dignity (and human rights) complicates ethical reasoning and decision making in end-of-life cases, organ sales, genetic engineering/enhancement, design babies, cloning, and human-animal chimera.

The main goal of this chapter is to facilitate and enhance the debate with regard to a better understanding of the nature of human dignity in bioethics. The notion of human dignity is still vastly undervalued in particular by bioethicists in the English-speaking bioethics discourse (most notably in the United States) and should be examined in more detail in order to disclose its full potential. This chapter focuses on the potential contribution of the concept of human dignity (and human rights) in cross-cultural bioethics or global bioethics. The first part presents Ruth Macklin's famous and acute critique on the (mis)use of the notion of human dignity in bioethics, while the second part provides different and challenging responses to her viewpoint.

Here, the crucial point is that human dignity is not equivalent to the principle of autonomy and respect for persons as Macklin claims but contains more features than she acknowledges (e.g., Killmister 2010). The third part deals with the vital issue of how the notion of human dignity and human rights can be used for bridging the gap between different and—sometimes very—diverse cultures. The chapter ends with some final remarks.

A CRITIQUE OF HUMAN DIGNITY: IS DIGNITY A USELESS CONCEPT?

The appeal to the notion of human dignity in bioethics has not been unquestioned by philosophers and bioethicists alike. The well-known bioethicist Ruth Macklin has argued in her famous editorial "Dignity Is a Useless Concept" in the *British Medical Journal* (2003) that "appeals to dignity are either vague restatements of other, more precise, notions or mere slogans that add nothing to an understanding of the topic" (1419).

Dignity is a useless concept and "seems to have no meaning beyond what is implied by the principle of medical ethics, respect for persons: the need to obtain voluntary, informed consent; the requirement to protect confidentiality; and the need to avoid discrimination and abusive practices" (2003: 1419). All in all, dignity can be regarded as equal to the principle of respect for autonomy. To support her hypothesis, Macklin refers to the following example:

> An altogether different use of dignity in relation to death occurs when medical students practise doing procedures (usually intubation) on newly dead bodies. Some medical ethicists charge that these educational efforts violate the dignity of the dead person. But this situation clearly has nothing to do with respect for autonomy since the object is no longer a person but a cadaver. There may be reasonable concern about how the dead person's relatives would feel if they knew that the body was being used in this way. But that concern has nothing to do with the dignity of the dead body and everything to do with respect for the wishes of the living. (Macklin 2003: 1419–20)

In her book, *Against Relativism: Cultural Diversity and the Search for Ethical Universals in Medicine* (1999), Macklin defends a human-rights approach based on her particular idea of moral progress. Even though she believes that "appeals to human dignity are not intuitively more clear than appeals to human rights. If anything, they are more obscure" (220), she also claims that "although the concept of human dignity can have a legitimate place in ethical discourse in connection with cloning, genetic manipulations, and other biomedical activities, more precision is required than simply asserting that 'human dignity is violated'" (221). These statements seem—in general—more conciliatory than the pithy and rather pessimistic or negative in her editorial.

Admittedly, more work needs to be done in order to provide a more satisfactory definition of the notion of human dignity to enhance and facilitate bioethical discourses. The many rapid responses to Macklin's editorial, however, show that her view has not been unchallenged for different reasons posed by laypeople, professionals, and well-known medical ethicists such as Arthur L. Caplan and Ann Gallagher. The following section examines various responses to Macklin's position.

HUMAN DIGNITY IN BIOETHICS:
A VALUABLE CONCEPT AFTER ALL?

Immediate Responses to Macklin's Editorial

Admittedly, appeals to human dignity are often *vague* and *unclear*, so that medical ethicists might have the feeling that this concept is rather *useless* to facilitate and enhance debates in bioethics. Practically speaking, physicians and health care workers seem to know what human dignity means, even though they cannot define it in detail. For example, William H. Konarzewski, a consultant anaesthetist, claims that he is:

> astonished that Ruth Macklin believes dignity is an unhelpful concept. It is regularly used on our intensive care unit and our doctors, nurses and the patients' relatives have no problem understanding that a death with dignity means a death in which the patient is allowed to pass away naturally without unnecessary suffering or anxiety and without the encumbrance of tubes and catheters that distort the appearance of the face and body. We shall continue to allow our patients to die with dignity when it is plain that they are beyond the help of modern medicine. (Konarzewski 2003[2])

Stanley M. Giannet, an affiliate assistant professor of psychiatry and behavioral medicine, argues:

> The shocking reality is that without dignity, clinicians often develop a sterile stoicism towards the suffering and a needless aloofness or alienation from those they serve. Even worse, the absence of dignity as a core value in medical practice can lead to depersonalization where the patient's identity and personhood are reduced to an insurance account number, hospital room number or a diagnosis. For instance, one of the most shocking

examples of this is when I overheard a nurse refer to a patient as "The urinary tract infection in room 306." (Giannet 2003[3])

Even if one is unable to provide a "perfect" definition of what human dignity really is, it is certainly true that one notices when people act without dignity.[4] With regard to the cadaver example, Macklin claims that dignity would be the wrong concept on which to rely, since it has nothing to do with the autonomy of the person concerned because there is no person to be concerned with. Rather, there is a "reasonable concern" to consider the feelings and wishes of the relatives with regard to the proper use of the dead family member. I agree with Macklin that the appeal to autonomy is inappropriate in this case, but the important point is that it is not about autonomy but about the dignity of the dead.

It is widely accepted among people within living memory that cadavers can be violated in a way that their dignity is lost—for example, when they are not buried appropriately but exhibited in a degrading way such as in public display. The point simply is that there is a meaningful sense of dignity that has nothing to do with autonomy—for instance, the long history of funeral practices of humankind (see also Killmister 2010).

Arthur Caplan claims that nonautonomous persons (e.g., cadavers) and probably objects have dignity, if dignity reflects a moral status that moral agents assign to others. His general idea, however, is based on social contract theory in the sense that morality itself is based on a mutual contract between people. Dignity is a "moral creation" that concerns only "autonomous moral agents" (if one does not assign a special moral status to, for example, other nonautonomous beings such as fetuses, small children, comatose people, or the infirm elderly).[5] Whether the notion of human dignity is entirely bound to a decision made by people, as Caplan claims, is not obvious and can be questioned as well. A brief response could be, as Gallagher puts it, that dignity acknowledges the worth of:

> humans qua humans regardless of competence, sentience or body form. Without dignity, it seems, there can be little (if any) meaningful discussion about the rights and wrongs of the treatment of those deemed non-autonomous or non-persons. Dignity is not only a useful value it is, in fact, an essential one. (Gallagher 2004[6])

Why Human Dignity Is Still a Useful Concept After All

Human Dignity Is a "Vague" Concept. Macklin (2003), and most recently Pacholczyk and Schüklenk (2010), believe that the notion of dignity is useless and should be avoided. Pacholczyk and Schüklenk claim in their 2010 editorial in the journal *Bioethics* that "despite the pervasive presence of appeals to dignity in medical ethics and the common use of this term in professional codes, constitutional texts and various human rights instruments, both the moral basis as well as the meaning of this term continue to remain nebulous at best" (Pacholczyk and Schüklenk 2010; Cochrane 2009).

Indeed, much of what has been proposed in the debate about human dignity is problematic by virtue of appealing to unjustified claims, but this does not mean that there is no valid argument that could justify to appeal to the notion of human dignity in bioethical discourses. Even if the notion is still "vague," it does not necessarily mean that this is a disadvantage given that people usually have a good intuition or awareness about what is at stake without necessarily being in the position to explain the notion(s) they use in a precise way.

For example, to display the dead bodies of soldiers in a degrading way concerns the dignity of these cadavers because we *feel* that something is wrong to treat cadavers in such a way, even if they are not living beings. This line of argumentation has its root in common sense, which is more intuitive and often more vague than (analytical) approaches that use technical, precise, and defined terms and language.

The notion of human dignity, like most normative concepts, is to some extent "vague" and open to distortion. But it is far from being *useless*. Vagueness is not emptiness—it is possible to resist wholesale extensions of important notions, for instance, by using the language of rights, in particular human rights, in connection with dignity (see below). Macklin believes that "if human dignity is a vague concept, its basis for claims about human rights is even more obscure" (1999: 221).

Her point of view is not surprising, but I do think that her claim is premature and needs to be addressed in more detail by virtue of the importance of both notions in current bioethical discourses. A quick response could refer to her own approach with regard to her concept of moral progress. Here, she is more faithful concerning the problem of vagueness. Macklin states the following:

> Admittedly, most of the key terms in the principles of humaneness and humanity are vague or denote qualities that are hard to measure, such as "sensitivity to" or "tolerance of" pain and suffering and "recognition of the universal worth or basic autonomy" of every human being. But even if the terms in which these two principles are couched are rather vague, the signs by which we know them in social and political life are clear and unmistakable. Behavioural and contextual evidence, as well as laws and rules that govern behaviour, are the signs. (Macklin 1999: 252)

The notion of human dignity can be known by exactly the same signs, and it seems arbitrary to be generous toward one's own approach in dealing with vagueness while refusing to show the same patience toward other approaches. Even though this kind of behavior is quite common among scholars and is psychologically understandable to some extent, it is nonetheless inappropriate in a philosophical analysis. Furthermore, "vagueness" can be a true strength by being a universal tool or picklock that can be applied to different ethical contexts when it is done in a reasonable way—that is, by appealing to the notion of prudence (see below).

Human Dignity as "Respect for Persons." The notion of human dignity is not limited to the idea of respect for persons (or autonomy), even though it is certainly one main point in describing the concept in more precise terms. But, as the above-mentioned example of treating cadavers with dignity shows, the idea of respect for persons is too restrictive to cover our basic intuitions appropriately.[7]

James Griffin claims, instead, that human dignity consists in personhood or autonomy (and practicalities):

What seems to me the best account of human rights is this. It is centered on the notion of agency. We human beings have the capacity to form pictures of what a good life would be and to try to realise these pictures. We value our status as agents especially highly, often more highly even than our happiness. Human rights can then be seen as protections of our agency—what one might call our personhood. (Griffin 2000)

James Nickel (2007) has rightly criticized Griffin for using a too-restrictive notion of human dignity. He argues that it seems unlikely to generate, for instance, due process rights, rights of nondiscrimination, and equality before the law on the basis of personhood (Nickel 2007: 54). Therefore, Nickel "rejects the view of many that human dignity is found exclusively in human agency or autonomy" (66). He argues:

We can speak of dignity with reference to any particular feature of persons that has distinctive value (for example, their ability to suffer, their lives, their agency, their consciousness and reflective capacities, their use of complicated languages and symbolic systems, their rationality, their individuality, their social awareness). (Nickel 2007: 66)

Indeed, there is no methodological argument why the notion of human dignity should be restricted to the idea of respect for persons. As Robert Andorno puts it:

Beyond all the abusive rhetoric that may surround this notion, a careful analysis of intergovernmental policy documents relating to bioethics, and of the discussion that led to their adoption, puts in evidence that the recourse to human dignity reflects a real concern about the need to ensure respect for the inherent worth of every human being. The concern is far broader than simply ensuring "respect for autonomy" for the simple reason that it also includes the protection of those who are not yet, or are no more, morally autonomous (newborn infants, senile elderly, people with serious mental disorders, comatose patients, etc.). (Andorno 2009: 230)

Whether or not human beings have "an inherent worth" is a question of much debate in philosophy and remains open. The important point that Andorno rightly mentions is that human dignity cannot simply be replaced by "respect for persons" because "respect for persons is just the *consequence* of human dignity, not dignity itself" (Andorno 2009: 230).

Human Dignity and the Task of Sisyphus. The Utilitarian bioethicist Udo Schüklenk—one of the contributors to this volume—poses two main objections against the use of the notion of human dignity in bioethical discourses that can be seen as a fundamental attack regarding concepts such as human dignity and human rights in general and particularly in bioethics (unpublished article). Even though I do not share his extreme view, I do acknowledge that his arguments need to be taken seriously in order to enhance and facilitate the debate in more proper ways to avoid "dignity's wooly uplift" (Pacholczyck and Schüklenk 2010).

His first argument,[8] however, concerns the variety of diverse and different definitions of human dignity in, for example, end-of-life decision making or reproductive cloning. According to Schüklenk, it seems unreasonable to use a notion such as human dignity that is used as a pro *and* contra argument to justify oppositional points of view in (bioethical) debates. It simply does not make any sense to appeal to the same notion and thereby to defending opposite goals.

In this respect he is critical that there is no uniform reading or interpretation of the notion of human dignity. Schüklenk claims that it is rather a placeholder for different definitions and therefore can be avoided altogether. If human dignity means, for example, respect for persons, then one should use the latter term instead of the former.

It is certainly true that there is no uniform reading of the notion of human dignity, but this objection concerns not only the concept of human dignity but also concerns most normative concepts in ethics (e.g., good life, equality, justice, utility). The vital question is not whether the variety of different definitions undermines the whole idea of a particular normative notion such as human dignity, but rather whether there is a proper definition of the normative term that contains objective criteria that are (more) binding.

The differing definitions with regard to the notion of human dignity can, then, be seen as different responses in the search of a more binding definition (see method of specification). Whether this is a so-called wild-goose chase as Schüklenk believes or whether one will find a proper general definition remains to be seen. Giving up the important search in determining proper definitions for normative concepts would finally mean giving up our *moral language* itself, which is a consequence few people might accept. Thus, one should not give up the notion of human dignity but simply be asked to try harder to find (some) objective criteria.

Schüklenk's second main argument questions the use of human dignity as: (1) a means of ethical guidance and (2) a means of justification. He argues that it is futile to use human dignity as a means of ethical guidance simply because opposite points of view claim to rely on the same notion. This, however, would undermine the very function of a proper ethical guidance (see above). The second point is related to two different possibilities with regard to the idea of justification itself.

This means that human dignity, as a (means of) justification, is either a *primitive* term or a *derived* term. If it is the latter possibility (Schüklenk), one should completely give up the notion of dignity and simply use the definition as, for example, respect for persons (i.e., dignity is redundant). If human dignity is a primitive term, one should be able to provide a proper example. So far, according to Schüklenk, this has not been done successfully: Religion (human beings possess human dignity because of *imago dei*) or Kantian approaches (human beings have dignity because of their rational nature) fail to be adequate candidates—there is currently no (convincing) theory of human dignity.

I agree that both ethical approaches are doomed to failure, but I do think that there is a solution to this problem that Richard Ashcroft briefly addresses in "Making Sense of Dignity" (2005: 680). He refers to a cognitive theory of dignity. That means that the notion of dignity is a "thick" concept that contains a descriptive and an evaluative meaning whose "understanding requires a grasp of both the descriptive and the evaluative components" (2005: 680). Ashcroft rightly points out that the vital point is that the evaluative component of a statement in a cognitivist theory of dignity is not (or not purely) subjective but can be true or false irrespective of what the person believes. He convincingly states:

> Nevertheless, such a theory should be able to give us some account of the relationship between moral knowledge and moral argument, and show how claims about moral knowledge can be corrigible or falsifiable. Too much actual argument about dignity tends to collapse into claim and counterclaim about moral intuitions concerning what dignity is, or what has it, or what would affect it. (Ashcroft 2005: 680)

Such a cognitivist theory of dignity would be an adequate example with regard to Schüklenk's point concerning the idea of dignity as a *primitive* term. Do we currently have such a (sophisticated) cognitivist theory of dignity that is convincing? It seems not; however, this does not mean that it is impossible to develop such a theory in the first place. The following section of this chapter contains some preliminary aspects of such a theory.

Human dignity is *a complex and multifaceted notion* that needs to be thoroughly examined; Beyleveld and Brownsword (2004: 42) refer to a list provided by Rendtorff and Kemp (1999: 31) that contains the following six strands:

1. Human dignity emerged "as a virtue of recognition of the other in an intersubjective relationship" and constitutes "a capacity that the person has because of his or her social position."
2. Human dignity indicates "the intrinsic value and moral responsibility of every human being."
3. If human beings have dignity a person must "be considered as without a price" and hence "cannot be objects for trade or commercial transactions."
4. Human dignity is "based on self-other relations of shame and proudness, e.g., in degradation and self-esteem."
5. Human dignity indicates "that there are certain things that a [civilized] society should just not do."
6. Human dignity "includes the individual's openness to the metaphysical dimensions of life, referring to dignified behaviour at the limit-situations of existence such as birth, sufferance, death of a beloved other, one's own death, etc."

We have already encountered some of the above-mentioned descriptions, and given the short history of the term in bioethics it is no wonder that there is still much to be discovered. To claim prematurely that the term is too vague and should be avoided is too simple and a rather lame excuse for not digging deeper. Time will show and recent publications already indicate that the notion of human dignity is useful and will gain a prominent and valuable place in bioethics (Killmister 2010). One point, however, seems crystal clear—even if one cannot currently provide a perfect definition of what dignity actually is, when people act without dignity one has the strong feeling that something is wrong with them.

HOW HUMAN RIGHTS AND HUMAN DIGNITY BRIDGE CULTURAL GAPS IN BIOETHICS

The Concept of Human Rights

Human rights are universal moral rights of high priority that bind all people in all places at all times; they are basic[9] moral rights, irrespective of whether they are enforced by local laws or not. Furthermore, they are international legal rights, which should be integrated into local law in order to be most effective for human beings. Human rights are usually seen as minimal standards to secure the basic interests and needs of human beings (e.g., Orend 2002, Nickel 2007, Griffin 2008).

Generally speaking, they are concerned with avoiding the terrible rather than achieving the best by being a utopian ideal to create a morally perfect society. To provide a thorough response to all ontological and epistemological problems concerning the notion of human rights is certainly one of the most challenging tasks in philosophy and is definitely beyond of the scope of this chapter (see Gordon 2011). The general idea, however, is to argue in the following that human rights can be seen as a *lingua franca* that is deeply interwoven with the notion of human dignity and is widely shared and best equipped to solve cases in ethics and bioethics.

Some Brief Remarks on the History of Human Rights in Bioethics

Historically speaking, human rights began to play an important role in the bioethical discussion for the first time in the late 1940s and could be seen as the immediate response to the abuse of human beings in medical research during the Nazi regime. The Nuremberg Code (1947), the Declaration of Human Rights (1948), and the Declaration of Helsinki (1964) and its revised versions form the starting point for the implementation of universal moral rights in international law.

The general idea was to prevent misconduct in the area of medicine by international law in the future. Hence, the reason for appealing to the concept of human rights in the first place was to identify questionable practices or experiments on human beings and to punish the responsible people.[10] Again and again during the last century it was revealed that human rights do not offer an absolute protection against abuses (even with regard to those countries that had signed the relevant international treaties, such as the United States) and that some people who were responsible for atrocities have not always been punished for their immoral deeds. Striking examples are as follows:

Research on human beings in the past

- Medical research during the Nazi regime in Germany
- Tuskegee syphilis study from 1932 to 1972 in the United States
- Human radiation experiments in the United States during the Cold War

Current problems

- Research on human beings (especially in developing countries)
- Female genital circumcision
- Organ sales
- Cloning of human beings; human-animal hybrids
- Poverty and public health
- Informed consent (individual versus community or family consent)
- Pandemia

Following the above-mentioned problems and in the course of the technological development of medicine (e.g., new biotechnology), international agreements have been continually modified, actualized, and extended. The most important documents concerning bioethics in recent history are as follows:

- The Proposed International Guidelines for Biomedical Research involving Human Subjects (1982)[11]
- The Declaration concerning the Human Genome and Human Rights (1997)
- The European Convention on Human Rights and Biomedicine (1997)
- The additional protocol of the European Convention with regard to the Prohibition of Cloning Human Beings (1998)
- The Universal Draft Declaration on Bioethics and Human Rights (2005)[12]

The basic idea to establish human rights as a universal standard for determining and solving international conflicts or problems did not stem from philosophers but mainly from lawyers, who were influenced by the traditional role of human rights.

Many philosophers (and in particular ethicists) at that time had serious reservations about the use of this concept because the ontological, legal, and moral status of human rights had not been determined appropriately prior to their application. However, in the following decades, authors discussed the concept of human rights in bioethics in more detail (e.g., Bandman and Bandman 1978, Annas and Grodin 1995, Baker 1998, Macklin 1999, Mann et al. 1999, CQHE 2001, Baker 2001, Beyleveld and Brownsword 2004, Annas 2005, DWB 2005, Pogge 2007).[13]

Why Human Rights in Bioethics?

There are many different reasons why it is of great advantage to appeal to human rights in bioethics, in particular in global or cross-cultural bioethics when dealing with vital issues that concern all people. *Globalization* is as old as humankind and is a vital reason why human beings share common problems due to mercantilism (e.g., global capitalism) and religious and cultural exchanges and are facilitated by new methods of transportation and technological developments in the media, such as the Internet, books, newspapers, and more that deeply influence and shape our social life.

The world—virtually speaking—has become a village. This is the reason why local problems transcend national borders that also concern the field of bioethics. Pandemics (e.g., HIV), global public health issues, environmental issues of global extent (e.g., global warming), the rise of biotechnology, and more arouse concerns that are universal in nature and need to be addressed by all people.

One promising way to deal with these issues and to find a global solution is by appealing to human rights as a starting point and constraining framework that can be seen as a "lingua franca that can both facilitate and broaden international bioethics discourse" (Knowles 2001: 253). The following incomplete list contains some main reasons why one should use a human rights approach in bioethics:

1. Force of language: The language of human rights has a great *rhetorical, moral,* and *popular* force (Baker 2001, Knowles 2001). Human rights violations are seen as serious incidents that call for immediate actions. Because of the vulnerability of human beings, bioethical and health-related issues are of great importance; therefore, human beings need special protection.
2. Established legal framework: Human rights instruments already exist within the established framework of international law, including treaties, agreements, and conventions (Baker 2001, Knowles 2001). That means an international so-called biolaw could help to solve ethical conflicts on an international and national level (Beyleveld and Brownsword 2002).
3. Universality: The universality of human rights facilitates the establishment of universal moral norms in bioethics "for analysing and responding to modern public health challenges" (Mann 1996: 924–25, Andorno 2008). A global bioethics necessarily needs to appeal to a (minimal) universal standard or *lingua franca* in order to solve cross-cultural problems.
4. Relation of rights and health: There is a close relationship between biomedicine and the most basic human rights such as the right to life, the right to physical integrity, and the rights to health care and health care resources (Ashcroft 2008; Gordon 2008, 2012; Arras and Fenton 2009; Ram-Tiktin 2012).
5. Additional principles: The notion of human dignity is often unable to provide clear answers in bioethics. Additional and more precise reasons are needed; this can be done by appealing to more concrete principles, that is, patient autonomy, confidentiality, privacy, and protection from discrimination. These principles are usually formulated in terms of rights (Andorno 2008, Baranzke 2012).

The Cultural Gap: The Claws of Ethical Relativism

The first paragraph of Ruth Macklin's book *Against Relativism* (1999) gets to the heart of the problem of ethical relativism. She writes:

> A long-standing debate surrounds the question whether ethics are relative to time and place. One side argues that there is no obvious source of a universal morality and that ethical rightness and wrongness are products of their cultural and historical setting. Opponents claim that even if a universal set of ethical norms has not yet been articulated or agreed upon, ethical relativism is a pernicious doctrine that must be rejected. The first group replies that the search for universal ethical precepts is a quest for the Holy Grail. The second group responds with the telling charge: If ethics were relative to time, place, and culture, then what the Nazis did was "right" for them, and there is no basis for moral criticism by anyone outside the Nazi society. (Macklin 1999: 4)

The *descriptive* thesis that particular moralities differ from culture to culture or within one multicultural society is certainly true (i.e., descriptive ethical relativism or cultural relativity). However, the vital question is whether this has any influence on *normative* ethics.

Normative ethical relativists argue "that different basic moral requirements apply to (at least some) different moral agents, or groups of agents, owing to different intentions, desires, or beliefs among such agents or groups" (Carson and Moser 2001: 2). The most common form of normative relativism is *social normative relativism,* which holds "that an action is morally obligatory for a person if and only if that action is prescribed by the basic moral principles accepted by that person's society" (Carson and Moser 2001: 2). In other words, there are no universal moral norms that apply to people of different cultures or societies.

That means that the racist system of Nazi Germany, the apartheid system in South Africa, the caste system in India, and the Taliban system in Afghanistan, for instance, cannot be evaluated and disapproved by universal moral standards because there are no such standards. According to ethical relativists, one has to *tolerate* different and diverse moral norms, even if one wholeheartedly disapproves of the moral norms of a particular culture or society. The fact that descriptive ethical relativism is correct and helps *to explain* why people behave the way they behave is nonetheless inappropriate for being a *moral justification.* Explanation is not justification.

Despite the fact that the relativists' claim of tolerance is itself a *universal* moral norm—and therefore undermines the very idea of ethical relativism—one should give up the view of ethical relativism by appealing to other good reasons that I briefly examine in the following by focusing on the notion of human rights as a paradigm case against ethical relativism (see also Nickel 2007: 168–84).[14]

First, the idea of universal moral norms—in particular the idea of human rights— is of Western origin and hence biased in a way that would lead to a *cultural or ethical imperialism,* if other cultures or societies are forced to adapt to the Western standard. This line of argumentation is misleading because of the so-called genetic fallacy that refers to a flaw in reasoning.

The flaw is as follows: "Rejecting an argument, or theory, not on the basis of its own merits but, rather, on the basis of the irrelevant personal characteristics of the person or group who invented it" (Orend 2002: 158). That means that even if the idea of universal human rights is of Western origin, it has nothing to do with the validity of its universal applicability.[15]

Secondly, the idea of multiculturalism to respect the traditions, ways of life, beliefs, and more of other cultures is certainly a valuable goal, but it does not follow from this point of view, however, that one is necessarily committed to the (more) extreme claim that *all* beliefs and practices of *all* cultural groups and subgroups must be equally respected. It is more reasonable to assume that some things are relative and others are not.

Macklin is right in claiming that "a convincing argument against ethical relativism need not conclude that *nothing* is relative, only that certain types of actions or practices—chiefly, those that violate human rights—are not" (Macklin 1999: 24). The vital point is, then, that one has to show that some moral considerations from outside the culture's own value framework are relevant or should be relevant with regard to some traditions and practices within that culture. This is the domain of cross-cultural ethical judgments.[16]

Thirdly, I have recently argued in my article "On Justifying Human Rights" (Gordon 2011) that the connecting bond of all human beings consists in universally shared basic needs which, in turn, are related to a small set of human rights that protect these basic needs. My approach is based on a revised version of Kant's notion of rationality and Rawls's idea of the veil of ignorance.

The main claim is that one is able to derive moral rights—in particular human rights—from a proper understanding of the notion of rationality. "Rationality itself commands the fulfilment of the basic needs (. . .) All contraventions concerning the fulfilment of the basic needs carry the burden of proof for the particular exception" (Gordon 2011). If traditions and practices violate basic human needs such as the physical integrity of the body (e.g., female genital circumcision), then this particular practice should be abolished (Gordon 2008). Not all traditions and practices of all cultures and subcultures are appropriate—for example, the institution of slavery, gender inequality, *ius primae noctis*.

It might be, at first sight, that (some) cultures seem to be so different and diverse in their traditions and practices that one could hardly believe that there is any connecting bond between the peoples. On second glance, however, one realizes that this is not the case (e.g., Rachels 2001). It is possible to criticize other cultures legitimately and to bridge cultural gaps by appealing to human rights and the idea of human dignity. Eventually, the claws of ethical relativism become dull. In the following section, I examine the relation between human rights and human dignity and answer the question why it is reasonable to use both notions in bioethics, in particular in cross-cultural bioethics or global bioethics.

Human Rights and Human Dignity

The general idea of an ethical approach is to guide people in their decision making and to provide them with a sound justification for why one should use this particular approach. This explains why a global bioethics or cross-cultural bioethics must also be able to respond to both challenges. In this respect, a *global* bioethics must be universal in its nature because it addresses global problems—such as pandemics, research on human beings in developing countries, (international) organ sales, and female genital circumcision—that people face around the world.

A global bioethics, then, should be able to consider both universal moral claims and cultural differences in such a way that it enriches bioethical discourses (see below). Therefore, it seems reasonable to assume that a global bioethics should appeal to a universal standard or *lingua franca* in order to warrant sound cross-cultural bioethical statements. I have argued in this chapter that a global bioethics should use human rights and the notion of human dignity in order to solve cross-cultural bioethical problems (e.g., Knowles 2001, Thomasma 2001, Andorno 2009).

The notion of human dignity, however, could be seen as an overarching principle by being the starting point and constraining framework of global bioethical discourses. In the following, I hope to clarify further both notions with regard to their potential for global bioethics. But before I examine the notion of human dignity in more detail, I want to briefly introduce six ways in which human dignity and human rights have been related to one another:[17]

1. Human dignity as the source of human rights.

According to this common view, human beings have intrinsic worth that should be maintained, respected, and protected by other people. Human beings are vulnerable, and therefore their intrinsic worth might sometimes be in jeopardy. Hence, it follows that their dignity needs to be protected by appealing to strong rights—human rights from those fellow members who disrespect the other person's dignity and the (unlawful) state. In this context, "human dignity, thus, justifies a protective regime of human rights in a very straightforward way" (Beyleveld and Brownsword 2004: 22).

2. Human dignity—as a species of human rights—is concerned with conditions of self-respect.

Beyleveld and Brownsword convincingly claim that there is a right to the conditions in which human dignity can flourish (2004: 18–21). They believe that the capacity for autonomous action is a distinctive human capacity that should be protected. The institutions of slavery and apartheid, so they argue, are undermining the self-respect and hence dignity of those individuals who are affected by these institutions. They claim: "Over and above such matters, the right to the conditions in which human dignity can flourish presupposes a certain level of self-respect or self esteem. The deep problem with the institution of slavery, however, is that it invites precisely the opposite perception of oneself—far from cultivating self-respect, this is an institution that brands a section of humans as mere property" (2004: 19).

3. Human dignity defining the subjects of human rights.

By claiming—as it is commonly done—that *only* human beings have human dignity, one is thereby committed to the claim that *only* human beings are protected by human rights. One might rightly object that this kind of reasoning is fallacious by virtue of its contingency on human commitment and acceptance (i.e., the charge of speciesism). Why should only human beings have dignity and thus should be protected? A supposed way out of this problem was to identify the dignity of human beings with their capacity for autonomous actions; that is, their rationality. By adhering to this view, one—at the same time—extends and limits the group of subjects of beings who are protected by human rights. One extends the protected group by considering other beings that are *rational* beings and are not necessarily humans in the first place. One limits the group of human beings by omitting human beings who lack rationality. In this sense human dignity defines the subjects of human rights.

4. Human dignity defining the objects to be protected by human rights.

Peter Kemp concedes that the (new) extended sense of human dignity is "not obvious" and explains that "if one transforms the idea of dignity as a virtue of the other into a universal principle for understanding the worth of human being as such, then dignity can be ascribed not only to men and women as rational beings, but also to the human being who has not yet, or has no longer, an autonomous will, and who is therefore unable to be a master of his or her own life" (quoted by Beyleveld and Brownsword 2004: 32). If embryonic and fetal life is directly protected by human dignity, then the indirect human-rights-based protection is out of date by having been replaced by a direct dignity-based justification. Beyleveld and Brownsword are correct in claiming that if this were the case, then "it almost certainly signals a much more restrictive approach to early-stage biomedical interventions" (2004: 33).

5. Human dignity as reinforcing rights of individual autonomy and self-determination.

Beyleveld and Brownsword discuss the famous French dwarf-throwing case as an example in which both parties—the dwarfs and legal authorities—appeal to the notion of human dignity (2004: 25–27). To put it in a nutshell, dwarf throwing in local clubs was banned in France, and several people challenged the ban. In particular, one dwarf (Manuel Wackenheim) claimed that he freely participated in the dwarf throwing without being reduced to a mere thing since he was always in control of the situation and it was his profession, providing him with a monthly income. If the ban makes him and others unemployed again, it would undermine the very condition in which he (and others) experienced a sense of dignity by being employed. It was their individual, autonomous decision to participate in this activity (*human dignity as empowerment*). The legal authorities, instead, argued that the dwarf "compromised his own dignity by allowing himself to be used as a projectile, as a mere thing, and that no such concession could be allowed" (Beyleveld and Brownsword 2004: 26). The latter view is called *human dignity as constraint* and limits a person's autonomy and self-determination.

6. Human dignity as limiting rights of individual autonomy and self-determination.

Several (prominent) bioethicists such as Leon R. Kass in *Life, Liberty and the Defense of Dignity* (2002) and Francis Fukuyama in *Our Posthuman Future: Consequences of the Biotechnology Revolution* (2002) argue that the vast possibilities of the new biotechnology are dangerous and will likely undermine human dignity in various fields (e.g., human-animal chimera, cloning, design babies, genetic engineering and enhancement, and prolongation of life). In this context, people appeal to human dignity as constraint by limiting other people's autonomous and self-determined decisions in research and public policy. The freedom of research is restricted by virtue of the supposed undermining effects to human dignity. Here, human dignity has a negative function and serves as a bulwark against abuse.

Despite this list of various ways to determine the relation between human dignity and human rights, I present an alternative account in the following. The notion of human dignity is a twofold "thick" concept. It is twofold because it can be (1) applied to single cases and (2) functions as an important ethical key term concerning the justification of human rights. It is a "thick" concept because it entails a *descriptive* and a *normative* or *evaluative* component.

The following example of a thick concept is illustrative: the notion of *cruelty* or *being cruel*. When people say that a particular action or person is cruel, then they mean: first, that the action or person corresponds with a particular empirical description that is, secondly, conceived of as *abhorrent* or *detestable*. Therefore (a) the action should not be performed or (b) the person should be morally criticized (and possibly be shunned, if not sent to prison, depending on the particular case). To put it in a nutshell, there seems to exist some *empirical features* that (can) make an action or person morally blameworthy.

In this section, I briefly present one argument for each part of the twofold notions of dignity by appealing to a cognitivist reading and show how this interpretation can be valuable for global bioethics.

(1) *Human Dignity Applied to Single Cases*

The notion of dignity is a complex and multifaceted concept that can be described in a much better way by appealing to its "negative" counterpart—the notion of indignity. What does this mean? The basic idea concerns *how* we generally *use* the notion *dignity*. It turns out that *the notion of indignity* is more fundamental than the concept of dignity because cases of indignity and *not* cases of dignity—strictly speaking—are most relevant in ethics and hence bioethics. It is about avoiding and ending cases of indignity and consequentially reestablishing dignity once it has been undermined or jeopardized. This line of reasoning is a better way to understand the complex dynamics of "dignity talk" because it makes it easier to understand how one should act in a particular case.

To torture people for fun, to rape and abuse women and men, to treat cadavers in a degrading way (e.g., to cut off the ears and stitch them to the buttocks) and more are clear cases of indignity and hence such and alike cases should be avoided and the people in question morally criticized and legally punished. Additionally, there are cases in the *penumbra* that make it very difficult to determine whether the notion of (in)dignity can be successfully applied. Examples of the latter type of cases are end-of-life decision making and reproductive cloning. It is unclear how one should act in these cases by appealing to human dignity (e.g., Schüklenk). The vital question is not whether the notion of (in)dignity should be applied or not, but rather whether a particular case belongs to the first group of cases (clear cases) or the second group of cases (cases in the penumbra).

Common morality theorists such as Beauchamp and Childress (2009) argue that there is a universal moral core (common morality) that can be distinguished from nonuniversal particular moralities of different societies that stem from different cultures, traditions, and diverse religious beliefs. (e.g., Gordon 2011). I believe that common morality theories try to bridge the gap between ethical relativism and universalism.

In *Principles of Biomedical Ethics*, fifth edition (2001), Beauchamp and Childress refer to the idea of "morally serious persons" in order to determine the content of common morality. Even though they later abandoned this idea with regard to their revised approach (Beauchamp and Childress 2009), I do think, however, that one is able to determine which case belongs to which group of cases by appealing to a line of reasoning in which the notion of prudence is of vital importance by using it as an ethical method in order to determine the relevant factors for each case, so that one is able to decide whether a case belongs to the group of clear cases or to the group of cases in the penumbra. The general idea is that cases in the penumbra are special in the following way.

First, they cannot be solved by appealing to the notion of human dignity, because it is very unlikely that people would agree on a uniform definition in a pluralistic society. What they certainly all would agree upon—despite their different definitions of what *dignity* is—is that all are cases of *indignity* and one should try everything to reestablish dignity, whether this means that in cases of end-of-life decisions *active euthanasia* or *palliative care* are different issues and need to be addressed separately.

It seems, however, that the notion of human dignity is with regard to cases in the penumbra—rather a butcher's knife than a surgeon's scalpel—because the relevant empirical features of these cases are normatively less binding concerning a particular outcome by virtue of their nonuniversal nature (e.g. traditional, cultural, and religious beliefs). Here, additional factors are needed in order to make an informed decision in addition to a human dignity approach. Simply to claim that "dignity" will do the job and to hope that everything is clear is inappropriate and should be avoided. One has to make sure that one does not end up in opaque and confusing statements.[18] This would severely jeopardize the human dignity approach in the first place.

Secondly, one should not give up the notion of dignity but simply try harder in order to find some objective criteria that can be vital for a well-informed decision concerning cases in the penumbra. Whether the latter option, however, is feasible remains to be seen.

(2) *Human Dignity as a Foundation of Human Rights—Obscurum per Obscurius?*

It is unquestionable that the human rights movement in bioethics has been challenged despite its successful practical application—for example, in research on human subjects around the world in recent decades.

With regard to the theoretical foundation of human rights, things look a bit different, even though it seems that, step by step, we will arrive at a more informed view about how one should understand the nature of human rights and its connection to human dignity. According to some bioethicists such as Ruth Macklin, it would be a mistake to ground human rights on human dignity because it "is a vague concept" and "its basis for claims about human rights is even more obscure" (Macklin 1999: 221). Without any doubt, the notion of human dignity—by being an important ethical key term—plays a vital part concerning the justification of human rights, although I do think that one should not ground human rights on human dignity itself (see Gordon 2011, Schroeder 2012).

Roberto Andorno has rightly mentioned that the notion of human dignity is used by international law—and hence also "biolaw"—as an *unconditional* or *absolute* worth that every human being has simply by virtue of being human and that it is the foundation of human rights—even though it remains somewhat unclear what the term really means because there is no precise definition in international law (Andorno 2009: 229). According to Schachter—to whom Andorno is referring—the meaning of human dignity is "left to intuitive understanding, conditioned in large measure by cultural factors" (Schachter 1983: 849). Is this a case of *obscurum per obscurius*?

To avoid this unfortunate consequence, one should give up the idea of grounding human rights on human dignity. This does not mean, however, that the notion of human dignity is futile; on the contrary, it offers many insights in bioethical discourses as we have already seen. Methodologically speaking, both notions are intimately interwoven with each other—for example, all human dignity violations are also human rights violations but not vice versa.

In this sense, human rights can be seen as an instrument or tool in order to protect human beings' dignity from any kind of practices that degrade and humiliate human beings as such. To be accused of violating a human right is a serious issue, and it should be clear that such conduct is absolutely unacceptable, at least, within decent societies.

CONCLUSION

The main goal of this chapter was to facilitate and enhance the debate with regard to a better understanding of the nature of human dignity in bioethics. To accomplish that goal, it was necessary to examine some important and influential approaches and to review the history of the notion of human dignity concerning its potential contribution for bioethics. Although I do think that the notion of human dignity, which is a complex and multifaceted concept, is an important ethical key term and can be (made) useful for bioethical discourses, I have the strong feeling that it still needs further analysis in order to justify its proper use.

The proponents of human dignity in bioethics and their opponents have provided valuable insights in the debate and pinpointed some challenging problems, in particular in recent publications. It seems obvious that more work needs to be done in order to convince the opponents that the notion of human dignity in bioethics is, indeed, valuable and not merely an "empty slogan."

Therefore, in the last part of the chapter, it is suggested that the notion of human dignity should be supported by the concept of human rights in order to establish a cognitivist theory of dignity that can be used in bioethical discourses. This new approach has merely been outlined in the most general terms so far, but it is my hope that this is the right track to deepen the analysis for debates to come.

ACKNOWLEDGMENTS

I would like to thank Wanda Teays and the anonymous reviewer for their helpful comments on earlier drafts of this article. Last, but not least, this work was envisaged in the context of my stay at Queen's University Kingston in Canada and was funded by the Heinrich Hertz Foundation (HHS, B41 No. 44/08).

NOTES

1. This work is funded by the Heinrich Hertz Foundation (HHS, B41 No. 44/08).

2. http://www.bmj.com/cgi/eletters/327/7429/1419#44475.

3. http://www.bmj.com/cgi/eletters/327/7429/1419#44696.

4. As Gallagher explains: "Criticisms of dignity apply also to other values in medical ethics. 'Autonomy' and 'respect for persons' are good examples. They also appear as vague, ill-defined and sometimes sloganistic in codes, reports and in legislation. Whilst theorists make laudable attempts to clarify these concepts, such clarification may fail to make its way into professional documents. This is also the case with dignity. There is now a good deal of theoretical and empirical work to draw on which makes vague references to dignity inexcusable. The rapid responses here are likely to advance thinking on this topic, most significantly, the response of Arthur Caplan. Fairly extensive previous work also deserves attention. See, for example, the work of Spiegelberg in Gotesky and Laszlo 1970; Mairis 1994; Haddock 1996; Moody 1998; Mann 1998; Pullman 1999; Seedhouse and Gallagher 2002; and Nordenfelt 2003." (Gallagher 2004, http://www.bmj.com/cgi/eletters/327/7429/1419#46594; accessed February 8, 2010).

5. Caplan claims "that dignity is a moral creation. It refers to the status conferred by those who are moral agents on others—both autonomous and not. It consists of a set of obligations, duties and restrictions on how others and even other objects may be treated by moral agents. There is no inherent property that confers dignity on a human being—it is a social and cultural decision to confer this status (not all human subgroups follow all parts of the Western view of dignity) as part of membership in a moral community. If there are no autonomous moral agents then there is no dignity for it takes a decision by moral agents to create moral standing in others who lack autonomy." (Caplan 2003, http://www.bmj.com/cgi/eletters/327/7429/1419#44646; accessed February 8, 2010).

6. http://www.bmj.com/cgi/eletters/327/7429/1419#46594 (accessed February 8, 2010).

7. Consider the following nonbioethical example of dwarf tossing concerning a nonautonomous reading of human dignity: People may claim that it is the *autonomous* decision of the particular dwarf to be tossed or not, and therefore other people who dislike and

disapprove it should not intervene. This is so because one has to respect or at least tolerate the informed consent of adult human beings, even though one wholeheartedly disagrees with the actions that might follow from it. This line of argumentation is flawed and can be questioned. It is not simply a matter of the autonomous decision of the particular dwarf, whether it is morally unproblematic that he or she can be tossed or not. If the dwarf tossing takes place in public, it is likely the case that this event could be seen by other people, including other dwarfs, who may feel great grief and despair when by accident they watch this humiliating scene (e.g., it simply hurts their feelings). Their self-esteem could be severely diminished by this public display, and most dwarfs would probably feel offended by it. If this is the case, then other dwarfs do have a right not to be insulted by such kind of public displays that diminish their human dignity. Generally speaking, the basic duty to oneself in terms of acting properly to oneself (e.g., Kant) is related to one's own and to other people's dignity (e.g., honor of the family, or group). If a person is diminishing her own human dignity by performing self-degrading actions, she not only fails to see herself as a moral agent but also thereby offends other people when they by accident watch the scene (see also Schroeder 2008: 233–34).

Human dignity can be lost or diminished in at least two ways. First, a person's dignity can be either humiliated by other people through atrocities or certain particular living conditions such as poor housing, poor clothing, or poor sanitation. Secondly, a person's dignity can be diminished or even lost by the person's own actions—for example, in the above-mentioned case of dwarf tossing, or by performing degrading actions that result in exposing oneself to extreme, embarrassing ridicule. The first type of cases concerns human rights, which protect the basic value of human dignity. In this respect, human rights are instrumental.

The second type of cases concerns the basic duty people have to themselves, that is, not to perform actions that are detrimental to one's own human dignity (e.g., Kant: To illustrate this claim Kant analyzes what the violation of four different types of duties would involve. (1) The perfect duty to oneself: The duty to preserve one's life; (2) The perfect duty to others: The duty to make only sincere promises; (3) The imperfect duty to oneself: The duty to promote one's talents; (4) The imperfect duty to others: The duty to help those in need). Duties are apparently not rights, but some basic duties imply human rights. Beyleveld and Brownsword also discuss a French case of dwarf tossing in their own approach on human dignity (e.g., 2004: 25–27 and 33–34).

8. For a discussion of this kind of argument, see also Schroeder (2008).

9. Security rights: They protect people against crimes such as murder, massacre, torture and rape. Due process rights: They protect people against abuses of the legal system such as imprisonment without trial, secret trials, and excessive punishments. Liberty rights: They protect freedoms in areas such as belief, expression, association, assembly, and movement. Political rights: They protect the liberty to participate in politics through actions such as communicating, assembling, protesting, voting, and serving in public office. Equality rights: They guarantee equal citizenship, equality before the law, and nondiscrimination. Social welfare rights: They require provision of education to all children and protection against severe poverty and starvation. Group rights: They include protection of ethnic groups against genocide and the ownership by countries of their national territories and resources.

10. For the ethical dimension, see Annas and Grodin (1995); for the history, see Ebbinghaus and Dörner (2002).

11. Council for the International Organization of Medical Sciences (CIOMS).

12. See Brownlie and Goodwin-Gill (2002).

13. There is now even a so-called philosophy of human rights, which underlines the great importance of this very concept and which foreshadows the possible establishment of a new subarea in philosophy (e.g., Gewirth 1982; Rorty 1993; Shue 1996; Gosepath and Lohmann 1999; Rawls 1999; Alexy 2002; Orend 2002; Reidy and Sellers 2005; Nickel 2007; Griffin 2008; Beitz 2009).

14. Macklin states: "If human rights is a meaningful concept, and if there are any human rights, then normative ethical relativism must be false. Human rights are, by definition, rights that belong to all people, wherever they may dwell and whatever may be the political system or the cultural traditions of their country or region of the world" (Macklin 1999: 243).

15. Orend provides an interesting example. He states: "Perhaps the most notorious real-world example of the genetic fallacy occurred in Nazi Germany, when it was briefly official policy to reject the theory of relativity because it was devised by a Jew, Albert Einstein. This is, obviously, an instance of poor reasoning, since the personal characteristics of Albert Einstein have no relevant bearing whatsoever on whether the theory of relativity he invented offers a true, or at least compelling, account of time, space and the movement of physical objects in the universe" (Orend 2002: 158).

16. See also Donnelly (1989: 109–42).

17. This list stems from Beyleveld and Brownsword (2004: 46).

18. Andorno rightly states: "Dignity alone cannot directly solve most bioethical dilemmas because it is not a magic word that provides immediate response to them. Some further explanations are usually required to indicate why some practices are considered to be in conformity (or not) with what is required by the intrinsic worth of human beings. Thus, to be *functional*, dignity needs other more concrete notions that are normally formulated using the terminology of 'rights' (e.g., informed consent, physical integrity, confidentiality, nondiscrimination, etc.)" (Andorno 2009: 234).

REFERENCES

Alexy, R., and J. Rivers. 2002. *A Theory of Constitutional Rights.* Oxford: Oxford University Press.

Andorno, R. 2008. "Global Bioethics and Human Rights." *Medicine and Law* 27 (1): 1–14.

———. 2009. "Human Dignity and Human Rights as a Common Ground for a Global Bioethics." *Journal of Medicine and Philosophy* 34 (3): 223–40.

Annas, G. J. 2005. *American Bioethics: Crossing Human Rights and Health Law Boundaries.* New York: Oxford University Press.

Annas, G. J., and M. Grodin, eds. 1995. *The Nazi Doctors and the Nuremberg Code: Human Rights in Human Experimentation.* New York: Oxford University Press.

Arras, J., and E. Fenton. 2009. "Bioethics and Human Rights: Access to Health-Related Goods." *Hastings Center Report* 29:27–38.

Ashcroft, R. E. 2005. "Making Sense of Dignity." *Journal of Medical Ethics* 31 (11): 679–82.

———. 2008. "The Troubled Relationship between Bioethics and Human Rights." In *Law and Bioethics*, edited by M. Freeman, 31–52. Oxford: Oxford University Press.

Baker, R. 1998. "Negotiating International Bioethics: A Response to Tom Beauchamp and Ruth Macklin." *Kennedy Institute of Ethics Journal* 8 (4): 423–53.

———. 2001. "Bioethics and Human Rights: A Historical Perspective." *Cambridge Quarterly of Healthcare Ethics* 10:241–52.

Bandman, E., and B. Bandman. 1978. *Bioethics and Human Rights: A Reader for Health Professionals.* Boston: Little, Brown.

Baranzke, H. 2012. "'Sanctity of Life'—A Bioethical Principle for a Right to Life?" In *Ethical Theory and Moral Practice*, Special Issue: "Human Rights in Bioethics," edited by J.-S. Gordon.

Beauchamp, T. L., and J. F. Childress. 2001. *Principles of Biomedical Ethics.* New York: Oxford University Press.

———. 2009. *Principles of Biomedical Ethics.* New York: Oxford University Press.

Beitz, C. R. 2009. *The Idea of Human Rights.* Oxford: Oxford University Press.

Beyleveld, D., and R. Brownsword. 2004. *Human Dignity in Bioethics and Biolaw.* Oxford: Oxford University Press.

Brownlie, I., and G. S. Goodwin-Gill. 2004. *Basic Documents on Human Rights.* New York: Oxford University Press.

Caplan, A. 2003. "Dignity Is a Social Construct." *BMJ Rapid Response.* http://www.bmj.com/cgi/eletters/327/7429/1419#44646 (accessed February 8, 2011).

Carson, T. L., and P. M. Moser. 2001. *Moral Relativism: A Reader.* New York: Oxford University Press.

Cochrane, A. 2009. "Undignified Bioethics." *Bioethics* 24 (5): 234–41.

Council of Europe. 1997. *The Convention for the Protection of Human Rights and Dignity of the Human Being with Regard to the Application of Biology and Medicine: Convention of Human Rights and Biomedicine*, Oviedo. http://conventions.coe.int/Treaty/en/Treaties/html/164.htm (accessed March 29, 2011).

———. 1998. *The Additional Protocol to the Convention for the Protection of Human Rights and Dignity of the Human Being with Regard to the Application of Biology and Medicine, on the Prohibition of Cloning Human Beings*, Paris. http://conventions.coe.int/Treaty/en/Treaties/html/168.htm (accessed March 29, 2011).

Donnelly, J. 1989. *Universal Human Rights in Theory and Practice.* Ithaca, NY: Cornell University Press.

D'Oronzo, J. 2001. "Special Section: Keeping Human Rights: An Appreciation of Jonathan M. Mann." *Cambridge Quarterly of Healthcare Ethics* 10 (3).

Ebbinghaus, A., and K. Dörner. 2002. *Vernichten und Heilen: Der Nürnberger Ärzteprozeß und seine Folgen.* Berlin: Aufbatb.

Fukuyama, F. 2002. *Our Posthuman Future: Consequences of the Biotechnology Revolution.* London: Profile Books.

Gallagher, A. 2004. "Defending Dignity." *BMJ Rapid Response.* http://www.bmj.com/cgi/eletters/327/7429/1419#46594 (accessed February 8, 2011).

Gewirth, A. 1982. *Human Rights: Essays on Justification and Applications.* Chicago: University of Chicago Press.

Giannet, S. M. 2003. "Dignity Is a Moral Imperative." *BMJ Rapid Response.* http://www.bmj.com/cgi/eletters/327/7429/1419#44696 (accessed February 8, 2011).

Gordon, J.-S. 2008. "Poverty, Human Rights and Justice Distribution." In *International Public Health Policy and Ethics*, edited by M. Boylan. Drodrecht: Springer.

———. 2009. *Morality and Justice. Reading Boylan's A Just Society."* Lanham, MD: Rowman & Littlefield.

———. 2011. "On Justifying Human Rights." In *The Morality and Global Justice Reader*, edited by M. Boylan, 27–49. Boulder: Westview Press.

———. 2012. "Human Rights in Bioethics—Theoretical and Applied." *Ethical Theory and Moral Practice* 15:283–94.

Gordon, J.-S., O. Rauprich, and J. Vollmann. 2011. "Applying the Four-Principle Approach." *Bioethics* 25 (6): 293–300.

Gosepath, S., and G. Lohmann, eds. 1999. *Philosophie der Menschenrechte.* Frankfurt am Main: Suhrkamp.

Gotesky, R., and E. Laszlo, eds. 1970. *Human Dignity: This Century and the Next. An Interdisciplinary Inquiry into Human Rights, Technology, War, and the Ideal Society.* New York: Gordon and Breach, Science Publishers.

Griffin, J. 2000. "Welfare Rights." *The Journal of Ethics* 4 (1): 27–43.

———. 2008. *On Human Rights.* Oxford: Oxford University Press.

Haddock, J. 1996. "Towards Further Clarification of the Concept 'Dignity.'" *Journal of Advanced Nursing* 24 (5): 924–31.

Kass, L. R. 2002. *Life, Liberty and the Defense of Dignity: The Challenge for Bioethics.* San Francisco: Encounter Books.

Killmister, S. 2010. "Dignity: Not Such a Useless Concept." *Journal of Medical Ethics* 36 (3): 160–64.

Knowles, L. 2001. "The Lingua Franca of Human Rights and the Rise of Global Bioethics." *Cambridge Quarterly of Healthcare Ethics* 10 (3): 253–63.

Konarzewski, W. H. 2003. "Dignity Is a Useful, Well-Understood Concept." *BMJ Rapid Response.*

Kuhse, H. 2000. "Is There a Tension between Autonomy and Dignity?" In *Bioethics and Biolaw*, Volume II, edited by P. Kemp and R. Brownsword, 61–74. Copenhagen: Rhodos International Science and Art Publishers and Centre for Ethics and Law.

Landman, W., and U. Schüklenk, eds. 2005. "Reflections on the UNESCO Draft Declaration on Bioethics and Human Rights." *Developing World Bioethics* 5 (3).

Macklin, R. 1999. *Against Relativism: Cultural Diversity and the Search for Ethical Universals in Medicine.* New York: Oxford University Press.

———. 2003. "Dignity Is a Useless Concept: It Means No More Than Respect for Persons or Their Autonomy." *British Medical Journal* 327 (7429): 1419–20.

Mairis, E. D. 1994. "Concept Clarification in Professional Practice: Dignity." *Journal of Advanced Nursing* 19 (5): 947–53.

Mann, J. 1996. "Editorial: Health and Human Rights." *British Medical* Journal 312 (7036): 924–25.

———. 1998. "Dignity and Health: The UDHR's Revolutionary First Article." *Health and Human Rights* 3 (2): 30–38.

Mann, J., M. A. Gordin, S. Gruskin, and G. J. Annas, eds. 1999. *Health and Human Rights: A Reader.* New York: Routledge.

Moody, H. R. 1998. "Why Dignity in Old Age Matters." In *Dignity and Old Age*, edited by R. Disch, R. Dobrof, and H. R. Moody, 13–38. New York: Haworth.

Nickel, J. 2007. *Making Sense of Human Rights.* Oxford: Blackwell.

Nordenfelt, L. 2003. "Dignity and the Care of the Elderly." *Medicine, Health Care and Philosophy* 6 (2): 103–10.

Orend, B. 2002. *Human Rights.* Peterborough, Ontario: Broadview.

Pacholczyk, A., and U. Schüklenk. 2010. "Dignity's 'Wooly Uplift.'" *Bioethics* 24 (2): ii.

Pogge, T., ed. 2007. *Freedom from Poverty as a Human Right: Who Owes What to the Very Poor?* Oxford: Oxford University Press.

Pullman, D. *1999.* "The Ethics of Autonomy and Dignity in Long-Term Care." *Canadian Journal of Aging* 18 (1): 26–46.

Rachels, S. 2001. "The Challenge of Cultural Relativism." In *Moral Relativism*, edited by P. Moser and T. Carson, 53–69. New York: Oxford University Press.

Ram-Tiktin, E. 2012. "The Right to Health Care as a Right to Basic Human Functional Capabilities." *Ethical Theory and Moral Practice*, Special Issue: "Human Rights in Bioethics," edited by J.-S. Gordon.

Rawls, J. 1999. *The Law of Peoples*. Cambridge, MA: Harvard University Press.

Reidy, D. A., and M. N. S. Sellers et al. 2005. *Universal Human Rights: Moral Order in a Divided World*. Lanham, MD: Rowman & Littlefield.

Rendtorff, J., and P. Kemp. 1999. *Basic Ethical Principles in European Bioethics and Biolaw, Vol. I: Autonomy, Dignity, Integrity and Vulnerability*. Copenhagen: Centre for Ethics and Law.

Rorty, R. 1993. "Human Rights, Rationality, and Sentimentality." In *On Human Rights: The Oxford Amnesty Lectures 1993*, edited by S. Shute and A. Hurley (eds.). New York: Basic Books.

Schachter, O. 1983. "Human Dignity as a Normative Concept." *The American Journal of International Law* 77 (4): 848–54.

Schroeder, D. 2008. "Dignity: Two Riddles and Four Concepts." *Cambridge Quarterly of Healthcare Ethics* 17 (2): 230–38.

———. 2012. "Human Rights and Human Dignity: An Appeal to Separate the Conjoined Twins." *Ethical Theory and Moral Practice*, Special Issue: "Human Rights in Bioethics," edited by J.-S. Gordon.

Seedhouse, D., *and A.* Gallagher. 2002. *"*Undignifying Institutions." *Journal of Medical Ethics* 28 (6): 368–72.

Shue, H. 1996. *Basic Rights*. Princeton, NJ: Princeton University Press.

Spiegelberg, H. *1970.* *"*Human Dignity: A Challenge to Contemporary Philosophy." *In Human Dignity: This Century and the Next*, edited by *R.* Gotesky *and E.* Laszlo, 39–64. New York: Gordon and Breach.

Thomasma, D. 2001. "Proposing a New Agenda: Bioethics and International Human Rights." *Cambridge Quarterly of Healthcare Ethics* 10 (3): 299–310.

Trials of War Criminals before the Nuremberg Military Tribunals under Control Council Law. 1949. *The Nuremberg Code*, Nuremberg. http://www.ushmm.org/information/exhibitions/online-features/special-focus/doctors-trial/nuremberg-code (accessed March 29, 2011).

UNESCO. 1997. *The Universal Declaration on the Human Genome and Human Rights*, Paris: General Conference of UNESCO. http://portal.unesco.org/en/ev.php-URL_ID=13177&URL_DO=DO_TOPIC&URL_SECTION=201.html (accessed March 29, 2011).

———. 2005. *Universal Declaration on Bioethics and Human Rights, Paris: General Conference of UNESCO*. http://portal.unesco.org/en/ev.php-URL_ID=31058&URL_DO=DO_TOPIC&URL_SECTION=201.html (accessed March 29, 2011).

United Nations. 1948. *The Universal Declaration of Human Rights, Paris:* General Assembly of the United Nations. http://www.un.org/en/documents/udhr/ (accessed March 29, 2011).

World Health Organization (WHO), The Council for International Organizations of Medical Sciences (CIOMS). 1982. *Proposed International Guidelines for Biomedical Research involving Human Subjects*, Geneva: Council for International Organizations of Medical Sciences. http://www.cioms.ch/publications/layout_guide2002.pdf (accessed March 29, 2011).

World Medical Association. 1964. *The Declaration of Helsinki*, Helsinki: WMA General Assembly. http://www.wma.net/en/30publications/10policies/b3/index.html (accessed March 29, 2011).

2

Bioethics and Human Rights

A Historical Perspective

Robert Baker

ABSTRACT

Bioethics and human rights were conceived in the aftermath of the Holocaust, when moral outrage reenergized the outmoded concepts of "medical ethics" and "natural rights," renaming them "bioethics" and "human rights" to give them new purpose. Originally, principles of bioethics were a means for protecting human rights, but through a historical accident, bioethical principles came to be considered as fundamental. In this chapter I reflect on the parallel development and accidental divorce of bioethics and human rights to urge their reconciliation.

INTRODUCTION

The sacred rights of Mankind are not to be rummaged for among old parchments or musty records. They are written, as with a sunbeam, in the whole volume of human nature by the hand of Divinity itself, and can never be erased or obscured.

—Alexander Hamilton, 1987[1]

Philosophers like myself . . . see our task as a matter of making our own culture—the human rights culture—more self-conscious and more powerful.

—Richard Rorty, 1993[2]

92

THE 1948 UN DECLARATION:
FROM THE RIGHTS OF MAN TO HUMAN RIGHTS

The immediate precursor to "human rights" are the *droits de l'homme*, the "natural, inalienable, and sacred rights of man" to "liberty, security, property, and resistance to oppression" declared by the French Republic in 1789.[3] The rights, in turn, derive from the God-given inalienable rights to life, liberty, and the pursuit of happiness in the 1776 American Declaration of Independence. Yet despite this heritage, the rights of man were moribund in the first part of the twentieth century.

> All . . . attempts to arrive at a bill of human rights were sponsored by marginal figures—a few international jurists without political experience or professional philanthropists supported by the uncertain sentiments of professional idealists. The groups they formed, the declarations they issued, showed an uncanny similarity in language and composition to that of societies for the prevention of cruelty to animals. No . . . political figure of any importance could possibly take them seriously; and none of the liberal or radical parties in Europe thought it necessary to incorporate into their program a new declaration of human rights.[4]

Individual human rights began to receive attention only after the failure of the system of ethnically based *group* rights negotiated at the end of World War I. One of Woodrow Wilson's war aims had been to "make the world safe for democracy by render[ing] it a secure habitation for the fundamental right of man to be governed by rulers accountable to him."[5] Ethnic groups were to rule themselves.

In the treaties drawn up after World War I, the multinational Austro-Hungarian and Turkish empires and various Middle Eastern colonies were dissolved and reconstructed as ethnically and religiously cohesive nation states. This process of nation creation inevitably stranded some ethnic and religious minorities in the new nation states—Muslims in Europe, Christians in the Middle East, and Jews everywhere. These minorities, however, were recognized and protected in the treaties that created the new nation-states.

The nature of "human rights" was left unspecified until the 1948 Universal Declaration of Human Rights. Specification was prompted by the 1947 Nuremberg trials, at which doctors, lawyers, scientists, and soldiers were indicted for "crimes against humanity." The trials taught the world what it meant to strip a human of rights. Shortly after the Nuremberg trials commenced, Eleanor Roosevelt convened a committee to draft a declaration of human rights. Thus, Jews in Nazi Germany became surrogates for all humans without rights, and the details revealed daily at Nuremberg gave content to the rights recognized by articles 4 through 20 of the Declaration.

Articles 4, 5, and 9 prohibited the "slavery or servitude," "arbitrary detention or exile," and "torture, or cruel, inhuman, or degrading treatment or punishment" concurrently on display at Nuremberg. Articles 6, 8, 10, and 11 ensure that never again would Nazi-style laws strip individuals of citizenship: "Everyone has a recognition everywhere as a person before the law."

Article 12 prohibits future Kristallnacht, yellow Stars of David, and other stigmatizing actions by protecting individuals' privacy, family, and home against attacks on honor and reputation. Mindful of the Nazi Racial Purity laws and the laws stripping Jews of their nationality and their property, Article 16 declares that everyone has a right to marry freely and to found a family "without any limitations due to race, nationality, or religion."

Article 15 states that everyone has a right to a nationality, and Article 17 affirms that everyone has a right to own property. Finally, Article 13 guaranteed that, unlike the Jews of the 1930s and 1940s, victims of human rights abuse would have the right to flee from persecution. Article 14 grants a right of asylum. The Declaration proclaims nine additional rights—rights of participation, rights to social security, rights to education, and so forth—but the first twenty declarations of human rights were designed to prevent anyone from ever undergoing the treatment accorded to the Jews by the Nazis.[6]

The Universal Declaration of Human Rights was shaped, not only by the failure of minority rights and by outrage at the discovery of the Holocaust, but by the need, underlined by the events unfolding at Nuremberg, to make transcultural, transnational, and transtemporal moral and legal judgments. Unlike their precursors, the *droits de l'homme* and the God-given natural rights of Jefferson and Hamilton, human rights *had* to be globally acceptable.

They had to be neutral between all religious and secular worldviews. Individuals might still subscribe to Hamilton's view that rights are "written, as with a sunbeam, in the whole volume of human nature by the hand of Divinity itself," but, in laying claim to universality, the UN Declaration abandoned all claims to religious authority.

To protect an individual's right to practice religion, the emerging human rights culture had to be neutral about religion. As philosopher Charles Taylor observed, "The concept of human rights could travel better if separated from some of its underlying justifications."[7]

THE NUREMBERG CODE AND THE PRINCIPLIST PRECEDENT IN AMERICAN BIOETHICS

The Preamble to the Universal Declaration of Human Rights reminds the world that it originates as a reaction to "barbarous acts that have outraged the conscience of mankind." The same has been said of the Nuremberg Code: it is "impossible to analyze the origins of the Nuremberg Code apart from the historical setting of atrocities and murders committed in Nazi Germany."[8] Like the Declaration, the Code is a post-Holocaust document.

Why did the tribunal need to *invent* a code of ethics to condemn the Nazi researchers? To quote the defense for the Nazi doctors, at that time there was "an almost complete lack of written legal norms"[9] on human-subjects research. There were two notable exceptions: the 1931 German Health Ministry regulations, and the 1946 American Medical Association (AMA) research principles.

The Ministry regulations prohibited research on German *patients* without their informed consent. The AMA principles prohibited research on *persons* without their consent—it thus anticipated the bioethical turn by using the language of principles to expand the traditional protections of medical ethics from "patients" to "persons."[10]

Read literally, however, neither the regulation nor the principle was applicable to the German researchers. Physicians and scientists working at the camps dealt with *inmates*, not with *patients* covered by the German health insurance,[11] and, as *Germans*, they were not answerable to *American* ethics principles. The researchers' conduct thus seemed to elude the scope of extant medical ethical principles, legal standards, and applicable regulations.

To deal with these problems, the prosecution turned to two American physicians: Colonel Leo Alexander, a psychiatrist who had treated concentration camp survivors; and Professor Andrew Ivy, former scientific director of the Naval Medical Research Institute at Bethesda—and the official observer for the AMA. Both argued that unconsented human experimentation was impermissible, appealing to Hippocratic tradition.[12]

Ivy, however, also appealed to the "*laws of humanity* and the *ethical principles* of the medical profession."[13] The expression *laws of humanity* was the language of the Nuremberg indictment; "ethical principles" was the language of the AMA, which had parsed ethics as "principles" since its 1903 "Principles of Medical Ethics."[14] Ivy went further than the AMA, however, by grounding his principles in human rights: "The involved Nazi physicians and scientists ignored . . . ethical principles and rules . . . which are necessary to insure the *human rights* of the individual" (emphasis added).[15] Ivy's conception of ethical principles as mechanisms for protecting human rights circumvents the defense arguments about the time and place at which specific rules were formulated.

Human rights are inviolable irrespective of any principle, rule, or law stating their inviolability. Thus, even if no ethical principle or law accepted in Germany in the 1930s and 1940s was violated, "physicians and scientists whose conduct is contrary to the laws of humanity and human rights . . . should be prosecuted as criminals."[16] For, to reiterate, unlike laws and principles, human rights are inviolable regardless of whether a rule, principle, or law was formulated prohibiting a specific act of violation.

The Nuremberg judges incorporated aspects of both Alexander's and Ivy's testimonies into their judgment condemning the Nazi doctors. They accepted Ivy's principlist discourse but ignored his elegant suggestion that transcultural ethics could be grounded in human rights. Instead they fabricated a fiction or, if one prefers, a myth.

They claimed that, "*all agree*, that certain *basic principles* must be observed in order to satisfy moral, ethical, and legal concepts." Consequently, they argued, because the Nazi experiments were contrary to "the principles of the law of nations as they result from the usages established among civilized peoples, from the laws of humanity, and from the dictates of public conscience,"[17] Nazi doctors were guilty of crimes against humanity.

Because the Tribunal grounded its case on the myth of converging civilized opinion, the Nuremberg Code should be regarded conceptually, as well as chronologically, as an artifact of the prehuman rights era. This historical accident is significant because the research ethics decalogue promulgated at Nuremberg was appropriated by the American bioethics movement of the 1970s as a foundational document. Its *universally agreed basic principles*, thus, set a precedent for the language and justifications offered in American bioethics—and rights discourse was ignored.

THE REBIRTH OF HUMAN RIGHTS AND BIOETHICS IN THE 1970S

It was an accident of history that human rights and the principles of bioethics were reborn in the 1970s in government documents (The Final Declaration of Helsinki, the Belmont Report) in which they were presumed to serve symbolic functions—which is to say, no real function at all.

The Final Declaration of Helsinki was intended to legitimate the Soviet Empire. Yet as political theorist Michael Ignatieff notes, the human rights movements legitimated by the Declaration of Helsinki would eventually bring "the Soviet system crashing down."[18] For, unlike its precursor, "minority rights," "human rights" discourse served to unify. Appeals to "minority rights" tended to imply rights for *my* minority, not for yours; by contrast, no one's human rights came at the expense of anyone else's.

By 1966, evidence of the abuse of human subjects was apparent enough to prompt the National Institutes of Health (NIH) to mandate a system of peer review to protect research subjects.[19] In that same year an article published in the *New England Journal of Medicine* by Henry Beecher found that twenty-two research papers published in such leading journals as *Journal of the American Medical Association* and the *New England Journal of Medicine* between 1948 and 1965 were morally questionable.[20]

In the absence of substantive guidelines, however, peer review alone did not prevent research abuses. In 1973 Senator Edward Kennedy investigated a study by the U.S. Public Health Service on untreated syphilis in African American males—which was conducted without their informed consent. The public was outraged, and federal response was swift.

On July 12, 1974, President Nixon signed the National Research Act (NRA), forming a National Commission for the Protection of Human Subjects of Biomedical and Behavioral Research to develop substantive rules for protecting the human subjects of federally funded research. In the next four years the National Commission published several reports recommending regulations to protect research subjects. Internationally, there was a parallel move, starting with Helsinki II (Tokyo, 1975).

The most influential report issued by the National Commission concerned *principles*. In 1978, it issued the three-volume Belmont Report,[21] in which it asserted that three basic ethical principles should regulate research on human subjects—the principles of respect for persons, beneficence, and justice. Following the Nuremberg precedent, the Commissioners justified these principles in terms of convergence: The principles were deemed binding because "all agreed" that they ought to be binding.[22]

Convergence was a liberating concept. Tom Beauchamp and James Childress were perhaps the first to appreciate this point. In *Principles of Biomedical Ethics* (first published in 1979),[23] they construct bioethics[24] in terms of four "basic" principles—autonomy, beneficence, nonmaleficence, and justice—one more than the three used in the Belmont Report. These principles, in turn, are justified by a presumed *convergence* of reflective ethical thought.

By placing convergence at the level of principles, Beauchamp and Childress liberated bioethics from the ethical theories that happened to be in vogue, philosophically. By so doing, it not only unified the ethical analysis of researcher and clinician conduct, it also deprofessionalized medical ethical discourse. Thus, just as human rights discourse could become a public discourse only freed from conceptions of divine and human nature, so too, bioethics discourse could serve as a public discourse only if freed from conceptions of the medical profession, its nature and mission.

The new discourses open the domain of diplomats and doctors to ordinary people, who have no professional pretensions whatsoever. Bioethics and human rights are thus kindred democratizing and deprofessionalizing public discourses that transform the ethics of elites into everyday ethics.

BIOETHICS AND HUMAN RIGHTS: SOME PARALLELS

The parallels between bioethics and human rights as concepts, discourses, movements, and fields are striking. Both were conceived out of horror of the Holocaust; both draw strength from the resolve that "never again" would any vulnerable population be treated as the Nazis had treated the Jews; both support respect for persons; both stake claims to universality; both were born in governmental documents that explicitly justify transnational, transtemporal, and transcultural moral judgments; both became unfashionable in the era of Cold War realism; both are international, and thus (perhaps not surprisingly) both refer to Helsinki declarations; both were resurrected in the mid-1970s; both are supported by an unusual alliance of governmental and nongovernmental organizations; both became widely disseminated by disassociating themselves from earlier metaphysical and philosophical moorings; and both use a public discourse to democratize the domain of professional elites, although, ironically, both are supported by professional groups who consider themselves expert in the domain of the discourses. Yet despite these similarities—and even though one of the progenitors of the Nuremberg Code, Andrew Ivy, envisioned principles as mechanisms for protecting human rights, American bioethics has been ill at ease with the idea of human rights.

It is time to reconsider. Pandemics leap from continent to continent, companies peddle their cures around the world, biomedical experiments sponsored in the developed world are conducted in the developing world, and, in all corners of the globe, the new biology foments culture shock. Bioethical issues do not stop for border crossings. Thus, we need global bioethics. But the principlism that has served

American bioethics so well is too parochial to play on an international stage, and so to meet the challenges of global bioethics, we need to turn to the more cosmopolitan concept of human rights.

Once bioethics enters the international stage, the ideal of converging principles becomes unsustainable. Different cultures embrace different principles and differ in their interpretations of common principles. If principlism is to function internationally, it must be reconceptualized to shed its parochialism.

RECONCILING BIOETHICS WITH HUMAN RIGHTS

It is time to reconsider Ivy's proposal that we construe the principles of international bioethics as mechanisms for protecting human rights. Rights discourse is already the accepted language of international ethics. As members of the United Nations, virtually all the nations on Earth have pledged themselves to accept as "a common standard" that "all human beings are born free and equal in dignity and rights." As philosopher Richard Rorty has observed, ours is already a human-rights culture.

A global bioethics that envisions principles as mechanisms for protecting human rights will thus inherit an internationally accepted ethical discourse.[25] Rights discourse is the best means available for achieving the shared goal of both bioethics and human rights theory: the moral demand that never again will anyone be treated in the manner that Nazis treated Jews.

An international bioethics based on respect for human rights will also be free from the feckless dispute over whose principles are preferable. Principles are preferable insofar as they effectively protect human rights. Because effectiveness is partially a function of cultural experience, different societies may properly use different principles—respect for persons, respect for families, solidarity—insofar as they effectively protect human rights in the culture in question. The proposed reconciliation of human rights and bioethics thus recognizes cultural variation in principles and does not challenge American principlism within its home cultural sphere.

Grounding international bioethics discourse in human rights will not be a panacea. Human rights discourse may be the *lingua franca* of the international community, but the scope and limits of human rights should properly be subject to intense debate, as should the principles and rules that we create to protect these rights. The depth of the dilemmas that we must address will not dissipate merely because we use a common mode of moral discourse to address them. The transcultural scope of human rights discourse can, however, dissipate problems of moral parochialism.

Each culture has a deeply rooted predilection to treat its own conception of morality, its own moral concepts and principles, as primary. Human rights discourse was designed to be as cosmopolitan and international as the United Nations itself; it permits us to transcend our parochialism and thus to focus on the substance of the profound moral challenges that we face.

NOTES

1. A. Hamilton, *Nonsense upon Stilts: Bentham, Burke, and Marx on the Rights of Man*, edited by J. Waldron (London: Methuen, 1987), 18.

2. R. Rorty, "Human Rights, Rationality, and Sentimentality," in *On Human Rights: The Oxford Amnesty Lectures*, edited by S. Shute and S. Hurley (New York: Basic Books, 1993), 117.

3. French Assembly, Declaration of the Rights of Man and the Citizen, 1789, in *Nonsense upon Stilts*, 26.

4. H. Arendt, *The Origins of Totalitarianism* (New York: Meridian Books, 1958), 292.

5. E. Schwelb, *Human Rights and the International Community: The Roots and Growth of the Universal Declaration of Human Rights, 1948–1963* (Chicago: Quadrangle Books, 1964), 24.

6. J. Morsink, *The Universal Declaration of Human Rights: Origins, Drafting, and Intent* (Philadelphia: University of Pennsylvania Press, 1999).

7. C. Taylor, "Conditions of an Unforced Consensus on Human Rights," in *The East Asian Challenge for Human Rights*, edited by J. R. Bauer and D. A. Bell, 126 (London/New York: Cambridge University Press, 1999).

8. M. Grodin, "The Historical Origins of the Nuremberg Code," in *The Nazi Doctors and the Nuremberg Code*, edited by G. A. Annas and M. Grodin, 135–36 (London/New York: Oxford University Press, 1992).

9. J. Katz, *Experimentation with Human Beings* (New York: Russell Sage Foundation, 1972), 300.

10. The AMA adopted this principle, but only in 1946; that is, only at Ivy's insistence, and only *after* the Nazi researchers were indicted.

11. Although this point was not raised at the trial, Gypsies, Jews, and homosexuals had been stripped of German citizenship and were considered *Untermenschen*, subhumans, and thus were not protected by regulations covering *Menschen*, humans. For the 1931 regulations in English and German, see H. M. Sass, "Reichrundschreiben 1931: Pre-Nuremberg German Regulations concerning New Therapy and Human Experimentation," *Journal of Medicine and Philosophy* 8 (1983): 104–9.

12. L. Alexander, "Ethics of Human Experimentation," *Psychiatric Journal of the University of Ottawa* 1 (1–2) 1976: 40–46.

13. See also M. Grodin, "The Historical Origins of the Nuremberg Code," in *The Nazi Doctors and the Nuremberg Code*, edited by G. A. Annas and M. Grodin (London: Oxford University Press, 1992), 134–35.

14. A. C. Ivy, "Report on War Crimes of a Medical Nature committed in Germany and Elsewhere on German Nationals and the Nationals of Occupied Countries by the Nazi Regime during World War II," Document JC 9218, American Medical Association Archives, 1946, 9.

15. American Medical Association, "Principles of Medical Ethics (1903)," in *The American Medical Ethics Revolution*, edited by R. Baker, A. Caplan, L. Emanuel, and S. Latham (Baltimore: Johns Hopkins University Press, 1999).

16. Ivy, "Report on War Crimes of a Medical Nature," 11, 13–14.

17. J. Katz, *Experimentation with Human Beings* (New York: Russell Sage Foundation, 1972), 305, emphasis added.

18. M. Ignatieff, "Human Rights: The Midlife Crisis," *New York Review of Books*, May 20, 1999.

19. W. J. Curran, "Governmental Regulation of the Use of Human Subjects in Medical Research: The Approach of Two Federal Agencies," *Daedalus* 98 (2) (1969): 576–78.

20. H. Beecher, "Ethics and Clinical Research," *New England Journal of Medicine* 274 (1966): 1354–60.

21. National Commission for the Protection of Human Subjects of Biomedical and Behavioral Research. *The Belmont Report.* Washington D.C., 1978, DHEW Pub. no. OS 78-0014.

22. For a detailed critique of the convergence justification and replies, see: R. Baker, "A Theory of International Bioethics: Multiculturalism, Postmodernism, and the Bankruptcy of Fundamentalism," *Kennedy Institute of Ethics Journal* 8 (3) (1998): 210–31; R. Baker, "A Theory of International Bioethics," *Kennedy Institute of Ethics Journal* 8 (3) (1998): 233–74; R. Baker, "Negotiating International Bioethics: A Response to Tom Beauchamp and Ruth Macklin," *Kennedy Institute of Ethics Journal* 8 (4) (1998): 423–55; T. L. Beauchamp, "The Mettle of Moral Fundamentalism: A Reply to Robert Baker," *Kennedy Institute of Ethics Journal* 8 (4) (1998): 423–55; R. Macklin, "A Defense of Fundamental Principles and Human Rights: A Reply to Robert Baker," *Kennedy Institute of Ethics Journal* 8 (4) (1998): 403–22.

23. T. L. Beauchamp, and J. F. Childress, *Principles of Biomedical Ethics* (London: Oxford University Press, 1979, 1983, 1989, 1994).

24. Ironically, Beauchamp and Childress tend to avoid the term *bioethics*. The term was coined in the early 1970s, perhaps by Sargent Shriver, or by André Hellegers or by Van Rensselaer Potter. It achieved canonical status when the Library of Congress entered it as a subject heading, citing as its authority an article, "Bioethics as a Discipline," published by Daniel Callahan in the first volume of the *Hastings Center Report*—Callahan can thus also be credited with coining the term. See A. R. Jonsen, *The Birth of Bioethics* (London: Oxford University Press, 1998), 26–27; and W. T. Reich, "The Word 'Bioethics': The Struggle over Its Earliest Meanings," *Kennedy Institute of Ethics Journal* 4 (1994): 319–36; 5 (1995): 19–34.

25. Transnational medical ethics has already done this: Thus, in the Preamble to the Convention for the Protection of Human Rights and Dignity of the Human Being with Regard to the Application of Biology and Medicine: Convention on Human Rights and Biomedicine, adopted by Council of Europe in 1997, the term *rights* or *human rights* appears eight times—no mention is made of "principles." "Convention for Protection of Human Rights and Dignity of the Human Being with Regard to the Application of Biology and Biomedicine: Convention on Human Rights and Biomedicine," *Kennedy Institute of Ethics Journal* 7 (1996): 277–90.

I should like to thank Joseph d'Oronzio for inviting me to compare the historical development of bioethics and human rights, thereby providing me with an excuse to engage in an exceptionally illuminating exercise. This chapter draws on my earlier work on human rights, which has been enriched by discussions at the International Association of Bioethics (Tokyo), the Hastings Center, New York University, the Mount Sinai Medical Center (especially with Rosamond Rhodes and Stephen Baumrin), and by critiques by Tom Beauchamp and Ruth Macklin.

3

Rights of Persons with Disabilities from a Global Perspective

Akiko Ito

ABSTRACT

This chapter provides an overview of the implementation phase of the United Nations Convention on the Rights of Persons with Disabilities (CRPD). It discusses the issues most pertinent for policymaking to support national implementation of the CRPD, with a focus on cultural rights. I draw from my involvement in the UN processes as Chief, Secretariat for the Convention on the Rights of Persons with Disabilities at the UN, to demonstrate how the conception of disability rights is part of international human rights law and policy.

INTRODUCTION

In this chapter, I discuss divergent constructions of disability and diverse approaches to equalizing opportunities for persons with disabilities. There has been an important shift in conceptualizing disability from the medical model to the socioeconomic/minority rights model; this latter model recognizes principles of bioethics. This reformulation of disability is one of the key driving forces behind the development of conceptual frameworks and the establishment of the significant legal mechanisms related to disability and human rights.

The Convention on the Rights of Persons with Disabilities (CRPD) is a new and groundbreaking human rights tool that is designed to change society. The treaty, as will be discussed below, clearly applies to emerging issues such as mental health and psychological aspects of disability, as well as bioethics concerns related to disabilities. It is imperative that we pay more attention to cross-cultural or global dimensions of disability rights. I conclude with recommendations regarding the implementation of the CRPD, including mainstreaming disability rights into global priorities.[1]

DISABILITY, CULTURE, AND EMERGING ISSUES

Prior to 1970, the United Nations approached disability issues from the perspective of a social welfare model. In its first ten years of work, the United Nations focused on promoting the rights of persons with physical disabilities. Its primary concern was the establishment of international bodies and the development of suitable operational programs to deal with disability issues in cooperation with nongovernmental organizations. In the period from 1955 to 1970, the emphasis was on the goals of prevention and rehabilitation, but little attention was paid to obstacles created by specific institutions and society in general (UN Secretariat 1997: 14–15, Degener and Koster-Reese 1995).

The social welfare perspective emphasized helping those with disabilities fit into general societal structures. For example, a deaf person might only be taught how to read lips. New approaches stress modifications to the environment to promote the equalization of opportunities for persons with disabilities; for example, providing sign language interpreters at public events. This new formulation emphasizes society's responsibility to remove barriers that underpin the exclusion of persons with disabilities and denial of their basic citizenship rights (Finkelstein 1980; Oliver 1983, 1990).

This approach sees persons with disabilities as constituting a minority group. According to Harlan Hahn, discrimination has historically isolated persons with disabilities as a minority group. In his view, "people with disabilities are a minority group because they have been the objects of prejudice and discrimination" (Hahn 1997: 47). Because discrimination occurs over time, it reinforces attitudes that, in turn, reinforce discrimination—thus becoming a vicious cycle. He considers *public attitudes* rather than physical limitations to be the primary source of difficulties facing persons with disabilities.

The minority-group model specifies that public policy shapes all facets of the environment. It considers government policies to be reflecting societal attitudes and values. As a result, existing features of architectural design, job requirements, and daily life that have a discriminatory impact on disabled citizens can't be viewed merely as happenstance or coincidence (Hahn 1997: 46).

Other scholars contend that a true human rights approach toward the issue of disability differs from approaches focusing on the environment (e.g., Rioux 1997).[2] In contrast to the environmental adaptation approach, which looks at ecological barriers, human rights approaches look at the rights to which all people, regardless of disability status, are entitled. It analyzes how society marginalizes people with disabilities and considers ways that the social environment can be changed (Oliver 1992).

Given these different perceptions of disability, the CRPD establishes a major conceptual break from earlier approaches—as seen in the World Programme of Action as well as the Standard Rules. It exclusively focuses on guaranteeing the human rights of persons with disabilities.[3] The CRPD addresses disability prevention and rehabilitation as an aspect of full and comprehensive *human rights protection* for persons with disabilities. As a result, prevention and rehabilitation are directed at ensuring equal access and making all public health programs accessible to persons with disabilities.

Drafters of the CRPD signaled that public health issues are not appropriately addressed within the framework of disability rights. The framework of disability rights would thus exclude public health issues such protecting the general population from infectious diseases or implementing public safety policies such as road safety or industrial accident prevention. This tension is particularly pronounced in view of the CRPD. For that reason, its drafters explicitly adopted a comprehensive, rights-based understanding of disability rooted in the social context. The Convention wants to address the long-standing challenge of defining disability within a human rights and social model framework. Consequently, it does not specifically define disability.[4]

The CRPD Preamble took a different approach, by asserting:

> Disability is an evolving concept and that disability results from the interaction between persons with impairments and attitudinal and environmental barriers that hinders their full and effective participation in society on an equal basis with others.[5] . . . Persons with disabilities include those who have long-term physical, mental, intellectual or sensory impairments which in interaction with various barriers may hinder their full and effective participation in society on an equal basis with others.[6] (see Article 1)

The Convention thus adopts a broad categorization of persons with disabilities. This moves away from the World Health Organization's more *medical orientation* and embraces a *social model* of disability within which civil, political, economic, social, and cultural rights are enumerated and elaborated. Clearly, this is a major shift, with broad implications. In the next section, I will discuss cultural aspects that should be considered.

CULTURAL AND RELATED EMERGING DIMENSIONS IN DISABILITIES

Disability is closely associated with the environment according to the *social model*, as we saw in the discussion above. It is important to pay attention to cultural and anthropological aspects of disability, since they play key roles in the environment for persons with disabilities. This includes the culturally sensitive implementation of CRPD.

The United Nations has facilitated regional years and decades on disability mechanisms—as seen in Europe's Year of the Disabled, the Asian and Pacific Decade of Disabled Persons, and the African Decade of Disabled Persons. These mechanisms can be more culturally sensitive than those at the international level. They also provide culturally appropriate opportunities for intraregional cooperation and technical assistance.

CRPD recognizes the right of persons with disabilities to take part on an equal basis with others in cultural life (Article 30). This called for measures to ensure that persons with disabilities, such as access to: (a) cultural materials in accessible formats; (b) TV programs, films, theater, and other cultural activities, in accessible formats; (c) places for cultural performances or services, such as museums, cinemas, libraries, and tourism services, and, as far as possible; (d) monuments and sites of national cultural importance.

The CRPD calls for appropriate measures to enable persons with disabilities to have the opportunity to develop and use their creative, artistic, and intellectual potential. This is not only for their benefit but also for the enrichment of society. In addition, CRPD calls for State Parties to ensure that laws protecting intellectual property rights do not pose an unreasonable or discriminatory barrier to access by persons with disabilities to cultural materials. Persons with disabilities are entitled, on an equal basis with others, to the recognition and support of their specific cultural and linguistic identity, including sign languages and deaf culture. This article plays a key role in promoting culturally sensitive mainstreaming of disability into development priorities.

In the future, the mental, psychological, and emotional aspects of disability will be a key issue in development processes. Paying more attention to cultural, anthropological, and environmental determinants of disability will play a crucial role in determining the quality of life of persons with disabilities as well as the effectiveness of policy implementation. Because persons with mental, psychosocial, or intellectual disabilities are often much marginalized, it is critical that we attend to these aspects of disability.

BIOETHICS IN THE CONVENTION ON THE RIGHTS OF PERSONS WITH DISABILITIES (CRPD)

The CRPD asserts, "States Parties undertake to collect appropriate information, including statistical and research data, to enable them to formulate and implement policies to give effect to the present Convention." The process of collecting and maintaining this information "shall comply with internationally accepted norms to protect human rights and fundamental freedoms and ethical principles in the collection and use of statistics" (see Article 31.1.b). Given the importance of research and the protection of human subjects, not to mention the importance placed on the Nuremberg Code and the Declaration of Helsinki, attention needs to be directed to this area of the CRPD.

Similarly, CRPD's position on respect for the family, the right to decide freely and responsibly on the number and spacing of their children, and to have access to age-appropriate information and reproductive and family planning education are recognized. Moreover, the means necessary to enable them to exercise these rights are provided, and the right to retain their fertility on an equal basis with others is specifically addressed (see Article 23).

Finally, CRPD's statement on health holds that State Parties shall provide persons with disabilities with the same range, quality, and standard of free or affordable health care and programs as provided to other persons, including in the area of sexual and reproductive health and population-based public health programs (see Article 25).

IMPLEMENTATION: CULTURALLY SENSITIVE MAINSTREAMING INTO MILLENNIUM DEVELOPMENT GOALS

Prior to the successful adoption of the CRPD, the UN put other instruments into effect. At the global level, the United Nations has adopted the World Programme of Action as an international policy framework for disability-inclusive development. It has also adopted the Standard Rules for the equalization of opportunities reaffirming the principles of inclusive policies, plans, and activities in development cooperation and provided further guidance on disability-inclusive measures.

The World Programme of Action, marking a "slow shift towards a rights-based model" of disability, is a hybrid instrument using a human-rights-oriented approach. It clearly articulates some of the core human rights issues of concern for persons with disabilities. At the same time, it reflects some of the more traditional conceptions of disability by focusing on disability prevention and rehabilitation. That said, it captures the social context of disability in observing that "it is largely the environment which determines the effect of an impairment or a disability on a person's daily life."[7]

The Standard Rules, while not legally binding, remain a practical framework in defining obstacles and barriers to equal opportunities for person with disabilities. It also helps target areas of action. These rules should serve as a guide to states that have not yet signed and ratified the CRPD. They could also be used to foster the further integration of disability with the UN system against the fuller framework of the CRPD. This could then be used as an additional mandate for inclusion within and across the UN system.

SIGNIFICANCE OF THE CONVENTION ON THE RIGHTS OF PERSONS WITH DISABILITIES

The CRPD promotes both human rights and development—and is legally binding. It provides a comprehensive, normative framework for mainstreaming disability in the development agenda with new opportunities (Flynn 2011). Mainstreaming disability in development policies, processes, and mechanisms has been on the UN agenda for more than a quarter of a century. Since the mid-1990s, many development agencies, funds, and programs have taken significant steps to mainstream disability at the policy level. The Convention recognizes the importance of international cooperation and its promotion for the realization of the rights of persons with disabilities and their full inclusion into all aspects of life (see Article 32).

In particular, Article 32 stipulates that international cooperation measures should:

(a) Be inclusive of and accessible to persons with disabilities;
(b) Facilitate and support capacity-building, including through the exchange and sharing of information, experiences, training programs, and best practices;
(c) Facilitate cooperation in research and access to scientific and technical knowledge; and
(d) Provide technical and economic assistance, including by facilitating access to and the sharing of accessible and assistive technologies, and through the transfer of technologies.

As the president of the General Assembly noted, the CRPD represents "a great opportunity to celebrate the emergence of comprehensive guidelines the world so urgently needs" (Al Khalifa 2006).[8] The World Programme of Action and the Standard Rules were important milestones to developing a legally binding human rights convention that would apply human rights to persons with disabilities.

The Standard Rules contributed to the development of the CRPD in articulating accessibility as a priority area for targeted reforms. They also serve as a core component in achieving rights for persons with disabilities. The CRPD takes these and other concepts further. It situates them within a framework that is comprehensive in its coverage of specific substantive rights and provides principles and obligations applicable to the achievement of civil, political, economic, social, and cultural rights.

Following these significant advances, the UN agencies, funds, and programs have started to mainstream disability in their development policies. For example,

• UNFPA and WHO developed a guidance note on sexual and reproductive health of persons with disabilities for their headquarters and regional and country offices, after UNFPA's integration of disability in its Strategic Plan 2008–2013 as a crosscutting issue.
• UNAIDS developed a policy brief on HIV and disability with its ten cosponsors.
• UNDP has started developing a guidance note on integrating disability into its development activities.

Development of processes and mechanisms to implement these policies are still underway. In addition, some UN agencies have yet to fully address the policy and implementation issues of mainstreaming disability. So there is still more work to be done.

The mainstreaming of disability in development cooperation is relatively new to most development partners. The Nordic countries and the United States (through

USAID) began the process of mainstreaming disability into their development cooperation during the 1990s. Australia, Austria, Canada, European Union, Japan, New Zealand, and the United Kingdom have also started the integration of development in its policies. However, there has not been extensive experience in mainstreaming disability at the program level—and, so, there has been little opportunity to evaluate best practices or share information on implementation.

Persons with disabilities comprise an estimated 10 percent of the world's population, with 80 percent living in developing countries. It is, therefore, an urgent priority to mainstream disability as a crosscutting issue in development policies and in processes and mechanisms at the global, regional, subregional, and national level. In order to achieve this, it is necessary to pay more attention to the emerging aspects of disability, such as culture and mental well-being.

The CRPD approach to disability and human rights is not a simple addition to the international human rights mechanisms. It is groundbreaking in changing the global society with its social model perspective, its attention to accessibility for all, and its inclusion of persons with disabilities in all the processes of decision making and implementation.

Together with gender equalization efforts, and efforts to mainstream mental, psychological, and emotional aspects of development, the CRPD will play a key role in forming a new, sustainable community and a better quality of life of all people.

NOTES

1. For United Nations reports and policies, see http://www.un.org/disabilities/default. asp?id=23. See also the appendix to this text on Human Rights and Disability Rights.

2. Marcia H. Rioux, "Disability: The Place of Judgement in a World of Fact," *Journal of Intellectual Disability Research* 41 (2) (1997): 102–11.

3. The CRPD in article 1 provides: "The purpose of the present Convention is to promote, protect and ensure the full and equal enjoyment of all human rights and fundamental freedoms by all persons with disabilities, and to promote respect for their inherent dignity."

4. *See* CRPD, *supra* note 1 at Preamble, para. (e) and art. 1.

5. Ibid. at preamble, para. (e).

6. CRPD, *supra* note 1 at art. 1.

7. World Programme, para. 21.

8. Statement by H. E. Sheikha Haya Rashed Al Khalifa, president of the United Nations General Assembly, at the Adoption of the Convention on the Rights of Persons with Disabilities (December 13, 2006), available online at http://www.un.org/ga/president/61/statements/statement20061213.shtml.

REFERENCES

Al Khalifa, and H. E. Sheikha Haya Rashed. 2006. Statement by H. E. Sheikha Haya Rashed Al Khalifa, the President of the United Nations General Assembly at the Adoption of the Convention on the Protection and Promotion of the Rights and Dignity of Persons with Disabilities, December 13, 2006, www.un.org/ga/president/61/statements/statement20061213.shtml.

Comprehensive and Integral International Convention to Promote and Protect the Rights and Dignity of Persons with Disabilities, G.A. Res. 56/168, U.N GAOR, 56th Sess., Supp. No. 168, U.N. Doc. A/RES/56/168 (Dec. 19, 2001) [hereinafter CRPD]. An Optional Protocol was adopted at the same time.

Degener, Theresia. *Disabled Persons and Human Rights: The Legal Framework*, in Theresia Degener and Yolan Koster-Reese (eds,), *Human Rights and Disabled Persons*. Boston: Martinus Nijhoff Publishers, 1995.

Finkelstein, Victor. *Attitudes and Disabled People*. New York: World Rehabilitation Fund, 1980.

Flynn, Eilionóir. *From Rhetoric to Action: Implementing the UN Convention on the Rights of Persons with Disabilities*. New York: Cambridge University Press, 2011.

Hahn, Harlan. The political implications of disability definitions and data. *Disability Policy Studies*, Vol. 4, No. 3, p. 46, 1993.

Oliver, Michael. Changing the social relations of research production. *Disability, Handicap and Society*, Vol. 7, No. 2, pp. 101–114, 1992.

Oliver, Michael. *Social Work with Disabled People*. Basingstroke, UK: Macmillan, 1983.

Oliver, Michael. *The Politics of Disablement.Social Work with Disabled People*. Basingstroke, UK: Macmillan, 1990.

Optional Protocol to the Convention on the Rights of Persons with Disabilities, G.A. Res. 61/106 (2007) [hereinafter Optional Protocol].

Rioux, Marcia H. Disability: The place of judgement in a world of fact. *Journal of Intellectual Disability Research*, Vol. 41, No. 2, pp. 102–111, 1997.

United Nations. Convention on the Rights of Persons with Disabilities, retrieved January 17, 2014 from www.un.org/disabilities/convention/conventionfull.shtml.

United Nations Secretariat, Division for Social Policy and Development. *The United Nations and Disabled Persons—An Historical Overview: First Fifty Years*. New York: United Nations, 1997, p. 15.

United Nations, World Programme of Action Concerning Disabled Persons, retrieved January 17, 2014 from www.un.org/disabilities/default.asp?id=23.

4

Torturous Deeds

Crossing Moral Boundaries

Wanda Teays

When you cross over that line of darkness, it's hard to come back. You lose your soul. You can do your best to justify it, but it's well outside the norm. You can't go to that dark a place without it changing you. . . . You are inflicting something really evil and horrible on somebody.

—former CIA official, as quoted by Jane Mayer

If torture becomes inevitable it is necessary to humanise it and have an attending physician to moderate it.

—Vesti and Lavik (1991) on IRA interrogations

ABSTRACT

In this chapter I look at medical personnel who have enabled or participated in abuse, torture, or unethical medical experimentation. I start with an examination of caregivers who have directly or indirectly permitted abuses in such areas as forced-feeding, solitary confinement, sensory deprivation, and waterboarding. Next I look at medical personnel involved in nontherapeutic experimentation in which subjects did not or could not have given informed consent or where consent could hardly be informed. I call for doctors, psychologists, nurses, and other medical professionals to report abuses and for professional organizations to take a stronger role in stopping ethical violations by their members in order to effect systemic change.

INTRODUCTION

When U.S. Defense Secretary Leon E. Panetta confirmed news reports that Pakistani doctor Shikal Afridi participated in the CIA-led quest for al Qaeda leader Osama bin Laden, alarm bells sounded. According to Panetta, Dr. Afridi was "very helpful" to the bin Laden operation—thus his displeasure that Pakistan was charging the doctor with treason. "For them to take this kind of action against somebody who was helping go after terrorism," asserted Panetta, "I just think is a real mistake on their part" (Mazzetti 2012).

However committed a physician may be to fighting terrorism, duties that attend to being a medical caregiver should not be cast aside. Evidently, Afridi had been running a "phony hepatitis B vaccination program" as a ruse to obtain DNA evidence from members of bin Laden's family (Mazzetti 2012). That this could have deleterious consequences for vaccination efforts around the globe or patient-doctor trust did not appear to be given weight. As Heidi Larson (2012) of *The Guardian (UK)* notes,

> The news had a particularly strong impact on those working in polio eradication, where door-to-door vaccination is the norm. Anxieties and distrust about the polio vaccine and its western providers were rampant in some communities, and suspicions about CIA links with the polio vaccination campaigns, and rumours they were a front for the sterilising of Muslims, had been around for a decade after 9/11.

One of the consequences was that—after years of working to dispel myths about CIA links to the polio eradication efforts—"all of the work seemed fruitless" (Larson 2012). Those anxieties and distrust have not abated: The fallout from the doctor's participation has been significant. Salma Mosin reports that antipolio campaigns have been targeted by militants ever since U.S. intelligence used a fake vaccination program to collect DNA samples from residents of bin Laden's compound to verify his presence there. Since July 2012, at least twenty-two polio workers have been killed (Mosen 2013).

It is not always clear where to draw boundaries, and surely doctors, nurses, and other medical personnel know this as well as anyone else. At times it may seem prudent to use one's medical expertise as a patriotic gesture, with the short-term goals in much stronger focus than distant or long-term consequences. In the case of Dr. Afridi, the vaccination ruse may have played a role in the killing of bin Laden, but it was at the cost of the drive to eradicate polio. As Donald G. McNeil Jr. (2012) reports:

> After the ruse by Dr. Shikal Afridi was revealed by a British newspaper a year ago, angry villagers, especially in the lawless tribal areas on the Afghan border, chased off legitimate vaccinators, accusing them of being spies. And then, late last month, Taliban commanders in two districts banned polio vaccination teams, saying they could not operate until the United States ended its drone strikes.

Where should the moral boundaries be drawn? Should short-term gains take precedence over long-ranging goals? It's not always easy to arrive at a decision, and time does not always permit second thoughts. Because of that, medical caregivers face—and some opted to cross—moral boundaries.

With the "war on terror" a global effort, the constrictions against torture have loosened. The role of doctors as participants or enablers warrants examination in bioethics, whether we condemn or condone the use of abuse or torture as a tool of war. I will argue that such participation violates the most fundamental codes of the medical profession and raises serious human rights concerns.

LOSING THE MORAL HIGH GROUND

Expressing dismay at the many abuses at the prison at Guantanamo Bay, Marine Brigadier General Michael Lehnert remarked, "I think we lost the moral high ground" (Perry 2009). He added, "For those who do not think much of the moral high ground, that is not that significant. But for those who think our standing in the international community is important, we need to stand for American values. You have to walk the walk, talk the talk."

When those who have lost their way are in the medical profession, the harm extends from the individual to the society. When doctors, psychologists, and nurses fail to treat patients with respect and dignity, *trust* begins to crumble. Competing interests introduce an adversarial element and erode the patient-doctor relationship. We saw this with Dr. Afridi's vaccination ruse that has now undermined polio eradication attempts. It is one of many examples that we could point to. When a person's humanity is stripped away—as with torture and unethical medical experimentation—and the patient is merely a means to an end, the moral high ground has been left behind. Such transgressions know no national or cultural boundaries.

Bioethicists have issued calls for physicians to speak out against torture and abuse. Too many health professionals have been silent for too long. There are numerous forms of inhumane or degrading treatment in which doctors are either directly or indirectly involved. Transgressions include both acts of omission (the failure to act on behalf of a patient) and acts of commission (affirmatively enabling or participating in the abuse of a patient). Their role in abuse and torture, solitary confinement, non-consensual force-feeding, indefinite detention, and unethical medical experimentation merits closer scrutiny. It raises serious questions about the participants[1] as well as the medical profession as a whole.

Some physicians believe that "participation may be acceptable when no doctor-patient relationship has been established" (Sessums et al. 2009). This has come to pass. The U.S. Army's report on Detainee Medical Operations and the Fay Report both concluded that medical personnel were among the fifty-four personnel found responsible or complicit in the abuse at the Abu Ghraib prison in Iraq (Kiley 2005: 17; Fay 2004).

Throughout history are those who elevate state interests, national security, scientific progress, or social goals to the detriment of the individual. Sacrificing the few for the many is excused, even exalted. Physicians are not immune to this mind-set. Vesti and Lavik (1991) argue that, historically, doctors treated the sick but also participated in torture. This "is mentioned frequently enough in historical material to indicate it was a regular occurrence," they state; thus legitimizing torture (4). Patients became collateral damage for the higher objective.

Without the roles clearly defined, the duty to care erodes. One of the first things to go under such circumstances is *trust.* Edmund Pellegrino has written eloquently on its importance in the patient-doctor relationship.[2] Loss of trust in the African American community was palpable after the decades-long Tuskegee syphilis study, with its flagrant racism and abuse of poor black men in Alabama. Their trust in the nurses and doctors was their undoing. Patients who sought treatment were turned away, and doctors inside and outside of the study shielded the patient-subjects from the truth. The result was a cover-up—a grand deception—that left some men heading to an early and avoidable death and others to live for decades with untreated syphilis.

As with the racist aspects of the Tuskegee Study, there is a cultural and religious dimension to the moral depravity in torture. The fact that this is global in scope underscores its significance. After getting an overview, we will turn to two types of patients—detainees and human subjects.

Lack of transparency and restricted access by watchdog agencies like the International Red Cross add to the problem. Both victims of torture and subjects of unethical medical experimentation are members of a vulnerable population. Isolated from public view, they are at the mercy of individuals and institutions. Systemic problems are more likely to go unchecked when independent review boards (IRBs) are not part of the equation. Halting procedures when things go awry is then left to chance, and medical caregivers become a cog in the wheel of that machinery. Bioethicists have a role to play as ethical watchdogs. We can support those who act in morally defensible ways—and speak up against moral breaches.

ABUSE, TORTURE, AND THE
MEDICAL PROFESSION: A GLOBAL ISSUE

Among the countries that permit torture are the United States, Britain, Germany, Austria, Poland, Turkey, Algeria, South Africa, Brazil, Uruguay, Chile, Japan, China, Syria, Egypt, Lebanon, and Uzbekistan. The list goes on and on.

Even countries such as Canada that have avoided the hot seat are not above reproach. We see this in the failure to protect citizen Maher Arar from "extraordinary rendition," in which the suspect is sent to a country known to use torture. The United States nabbed him at the JFK Airport en route back to Canada after a vacation. He was "rendered" to Syria for nearly a year, where he faced solitary confinement and torture. The Canadian government did *not* stand by their citizen—a partial explanation for the out-of-court $10.5 million settlement with Arar. The United States has yet to apologize.

Some medical professionals fail to put fiduciary duties above political or other interests. The most extreme form is when the doctor is the *actual* torturer (Dowdall 1991: 52). Nazi "medicine" comes readily to mind. Unfortunately, the Nuremberg trials and the resulting code have had limited impact. It is lamentable when medical caregivers lose sight of the therapeutic dimension of their work. Conflicts of interest lead to less diligence in reporting malpractice and torture/abuse, as with dual loyalties on the part of medical personnel. The fact of conflicting allegiances does not bode well for the patient.

Robert Jay Lifton (2004) remarks on "doctors' vulnerability to being socialized to abusive environments and to engage in destructive behavior." In his view, "We need to learn all that we can about abuses by doctors everywhere, as a means of strengthening the healing commitment of medical institutions in a democratic society" (2004: 1574). Understanding the extent of the problem will help us determine what the next steps should be. Let's look at examples.

Doctors in apartheid South Africa may not have tortured anyone, but they collaborated with security police, reports T. L. Dowdall. They withheld treatment, pronounced detainees fit for further abuse, falsified medical and/or autopsy reports, and monitored abuses to protect the police (Dowdall 1991: 52). The result is that doctors played an integral part in the abuse.

Keeping quiet out of fear of reprisal takes its toll as well. After Zimbabwe's disputed general election in March 2008, for instance, there were "widespread mass beatings, intimidation, extra-judicial executions and torture." With few exceptions, the organized health profession in Zimbabwe was generally silent against the abuses (London et al. 2008).

Detainees' low moral status was sealed by the linguistic sleight of hand that replaced the term *prisoners* with *detainees* (Teays 2007). The U.S. Navy's Human Research Protection Program report defines *prisoner* as "any individual (other than Captured or Detained Personnel) involuntarily confined or detained in a penal institution" (2006: 4). Rita Manning examines how this plays out on the domestic front in the next chapter in this book.

That's not all. Instead of "doctors," we have "medically trained interrogators," as philosopher Fritz Allhoff calls them. "The interrogator's primary task is to facilitate the acquisition of information, not to heal," he declares (2008: 101). Similarly, some consider doctors in interrogations to be *combatants* to whom the Hippocratic Oath does not apply (Stephens 2005).

With these new concepts in place, other policies and protections, such as the Geneva Conventions, are seen as inapplicable. The 2011 case of Somali prisoner Ahmed Abdulkadir Warsame suggests the end is not in sight. Warsame was detained on the navy ship, USS *Boxer*, called a "floating Gitmo" by Spencer Ackerman, who considers this the future of terrorist detentions. Because "Obama administration lawyers couldn't tell reporters why detaining Warsame was legal," we have cause for concern (Ackerman 2011).

Journalists Dana Priest and Barton Gellman (2002) point to the "brass-knuckled quest for information, often in concert with allies of dubious human rights reputation, in which the traditional lines between right and wrong, legal and inhumane, are evolving and blurred." They note that "national security officials defended the use of violence against captives as just and necessary" and expressed confidence that the American public would concur. The assassination of political leaders such as Osama bin Laden brought cheers of jubilation, indicating how fertile the ground is for torture to be institutionalized and made systemic.

On the other hand, the public has not been privy to the fine details. Even the Red Cross has lacked full access to prisons. However, they had enough evidence to conclude, "We were dealing here with a broad pattern, not individual acts. There was a pattern and a system," as Pierre Krahenbuhl, the Red Cross operations director, said (Hanley 2010). Given the destruction of ninety-two interrogation tapes, we may never know the extent of the abuse (ACLU 2009). But we've seen enough to know that medical caregivers played a part.

THE ROLE OF MEDICAL PROFESSIONALS

Bioethicist Steven H. Miles asserts that doctors and other medical personnel have collaborated in abuse or torture by: (1) certifying prisoners as fit for harsh interrogation; (2) monitoring and treating them during interrogation; (3) concealing evidence of abuse; (4) conducting abusive research; (5) overseeing the systematic neglect of prisoners' basic health care; and (6) keeping silent while abuse is ongoing (Marks 2007, 41).

We could add (7): helping design and monitor interrogations that exploit the detainee's physical and mental vulnerabilities. Evidently behavioral scientists sought to control even minute details of the interrogations, leaving little to chance. "In one case, a psychologist told guards to limit a detainee to seven squares of toilet paper a day" (Tietz 2006).

Why the bizarre control tactics? If the goal is to break the spirit and achieve near-complete dependency ("learned helplessness"), this should do it. But the price is awfully high. "It is both illegal and deeply unethical to use techniques that profoundly disrupt someone's personality," says Leonard S. Rubenstein of Physicians for Human Rights (PHR), "but that's precisely what interrogators are doing" (Mayer 2005b). Detainee lawyer Baher Azmy agrees. "These psychological gambits are obviously not isolated events," he states. "They're prevalent and systematic. They're tried, measured, and charted. These are ways to humiliate and disorient the detainees" (Mayer 2005b).

Doctors and psychologists have assisted in initial psychological and physical assessments in the intake process (Keller et al. 2009: 4). A PHR report on the role of health professionals notes six techniques used on detainees:

- Forced shaving (for humiliation)
- Hooding (for sensory deprivation, isolation, and confusion)
- Restricted diet (for helplessness, dependency, and loss of self-control, as well as the deprivation of solid food)
- Prolonged diapering (for humiliation, loss of self-control)
- "Walling" (using a towel or plastic collar around the neck and thrusting a prisoner into a plywood wall, for psychological stress)
- Confinement in boxes (for sensory deprivation and stress)

Other abusive treatment includes forced nudity; force-feeding; stress positions; forced standing; sensory manipulation; temperature extremes; mock executions; use (or threatened use) of snakes, scorpions, insects, or other animals; threatened or actual rape/sodomy; solitary confinement; and waterboarding. Sleep deprivation has been widely used, as we see with the reports from the U.S. Department of Justice (Testimony 2008). The 2007 report of the International Committee of the Red Cross (ICRC) on the treatment of "high value" detainees clearly sets out the range and scope of tactics and abuses used that raise serious questions about their treatment.

Major General George R. Fay notes the systemic use of forced nudity in the 2004 Fay Report. It was seen by the Counter-Resistance Strategy as an "incentive" in detention operations and interrogations at Guantanamo Bay and then carried forward to Afghanistan and Iraq as an effective "ego-down" technique (122). Forced nudity has not *historically* been included in interrogations, but it was thought to be an "effective technique for which *no specific written legal prohibition existed.*" The Fay Report concludes that forced nudity was "employed routinely and with the belief it was not abuse" and that it contributed to an escalating "de-humanization" of the detainees (2004: 122, *my emphasis*).

Major General Fay rightly predicted that this set the stage for more severe abuses to occur. This we saw with nonconsensual medical experimentation and forced injections of unknown substances on unsuspecting detainees (Warrick 2008). For instance, American detainee Jose Padilla contended he was injected with psychotropic drugs (Cassel 2008). This violates the U.S. guidelines that "research involving any person captured, detained, held, or otherwise under the control of [Department of Defense] personnel (military and civilian, or contractor employee) is prohibited" (Department of Navy 2006: 6).

Although sleep deprivation and solitary confinement have longer-lasting effects, waterboarding has elicited the most concern. In 2008, Louise Arbour, UN High Commissioner for Human Rights, declared waterboarding a prosecutable war crime. "I would have no problems with describing this practice as falling under the prohibition of torture," she said (Reuters 2008).

That the U.S. government saw a role for medical personnel was made explicit in the so-called torture memos. In a 2005 memo, Deputy Assistant Attorney General Steven G. Bradbury noted waterboarding had risks and recommended "close and ongoing monitoring by *medical and psychological* personnel." Medical advisor Scott Allen said doctors and psychologists colluded with the CIA to keep observational records about waterboarding. In his view, it "approaches unethical and unlawful human experimentation" (Harmon 2009).

Mind you, it's not merely *American* doctors losing their moral grip; the issue is international in scope. Methods deemed effective in one country travel to others. Stress positions and hooding, used in Brazil, in apartheid South Africa, and on IRA prisoners by the British, became the norm in Iraq, Afghanistan, and Guantanamo Bay (Wead 2007). Linking Abu Ghraib to Central America, lawyer Jennifer Harbury remarked, "All of the Latin American torture survivors remembered the hoods, the constant beatings, the nakedness, the electrodes, and the rapes and sexual humiliations as well" (Sawyer 2008).

Ex-British ambassador Craig Murray cites horrific torture he became aware of while in Uzbekistan, including photographs of victims who were boiled. He contended that the partial boiling of an arm was common. At the other extreme is hypothermia. Like boiling, it must be carefully monitored to ensure the victim does not expire. Speaking of his stint in Afghanistan and Iraq, ex-interrogator Tony Lagouranis said, "We used it a lot." Navy SEALS induced hypothermia with ice water, using a rectal thermometer to make sure the captives didn't freeze to death, he said (Goodman 2005, Conroy 2007).

Another area where moral lapses occur is force-feeding. Special restraint chairs forcing the head back in a contorted position are now used to do the job, with doctors keeping the subjects from expiring. This violated medical codes granting competent patients the right to refuse medical treatment. In January 2009, Jamil Dakwar, ACLU Human Rights Program director, declared, "Force-feeding is universally considered to be a form of cruel, inhuman and degrading treatment." He agrees with the United Nations that it raises "grave and distinct human rights concerns" (Leopold 2011). Given April 2011 and March 2013 saw more hunger strikes of Guantanamo detainees, the issue still stands. As of October 2013, reports *al Jazeera*, there are seventeen hunger strikers and sixteen people being force-fed at Guantanamo Bay.

This is not just an issue regarding detainees—2013 saw 30,000 of 133,000 inmates in California also on a hunger strike in protest of solitary confinement at Pelican Bay (prison) (*Today Online* 2013). Prison officials won a court hearing to allow force-feeding of dozens of the strikers.

Dr. Otmar Kloiber, WMA Secretary General, insists that physicians should never be used to break hunger strikes through force-feeding. The WMA holds that "once the doctor agrees to attend to a hunger striker, that person becomes the doctor's patient," with all the responsibilities that incurs, including consent and confidentiality. It asserts that doctors working in prisons or the armed forces owe prisoners the same duty of care as other patients (Barratt 2006).

U.S. Air Force sociologist Albert Biderman found that physical torture doesn't provide actionable intelligence (Siems 2010). "Many detainees have nothing to tell," says Tom Parker, formerly of the British intelligence agency, the MI5 (Rejali 2007: 513; Mayer 2005a). High-profile suspect Khalid Sheikh Mohammed (KSM) claims,

"During the harshest period of my interrogation I gave a lot of false information in order to satisfy what I believed the interrogators wished to hear in order to make the ill-treatment stop" (ICRC 2007: 37).

Doctors are in the thick of it. This is not a problem of *one* country, one religion, or one ethnic group. Navin Narayan (1998) explains,

> Modern regimes throughout South America employ doctors' anatomical knowledge to monitor the effectiveness of torture and to develop new torture techniques. . . . The cooperation of the medical community in torture has become pandemic and a valuable asset for the world's most despotic regimes. . . . The contributions of doctors to undetectable forms of torture include refinements in electrical shock therapy that stop just short of arresting the heart, submersion in water and human excrement to the point of near-drowning and sleep and sensory deprivation . . . physicians have also bolstered torture's arsenal with a wider variety of psychoactive agents that induce nervous breakdowns and mental confusion.

Guantanamo senior psychologist, Major John Leso, reportedly helped plan al-Qahtani's fifty-day interrogation—from sexual humiliation and shackling to the use of dogs. "During one session, the medical staff injected the prisoner with three and a half IV bags of saline—[and they] wouldn't let him urinate until he provided satisfactory answers" (Sharrock 2009). This tactic was also used in Afghanistan and Iraq. The Taguba Report of May 2004 notes that military dogs (without muzzles) were used to intimidate and frighten detainees, and they bit and severely injured at least one detainee. See also Mark Danner's *Torture and Truth* (2004: 17, 31, and 43). Using dogs or other animals to terrorize suspects violates basic human rights and leaves a stain on the medical profession.

Once torture has been institutionalized, doctors and psychologists are vital. Ugur Cilasun, MD (1991), the executive director of the Turkish Medical Association, states that, "If doctors did not participate in, or contribute to these practices, systematic torture could never be realized" (21). When the CIA began its "increased pressure phase" on suspect Abu Zubaydah in 2002, psychologists, physicians, and other health officials helped design and implement the interrogation. "Their presence also enabled the government to argue that the interrogations did not include torture" (Warrick and Finn 2009a). Medical personnel get used in the bargain.

Doctors have given advice on how to maximize pain (physical and mental) without killing the victim (Forrest 1998). However, care must be taken, since death could turn the torture victim into a martyr—which is clearly undesirable politically. If the goal is information, staying this side of death is crucial. For that, torture needs an "informed assistant" to monitor bodily functions. "What better specialist than a doctor?" Cilasun asks (1991: 21).

Doctors assist interrogations by offering advice and monitoring the detainee/patient. This is not without risk for the participating doctor. Those who refuse to take part or who won't falsify death certificates are in danger of being detained, tortured, and killed, as Forrest (1998) reports.

Of course, at times there are few options. Many doctors and nurses "disappeared" in Central and South America after aiding dissidents. And of doctors in Syria who protested human rights abuses in 1980, "Over a hundred were arrested and remained in prison without charge or trial for up to fifteen years." Even speaking up can be perilous and may partly explain the widespread silence by medical professionals who witness abuse and torture (Forrest 1998).

Medical personnel can be swayed by national, ethnic, or cultural allegiances, making it difficult for medical *ethics* to stay in the forefront. Moreover, the presence of doctors adds credibility—legitimacy—to the proceedings. "We believe that doctors are used by torturers as a safety net," says Anat Litvin of Physicians for Human Rights. "Take them out of the system and torture will be much more difficult to enact" (Cook 2009).

From the victim's perspective, however, the participation of doctors is crushing. When those we trust fail us, hope slips through our fingers like grains of sand. When that involves doctors, it's hard not to be disillusioned about the entire profession.

TORTURE AND THE VIOLATION OF MEDICAL ETHICS

What's wrong with torture or with doctors and psychologists being direct or indirect enablers? Surely we want to stop terrorism, and the well-being of the society may demand sacrifices. The Principle of Utility to maximize benefits (the most for the most) has its appeal, but even card-carrying Utilitarians should not avert their eyes from long-term consequences. Short-term gains cannot be allowed to rule if the costs are too great.

Active participation in torture is a violation of medical ethics. Those failing to act are still culpable. Doctors have falsified documents and death certificates. They have concealed misdeeds and used deception to avoid implicating themselves or others. Look, for instance, at the innocent Afghani cab driver Dilawar, profiled in *Taxi to the Dark Side*. He was hooded, shackled, and suspended by his arms from the ceiling. Over a twenty-four-hour period, Dilawar was reportedly struck over one hundred times by soldiers (Shamsi 2006). His legs were "pulpified." The doctor stated that Dilawar died of *natural causes*, thus covering up the crime (Miles 2006, 69). The doctor enabled torture to continue.

"Torture practices diminish the moral clout of implicated military physicians and governments," professor Niyi Awofeso (2006) affirms. He adds, "Prison torture practices in which doctors are actively or passively involved diminish the standing of the medical profession, whose members are expected to be advocates for people at risk of torture."

Since 2002, psychologists and psychiatrists have enabled a strategy using "extreme stress, combined with behavior-shaping rewards, to extract actionable intelligence from resistant captives" (Bloche and Marks 2005). Torture expert Darius Rejali (2007) asserts that many torture techniques used in Afghanistan and Iraq were previously known (e.g., "The Vietnam," "The Scorpion," etc.); they are *not* recent inventions or the product of a few "bad apples." The techniques were the result of careful planning.

Torture has evolved into two categories. There is the classical pain-short-of-organ-failure variety, such as using electric shock, beating, and waterboarding—to maximize the *physical* effect. Think Inquisition. There is also torture that pushes mental and emotional endurance, as with hooding, solitary confinement, and sleep deprivation—to maximize the *psychological* effect. Think nightmare. One hypothesis is that there was a shift in the 1970s from physical to *psychological* torture.

> A historic view of torture techniques shows a clear change from physical to psychological torture . . . [which was] more effective in weakening and silencing the tortured than was physical torture. Furthermore, it is easier to hide the evidence of torture in this way. Isolation, sham executions, deprivation of sleep. . . . Without leaving any physical marks, these procedures can lead to serious psychiatric problems [. . .] and the readjustment of a torture victim to civilian life becomes almost impossible. (Vorbrüuggen and Baer 2007)

When patients are stripped of their autonomy, they are susceptible to exploitation and mistreatment. Ethicist Nancy Sherman (2006) points out, "Victims often are made to feel complicit in their own abuse." The result is "a compromised agency, of turning against oneself through the very exercise of one's own will." As Alfred McCoy warns, "There is no such thing as a little bit of torture" (Kennedy 2007).

Some suggest using medical and psychological personnel to monitor interrogations as a form of patient protection or insurance. Without their expertise, the situation would surely be worse. But will it lead to indifference? Detainee Necen Hambali testified that a "health person" told him, "I look after your body only because we need you for information." Others testified that medical care was made conditional upon cooperation with their interrogators (ICRC 2007: 22).

Medical caregivers have been implicated—for example, for monitoring a detainee's oxygen saturation used in waterboarding (ICRC 2007: 22). Bioethicist Arthur Caplan asserts, "The challenge to bioethics and indeed all of ethics, is to subject the beliefs that led to such horror to close critical scrutiny" (2007: 72). Human rights cannot be marginalized.

As the WMA states in its Declaration of Tokyo, "The physician shall not use nor allow to be used, as far as he or she can, medical knowledge or skills, or health information specific to individuals, to facilitate or otherwise aid any interrogation, legal or illegal, of those individuals." Physicians must retain their independence and not subvert their professional values to other interests. As the Declaration states, "The physician's fundamental role is to alleviate the distress of his or her fellow human beings, and no motive, whether personal, collective or political, shall prevail against this higher purpose."

Nobel laureate Elie Wiesel (2005) put it this way: "Shouldn't the prison conditions in Iraq have been condemned by the legal profession and military doctors alike?

Am I naïve in believing that medicine is still a noble profession, upholding the highest ethical principles? For the ill, doctors stand for life. And for us hope."

THE ROLE OF THE PROFESSIONS

In April 2009, the APA issued a condemnation of those who enable abuse or torture: "It is unthinkable that any psychologist could assert that stress positions, forced nudity, sleep deprivation, exploiting phobias, and waterboarding—along with other forms of torture techniques that the American Psychological Association has condemned and prohibited—cause no lasting damage to a human being's psyche" (Robinson 2009).

What more should be done? Along with prohibitions and guidelines, there should be channels for filing reports of abuse, so those suspected of wrongdoing could be investigated and sanctioned. One proposal is to make reporting *mandatory*, as with child abuse. Personnel and management of detention centers would then face penalties for failing to comply (Smith and Freeman 2005: 331). As Smith and Freeman point out, "Those who perpetrate torture rely upon the silence and complicity of their colleagues" (332). Perhaps some form of *mandatory reporting* would change that.

Jonathan Marks (2005) cites examples of professional organizations taking action against doctors enabling torture by setting down *sanctions* or even *expulsions*. Examples range from the Chilean Medical Society (for overseeing torture under Pinochet) and the National Medical Council of Uruguay (for abetting torture under a military junta) to South African sanctions (for failing to report/treat the torture of civil rights leader Steve Biko). Such sanctions may be an effective way for professional organizations to bring attention to the issue and discourage doctors from enabling torture.

Physicians for Human Rights' Alan Donaghue calls for psychologists and physicians involved to permanently lose their license. Peter Hall and David N. Tornberg (2005) think similarly: "Every one of the 139 countries that ratified the UN Convention against Torture is obligated to either prosecute suspects entering its territory or extradite them to a country that will." And so, in 1997, a Sudanese doctor working in Scotland was charged with aiding torture while in Sudan (Hall and Tornberg 2005: 1263). He could not escape his past—a warning to all who lose sight of the moral high ground.

THE CULTURAL DIMENSION

There is often a cultural dimension at work. In December 2008, Senator Carl Levin publicized a 2003 U.S. Central Command memo on "exploiting the Arab fear of dogs" (Levin 2008). In both Afghanistan and Iraq, dogs were used to terrify "Arab" detainees (See also Danner 2004: 49). Mind you, as ex-interrogator Tony Lagouranis observed, "Who *isn't* afraid of snarling dogs?"

There are other techniques based on cultural, religious, and ethnic stereotypes. Former State Department official Christopher Kojm says, "The CIA sometimes prefers Saudi interrogation sites and other places in the Arab world [for interrogation of detainees] because their interrogators speak a detainee's language and can *exploit his religion and customs*" (Priest and Stephens 2004, *emphasis mine*). Major General Taguba (2004) concluded in his report that psychological factors, such as the difference in culture, contributed to "the perversive atmosphere" at Abu Ghraib.

Health professionals helped develop, implement, and justify torture. They monitored interrogation techniques to determine their effectiveness. This turned detainees into human subjects without their consent and, according to Physicians for Human Rights, approached unlawful experimentation (2009: 4). Like torture, unethical medical experimentation has deep roots. It has been addressed by medical codes, such as the Geneva Conventions and the Declaration of Tokyo. Furthermore, Nigel S. Rodley looks at the application of international law to torture or cruel, inhuman, or degrading treatment or punishment (2009, chapters 1–5). In spite of the recognition of torture and abuse as a global problem, these codes and guidelines have not been given their due. We will look at this next.

HUMAN EXPERIMENTATION

Human subjects of nontherapeutic medical experimentation are also vulnerable to abuse. Subjects are drawn from hospitals (e.g., radiation studies), prisons (e.g., pharmaceutical studies), the military (e.g., mind control studies), civilian populations (e.g., pesticide studies), international populations (e.g., Depo Provera studies in Kenya, Thailand, and Mexico and HIV studies in South Africa), indigenous populations (e.g., the Human Genome Project studies of Native Americans), and so on. Marlene Brant Castellano looks at issues around Aboriginal research in part 3.

Peter F. Omonzejele examines serious issues around informed consent raised by pharmaceutical company Pfizer's 1996 clinical trials in Nigeria also in part 3. George Annas (2009) asks whether their failure to get informed consent violated a substantially similar international human rights law to those prohibiting torture.

Some experiments involve patient consent, others do not. Some factor in patient rights, others do not. Concepts like "self-determination" do not always carry much weight. But patient consent has little meaning if it is not "informed." As Allen M. Hornblum observes, "It is next to impossible to get informed consent from individuals in a dependent state. Prison inmates are very vulnerable" (1998: 66).

In addition, violating patient confidentiality has raised ethical concerns: M. Gregg Bloche and Jonathan Marks claim interrogators tapped clinical data to devise interrogation strategies, violating patient confidentiality. And Jonathan Moreno (2003) criticizes the use of detainee interviews by psychologists seeking personal data to assist interrogations and planning. "It seems a sure bet that there has been no IRB review within the Justice Department of the psychological profiling project," he asserts (2003).

The U.S. Navy sets out guidelines for experiments involving consciousness-altering drugs or mind-control techniques, prisoners, and "potentially controversial topics likely to attract media coverage" (2006: 9). Human experiments involving nuclear, biological, or chemical warfare agents is also addressed, but not how *informed* consent is possible.

With such nontherapeutic experiments, doctors may not be providing medical *care*. The social and cultural context foregrounds national security, political expediency, monetary benefits, weapons research, or scientific knowledge—and not the patient's best interests.

By subverting the patient's well-being to other goals, the ethical codes get left behind. At that point, the Hippocratic Oath loses its force. What is morally permissible in the moment may, in retrospect, fall short. For example, Arthur L. Caplan (2005) observes that most Nazi doctors thought it the right thing to do. They were not "either inept, mad, or coerced." We cannot assume, he says, that "those who know what is ethical will not behave in immoral ways" (394).

The APA is right to condemn such participation, given the recruitment of medical professionals for all sorts of nefarious experiments. Look, for example, at experiments involving biological and chemical weapons, including:

- Nerve agents, LSD, mustard gas, and sarin on British servicemen during/after after World War II (Eliott 2006), mustard gas and lewisite on American servicemen (*Health News Network*), and mustard gas and typhus by the Nazis (Lifton 1986: 301)
- Biological/germ warfare research and extreme-condition experiments (hypothermia, electric shock, etc.) on the Chinese by the Japanese during World War II (Yamaguchi 2000, Nie 2002)
- Malaria experiments on Chicago prisoners during World War II (Comfort 2009)
- Human radiation studies extending from the 1940s into the 1970s (Welsome 1999)
- Pesticide studies on human subjects in Scotland (Rogers 2003) and the United States—where informed consent forms failed "to disclose the potential risks involved" (Keim 2007)

Look, too, at research on white phosphorus, a biochemical warfare agent. "If particles of ignited white phosphorus land on a person's skin, they can continue to burn right through flesh to the bone" (BBC 2005). U.S. Marine Corps General Pace considers it a "legitimate tool" of the military (Miles 2005).

The Alliance for Human Research Protection warns that using human beings in toxic chemical experiments strips them of human dignity and reduces them to commodities, not to mention exploiting poor people by recruiting them as subjects (Reuters 2003). However, the September 2006 congressional compromise on torture *bars* biological experiments,[3] presumably because of actual or planned experiments.

Doctors involved in such experiments violate the Nuremberg Code by failing to obtain the subject's consent. "The medical research community found, and still finds, the stringency of the NC's first principle all too onerous," observes Jay Katz. In his assessment, many doctors consider the Nuremberg Code for barbarians and *not* for "ordinary physicians" (Cantwell 2001). Steven Miles finds it ironic that there was no trial of doctors working on biological warfare during World War II in Japan. He opined that the United States wanted access to their biological warfare data (Miles 2006).

Subjects of dubious medical experiments come from all quarters. For example, Steven Miles (2011) raises concerns about U.S. soldiers being given untested vaccines without obtaining consent. In his view, "dual loyalty ethics failed after military policy subordinated health interests to mission aims." There are lessons to be learned. As Jonathan Moreno (2003) reminds us, "History tends to be less forgiving when governments ride roughshod over those values that are supposed to be among their most cherished."

CONCLUSION

Denial and avoidance can look attractive when accountability rears its ugly head. Major General Taguba found this out when he urged a lieutenant general to look at the Abu Ghraib photographs of abuse and torture. He was told, "I don't want to get involved by looking, because what do you do with that information, once you know what they show?" (Hersh 2007).

As Taguba discovered, we may not want to know what is done "in our names." The torture memos claimed that the use of doctors in CIA interrogations was *morally distinct* from the practices of other countries accused of committing torture—doctors attending interrogations could stop them if medically indicated. This is not like a runaway train, but it assumes more independence of thought and absence of coercion than may be the case.

"I don't think we had any idea doctors were involved to this extent, and it will shock most physicians," Annas observes (Warrick and Finn 2009b). A psychologist and doctor were required to be present at the CIA's enhanced interrogations. They were there to calibrate harm—not to serve as protectors and healers (Keller et al. 2009: 6).

Chiara Lepora and Joseph Millum (2011) contend that doctors may be morally justified in assisting torture, particularly if the victim is in agreement (38). "If the state is going to amputate a limb as punishment," they argue, then it is surely better for the victim that the amputation be performed in a surgical theatre, under anesthesia, by a qualified surgeon (40). Doctors should provide competent medical service and act in the patient's best interest, and, so, participate in the atrocity rather than leave the victim in others' hands.

By that reasoning, doctors might feel compelled to put the victim out of his suffering to avoid a gruesome death. Once it's clear that torture will proceed no matter what, then the doctor should be a merciful agent as a cotorturer—so say Lepora and Millum.

However, once we cross that moral boundary with such consequentialist reasoning, doctors are no longer part of the *healing* profession, as Hopkins (2009) points out.

As a consultant psychiatrist and psychotherapist with the Medical Foundation for the Care of Victims of Torture, Hopkins (2009) is justified in raising doubts. He points to a 2004 CIA memo that a qualified physician would immediately intervene after an interrogation session to perform a tracheotomy if the detainee stopped breathing. Such intervention allows torture and abuse to be systemic. It also allows torturers the comfort in knowing that a doctor is standing by to make sure the victim doesn't die.

Jonathan Marks (2005) observes that, if we find doctors' participation in torture morally permissible, we will need to rethink medical training. We would then need "to embrace the interrogation ethos and its institutional sequelae, not just the practice." This would include teaching "interrogation medicine" and "interrogation psychiatry" courses (Marks 2005).

Reflecting on what transpired at Abu Ghraib, Army reservist Israel Rivera saw harms to *all* participants, not just the victims of abuse. His words resonate:

> It was a door that I was afraid to walk through. If you walk through it, at which point do you say it's enough? What's cruel enough? How do you get back from that? And I was afraid that I wouldn't come back, that I would get lost. (Kennedy 2007)

Once lost, there may be no road back. When Dante descended into Hell, at least he had a mentor and guide (Virgil) to help him return unscathed. Doctors and other caregivers have no Virgil to lead the way out of the moral turpitude into which they sink due to the harmful practices examined here. Once that threshold is crossed, it's hard to answer the question, "What's cruel enough?" As for, "How do you get back from that?" the truth, unfortunately, is that some never do. Not entirely.

Tony Lagouranis put it this way, "It takes a unique clarity to stand up and say what everyone thinks is so normal is actually abhorrent. I think I did well under the circumstances, but no one reported what they should have when they should have— including me." And, as he says, "It's a lonely road when everyone else is taking the other one" (Conroy 2007).

No one reported *what* they should have *when* they could have. We are paying the price for that moral failure now. But we can learn and go forward. Daniel Jacoby, MD (2004) calls for medical personnel to do more than *speak out* about abuse or torture. He also recommends that major medical organizations such as the American Medical Association establish a commission for the investigation of abuses by medical professionals and to set out specific recommendations to prevent further abuses.

To ensure better treatment of patients and a stronger moral spine on the part of medical caregivers, things have to change. When their actions fall below the standard of care and they cease to honor the ethical codes shaping professional conduct, they must be held accountable. Professional organizations must become proactive and hold their members to the standards they set. Bioethicists are already pointing out the need for change. Our continued efforts and attention to human rights can make all the difference.

NOTES

1. As stated by the Office of the Surgeon General of the (U.S.) Army (2005), "Medical personnel who assist in developing the plan of interrogation are not deemed to be 'participating in an interrogation.' Likewise, actual presence in the interrogation room may not constitute 'participating in an interrogation' . . . [if] to ensure the health and welfare of the detainee."

2. See, for example, *Ethics, Trust, and the Professions* (Georgetown University Press, 1991), which he wrote with Robert M. Veatch and John P. Langan, SJ.

3. See CNN, "Deal on Detainee Treatment Quells GOP Revolt," September 22, 2006, at www.cnn.com/2006/POLITICS/09/21/terror.bill/.

REFERENCES

ABC News [Australia]. 2002, August 20. "Biowarfare Experiments Reported in Northern Iraq: US Official."

Ackerman, Spencer. 2011, July 6. "Drift: How This Ship Became a Floating Gitmo." *Wired.* http://www.wired.com/dangerroom/2011/07/floating-gitmo/.

ACLU. 2005, May 25. "Guantánamo Prisoners Told FBI of Qur'an Desecration in 2002, New Documents Reveal." American Civil Liberties Union website. http://www.aclu.org/print/national-security/guantanamo-prisoners-told-fbi-quran-desecration-2002-new-documents-reveal.

———. 2009, March 2. "CIA Destroyed 92 Interrogation Tapes." American Civil Liberties Union website. http://www.aclu.org/national-security/cia-destroyed-92-interrogation-tapes.

Allhoff, F. 2008. "Physician Involvement in Hostile Interrogations." In *Physicians at War: The Dual-Loyalties Challenge,* edited by F. Allhoff, 91–104. New York: Springer.

Annas, G. J. 2009, May 14. "Globalized Clinical Trials and Informed Consent." *New England Journal of Medicine* 360:2050–3. http://www.nejm.org/doi/full/10.1056/NEJMp0901474.

Awofeso, N. 2006, June 5. "Doctors, Prison Torture and the 'War on Terror' [Letter to the editor]." *Medical Journal of Australia* 184:588–9. http://www.mja.com.au/public/issues/184_11_050606/letters_050606_fm-2.html.

Barratt, K. 2006, February 25. "The Sanitized Horrors of Guantanamo Bay." *ePluribus Media.* http://www.epluribusmedia.org/archives/columns/2006/0221barratt.html.

BBC. 2002, August 20. "US knew of bioterror tests in Iraq," *BBC News* World Edition, http://news.bbc.co.uk/2/hi/americas/2294321.stm.

BBC. 2005, November 16. "Q&A: White Phosphorus." *BBC News.* http://news.bbc.co.uk/2/hi/middle_east/4441902.stm.

Bloche, M. G., and J. H. Marks. 2005. "Doctors and Interrogators at Guantánamo Bay." *New England Journal of Medicine* 353:6–8. http://www.nejm.org/doi/full/10.1056/NEJMp058145.

Bradbury, S. G. 2005, May 10. "Memorandum Regarding Application of 18 USC. §§ 2340-2340A to Certain Techniques That May Be Used in the Interrogation of a High Value al Qaeda Detainee." http://www.justice.gov/olc/docs/memo-bradbury2005-3.pdf.

Cantwell, Jr., A. R. 2001, September–October. "The Human Radiation Experiments." *New Dawn* 68. http://www.newdawnmagazine.com/articles/the-human-radiation-experiments.

Caplan, A. 2005. "Too Hard to Face." *Journal of the American Academy of Psychiatry and the Law* 33 (3): 394–400.

———. 2007. "The Ethics of Evil: The Challenge of Nazi Medical Experiments." In *Dark Medicine*, edited by W. R. LaFleur, G. Böhme, and S. Shimazono, 63–72. Bloomington: Indiana University Press.

Cassel, D. 2008, February 14. "Jose Padilla Brings Torture to Trial." *In These Times*. http://www.inthesetimes.com/article/3536/jose_padilla_brings_torture_to_trial.

Center for Constitutional Rights. 2006, July. *Report on Torture and Cruel, Inhuman, and Degrading Treatment of Prisoners at Guantánamo Bay, Cuba*. http://ccrjustice.org/files/Report_ReportOnTorture.pdf.

Cilasun, U. 1991. "Torture and the Participation of Doctors." *Journal of Medical Ethics 17 Supplement*:21–22. http://www.ncbi.nlm.nih.gov/pmc/articles/PMC1378166/pdf/jmedeth00280-0023.pdf.

Comfort, N. 2009, September. "The Prisoner as Model Organism: Malaria Research at Stateville Penitentiary," *Studies in History and Philosophy of Biology and Biomedical Sciences* Vol. 40, no. 3: 190–203.

Conroy, J. 2007, March 2. "Confessions of a Torturer: An Army Interrogator's Story." *Chicago Reader*. http://www.chicagoreader.com/chicago/confessions-of-a-torturer/Content?oid=924419.

Cook, J. 2009, June 29. "Israeli Doctors Accused of Flouting Ethics." *The National (United Arab Emirates)*. http://www.thenational.ae/news/worldwide/middle-east/israeli-doctors-accused-of-flouting-ethics.

Danner, M. 2004, June 10. "Torture and Truth." *The New York Review of Books*, http://www.nybooks.com/articles/archives/2004/jun/10/torture-and-truth/.

Department of Justice. 2008. FBI Observations Regarding Detainee Treatment in Guantanamo Bay: Conclusion. *Center for the Study of Human Rights in the Americas*. http://humanrights.ucdavis.edu/projects/the-guantanamo-testimonials-project/testimonies/testimony-of-the-department-of-justice/fbi-observations-regarding-detainee-treatment-in-guantanamo-bay-conclusion.

Department of Justice, OIG. 2008. "A Review of the FBI's Involvement in and Observations of Detainee Interrogations in Guantanamo Bay, Afghanistan, and Iraq." http://www.justice.gov/oig/special/s0805/final.pdf.

Dowdall, T. L. 1991. "Repression, Health Care and Ethics under Apartheid." *Journal of Medical Ethics 17 Supplement*:51–54. http://www.ncbi.nlm.nih.gov/pmc/articles/PMC1378176/pdf/jmedeth00280-0053.pdf.

Eggen, D. 2007, January 3. "FBI Reports Duct-Taping, 'Baptizing' at Guantanamo." *Washington Post*.

Elliott, F. 2006, July 9. "Chemical Warfare: Inside Britain's Toxic House of Horrors." *The Independent* (UK). http://www.independent.co.uk/news/uk/politics/chemical-warfare-inside-britains-toxic-house-of-horrors-407244.html.

Fay, Major General G. R. 2004, August 25. "AR 15-6 Investigation of the Abu Ghraib Detention Facility and 205th Military Intelligence Brigade (u) (*Fay Report*)." Find Law website. http://news.findlaw.com/hdocs/docs/dod/fay82504rpt.pdf.

Forrest, D. 1998, March. "Doctors and Torture." *The Hoolet*. http://www.freedomfromtorture.org/sites/default/files/documents/Forrest-Doctors%26Torture.pdf.

Gawande, A. 2009, March 30. "Hellhole." *New Yorker*. http://www.newyorker.com/reporting/2009/03/30/090330fa_fact_gawande.

Goodman, A. 2005, November 25. "Former U.S. Army Interrogator Describes the Harsh Techniques He Used in Iraq." *Democracy Now.* http://www.democracynow.org/2005/11/15/former_u_s_army_interrogator_describes.

Goodman, A. (executive producer and host) and J. Gonzalez (cohost). 2006, October 26. "Abu Ghraib at Home: New Human Rights Watch Report Says US Using Dogs to Terrify Prisoners." Interview with J. Fellner. *Democracy Now!* [television broadcast]. http://www.democracynow.org/2006/10/12/abu_ghraib_at_home_new_human.

———. 2009, July 31. "Exclusive: John Walker Lindh's Parents Discuss Their Son's Story, from Joining the US-Backed Taliban Army to Surviving a Northern Alliance Massacre, to His Abuse at the Hands of US Forces." *Democracy Now!* [television broadcast]. http://www.democracynow.org/2009/7/31/exclusive_john_walker_lindhs_parents_discuss.

Hall, P., and D. N. Tornberg. 2005, October 8. "A Stain on Medical Ethics [Letter to the editor]." *Lancet* 366:1263. http://download.thelancet.com/pdfs/journals/lancet/PIIS0140673605675204.pdf.

Hanley, C. J. 2004, May 8. "Early Iraq Abuse Accounts Met with Silence." http://www.rath.us/random-stuff/interesting-articles/prisoner_mistreatment.txt.

Harmon, K. 2009, September 1. "Role of Physicians and Psychologists in Interrogation of Terrorism Suspects Reexamined." *Scientific American.* http://www.scientificamerican.com/blog/post.cfm?id=role-of-physicians-and-psychologist-2009-09-01.

Health News Network. n.d. "A History of Secret Human Experimentation." http://www.rense.com/general36/history.htm.

Hersh, S. M. 2007, June 25. "The General's Report." *New Yorker.* http://www.newyorker.com/reporting/2007/06/25/070625fa_fact_hersh?printable=true.

Hopkins, W. 2009, August 6. "Doctors Who Assist in Torture Should Be Brought to Justice." *The Telegraph (U.K.).* http://www.telegraph.co.uk/health/5984212/Doctors-who-assist-in-torture-should-be-brought-to-justice.html.

Hornblum, A. M. 1998. *Acres of Skin: Human Experiments at Holmesberg Prison.* New York: Routledge.

Human Rights Watch. 2006. "Cruel and Degrading: The Use of Dogs for Cell Extractions in US Prisons." http://www.hrw.org/en/reports/2006/10/09/cruel-and-degrading.

International Committee of the Red Cross. 2007, February 14. "ICRC Report on the Treatment of Fourteen 'High Value Detainees' in CIA Custody." http://www.nybooks.com/media/doc/2010/04/22/icrc-report.pdf.

Jacoby, D. 2004, October 7. Letter to the editor. *The New England Journal of Medicine* 38. http://www.nejm.org/doi/pdf/10.1056/NEJM200410073511518.

Keim, B. 2007, August 3. "Human Pesticide Testing's Greatest Hits." http://www.wired.com/wiredscience/2007/08/human-pesticide/.

Keller, Allen, Scott Allen, Steven Reisner, and Vincent Iacopino. Physicians for Human Rights. 2009, August. "Aiding Torture." http://physiciansforhumanrights.org/library/reports/aiding-torture-2009.html.

Kennedy, R. (producer and director) and L. Garbus, J. Youngelson, D. Barrett, S. Nevins, and N. Abraham (producers). 2007. *Ghosts of Abu Ghraib* [motion picture]. United States: HBO Home Video.

Kiley, K. C. 2005, April 13. "Detainee Medical Operations Report." http://dspace.wrlc.org/doc/bitstream/2041/85008/02920_050413.pdf.

Kupers, T. 2011, March 16. "Cruel and Unusual Treatment of WikiLeaks Suspect." *CNN.com.* http://articles.cnn.com/2011-03-16/opinion/kupers.bradley.manning.prison_1_solitary-confinement-prisoners-mental-illness?_s=PM:OPINION.

Larson, H. 2012, May 27. "The CIA's Fake Vaccination Drive Has Damaged the Battle against Polio." *The Guardian* (UK) http://www.guardian.co.uk/commentisfree/2012/may/27/cia-fake-vaccination-polio.

Leopold, J. 2011, April 29. "Guantanamo Detainees Stage Hunger Strike to Protest Confinement Conditions." http://www.truth-out.org/guantanamo-detainees-hunger-strike-protest-confinement-conditions/1304092655.

Lepora, C., and J. Millum. 2011, May–June. "The Tortured Patient." *The Hastings Center Report*:38–47. www.thehastingscenter.org/Publications/HCR/Detail.aspx?id=5360.

Levin, Senator Carl. 2008, December 11. "Statement of Senator Carl Levin on Senate Armed Services Committee Report of Its Inquiry into the Treatment of Detainees in US Custody." http://levin.senate.gov/newsroom/press/release/?id=dfe6e48a-6900-42e6-852c-ae9046748bdf.

Lewis, N. A. 2005, September 18. "Guantanamo Prisoners Go on Hunger Strike." *The New York Times.*

———. 1986. *The Nazi Doctors: Medical Killing and the Psychology of Genocide.* New York: Basic Books.

Lifton, R. J. 1986. *The Nazi Doctors: Medical Killing and the Psychology of Genocide.* New York: Basic Books.

———. 2004, October 7. "Reply to Letters to the Editor." *New England Journal of Medicine 351*:1574. www.nejm.org/doi/pdf/10.1056/NEJM200410073511518.

London, L., D. Ncayiyana, D. Sanders, A. Kalebi, and J. Kasolo. 2008, October. "Editorial. Zimbabwe: A Crossroads for the Health Professions." *South African Medical Journal* 98:77–78. www.samj.org.za/index.php/samj/article/view/2735/2138+Rayner+M.+Turning+a+blind+eye%3F&cd=5&hl=en&ct=clnk&gl=us&client=safari.

Marks, J. H. 2005, July–August. "Doctors of Interrogation: The Contours of Physician Participation." *The Hastings Center Report* 35:17–22.

———. 2007, March–April. "The Bioethics of War." *The Hastings Center Report* 37:41–42.

Mayer, J. 2005a, February 14. "Outsourcing Torture." *New Yorker.* http://www.newyorker.com/archive/2005/02/14/050214fa_fact6.

———. 2005b, July 11. "The Experiment: A Reporter at Large." *New Yorker*: 65–66.

Mazzetti, M. 2012, January 28. "Panetta Credits Pakistani Doctor in Bin Laden Raid." http://www.nytimes.com/2012/01/29/world/asia/panetta-credits-pakistani-doctor-in-bin-laden-raid.html.

Mazzetti, M., and S. Shane. 2008, March 13. "Pentagon Cites Tapes Showing Interrogations." *The New York Times.*

McNeil, Jr., D. G. 2012, July 9. "C.I.A. Vaccine Ruse May Have Harmed the War on Polio." *The New York Times.* http://www.nytimes.com/2012/07/10/health/cia-vaccine-ruse-in-pakistan-may-have-harmed-polio-fight.html?pagewanted=all.

Miles, D. 2005, November 30. "Chairman Calls White Phosphorous Legitimate Military Tool." *Defense Link.* http://www.defense.gov/news/newsarticle.aspx?id=18195.

Miles, S. H. 2006. *Oath Betrayed: Torture, Medical Complicity, and the War on Terror.* New York: Random House.

———. 2011, July 13. "The New Military Medical Ethics: Legacies of the Gulf Wars and the War on Terror." *Bioethics.* http://onlinelibrary.wiley.com/doi/10.1111/j.1467-8519.2011.01920.x/full.

Mohsin, S. 2013, October 9. "In Pakistan, Vaccinating Children against Polio Can Be a Deadly Job." *CNN.* http://www.cnn.com/2013/10/09/world/asia/pakistan-polio-workers/index.html.

Moreno, J. D. 2003. "Detainee Ethics: Terrorists as Research Subjects." *The American Journal of Bioethics* 3 (4): W32–W33.

Murray, C. 2010, October 29. "Lib. Dem. Ministers Complicit in Torture." http://www.craigmurray.org.uk/archives/2010/10/lib_dem_ministe/.

Narayan, N. 1998, Summer. "Bad Medicine." *Harvard International Review* 20 (4). http://hir.harvard.edu/bad-medicine.

Nie, J.-B. 2002, December. "Japanese Doctors' Experimentation in Wartime China." *The Lancet* 360:S5–S6. http://www.thelancet.com/journals/lancet/article/PIIS0140-6736(02)11797-1/fulltext.

Pawlaczyk, G., and B. Hundsdorfer. 2010, October 22. "Trapped in Tamms." *Belleville News Democrat*, http://www.bnd.com/trapped-in-tamms/.

Perry, T. 2009, September 25. "We Lost the Moral High Ground." *Los Angeles Times.*

Priest, D., and B. Gellman. 2002, December 26. "US Decries Abuse but Defends Interrogations." *The Washington Post.*

Priest, D., and J. Stephens. 2004, May 11. "Secret World of US Interrogation: Long History of Tactics in Overseas Prisons Is Coming to Light." *The Washington Post.*

Rejali, D. 2007. *Torture and Democracy.* Princeton: Princeton University Press.

Reuters. 2003, January 15. "Chemical Giant Paid Students to Drink Pesticide." http://www.ahrp.org/infomail/0103/15.php.

Reuters. 2008, February 8. "U.N. Says Waterboarding Should Be Prosecuted as Torture." http://uk.reuters.com/article/2008/02/08/uk-usa-torture-un-idUKN0852061620080208.

Richey, W. 2007, August 13. "US Terror Interrogation Went Too Far, Experts Say." *Christian Science Monitor.* http://www.csmonitor.com/2007/0813/p01s03-usju.html.

Robinson, E. 2009, September 4. "Medical Professionals Owe Torture Accounting." *The Washington Post.*

Rodley, N. S. 2009. *The Treatment of Prisoners under International Law*, 3rd ed. Oxford: Oxford University Press.

Sawyer, J. 2008, June 5, updated October 10, 2010. "Torture." http://www.westernoregonjournal.com/2.13057/torture-1.1698592.

Sessums, L. L., J. F. Collen, P. G. O'Malley, J. L. Jackson, and M. J. Roy. 2009. "Ethical Practice under Fire: Deployed Physicians in the Global War on Terrorism." *Military Medicine* 174:441–7.

Shamsi, H. 2006, February. "Detainee Deaths in US Custody in Iraq and Afghanistan." *Commands Responsibility.* http://www.humanrightsfirst.org/wp-content/uploads/pdf/06221-etn-hrf-dic-rep-web.pdf.

Sharrock, J. 2009, July–August. "First, Do Harm." *Mother Jones.* http://motherjones.com/politics/2009/07/first-do-harm.

Sherman, N. 2006. "Holding Doctors Responsible at Guantánamo." *Kennedy Institute of Ethics Journal* 16:199–203.

Siems, L. 2010, September 3. "Chapter 5, Part 2—The Battle Lab. The Torture Report." http://www.thettorturereport.org/report/chapter-5-part-2-battle-lab.

Smith, H. F., and M. Freeman. 2005. "The Mandatory Reporting of Torture by Detention Center Officials: An Original Proposal." *Human Rights Quarterly* 27:327–45.

Stephens, J. 2005, January 6. "Army Doctors Implicated in Abuse." *Washington Post.*

Taguba, Major General. 2004. Taguba Report. http://www.npr.org/iraq/2004/prison_abuse_report.pdf.

Teays, W. 2007. "Torture and Public Health." In *International Public Health Ethics and Policy*, edited by M. Boylan, 59–90. New York: Springer.

Tietz, J. 2006, August 24. "The Unending Torture of Omar Khadr." *Rolling Stone*. http://humanrights.ucdavis.edu/projects/the-guantanamo-testimonials-project/testimonies/prisoner-testimonies/the-unending-torture-of-omar-khadr.

Today Online. "California Prison Inmates Go on Hunger Strike." 2013, July 10. http://www.todayonline.com/world/americas/california-prison-inmates-go-hunger-strike.

U.S. Department of the Navy. 2006, November 6. "Protection of Human Subjects and Adherence to Ethical Standards in DoD Supported Research." http://www.fas.org/irp/doddir/navy/secnavinst/3900_39d.pdf.

Vesti, P., and N. J. Lavik. 1991. "Torture and the Medical Profession: A Review." *Journal of Medical Ethics 17 Supplement*: 4–8.

Vorbrüggen, M., and H. U. Baer. 2007. "Humiliation: The Lasting Effect of Torture." *Military Medicine 172*, 12 Supplement: 29–33.

Vries, Lloyd. 2002, August 1. "Al Qaeda Facility in Iraq Targeted?" *CBS News*, http://www.cbsnews.com/news/al-qaeda-facility-in-iraq-targeted/.

Wallach, E. 2007, November 4. "Waterboarding Used to Be a Crime." *Washington Post*.

Warrick, J. 2008, April 22. "Detainees Allege Being Drugged, Questioned." *Washington Post*.

Warrick, J., P. Finn, and J. Tate. 2009a, August 16. "CIA Releases Its Instructions for Breaking a Detainee's Will." *Washington Post*.

———. 2009b, April 18. "Interrogation Memos Detail Psychologists' Involvement; Ethicists Outraged." *Washington Post*.

Wead, Cdr. F. 2007, November 5. "Waterboarding: A SERE-ing Experience for Tens of Thousands of US Military Personnel." *Human Events*. http://www.humanevents.com/article.php?id=23220.

Welsome, E. 1999. *The Plutonium Files: America's Secret Medical Experiments in the Cold War*. New York: Dell Publishing.

White, J., and S. Higham. 2004, June 11. "Use of Dogs to Scare Prisoners Was Authorized: Military Intelligence Personnel Were Involved, Handlers Say." *Washington Post*.

Whoriskey, P. 2007, March 24. "Judge Refuses to Dismiss Padilla's Charges." *Washington Post*.

Wiesel, E. 2005, April 14. "Without Conscience." *New England Journal of Medicine* 352 (15): 1511–3. http://www.nejm.org/doi/full/10.1056/NEJMp058069.

World Medical Association. 2006. "WMA Condemns All Forced Feeding." http://www.wma.net/en/40news/20archives/2006/2006_10/index.html.

Yamaguchi, M. 2000, November 16. "Japanese Veteran Tells of Experiments Done on Chinese." *Milwaukee Journal Sentinel*.

———. 2011, February 22. "Medical Site Excavation Sees Japan Dig into Murky Period of Its History." *The Scotsman*. http://news.scotsman.com/worldwarii/Medical-site-excavation-sees-Japan.6722139.jp.

Yee, J. 2011, July 22. "Steven Miles: Call for Renewal of Bioethics in Military." http://www.bioedge.org/index.php/bioethics/bioethics_article/9647/.

5

Immigration Detention and the Right to Health Care

Rita Manning

ABSTRACT

There are now over 1.1 million people overseen by Immigration and Customs Enforcement (ICE), with about thirty-three detained in jails and federal detention centers around the country at any particular time. The average detention time is two months, but some are detained for much longer periods. Since its inception, 121 deaths and countless cases of medical neglect have occurred. Given its secrecy and lack of oversight, it is not clear how many of these deaths are the result of inadequate medical care. ICE is a branch of a government agency in a democratic country, thus citizens have an obligation to ensure that it operates in conformity with the fundamental principles of justice on which this nation was founded. ICE is a young and rapidly growing bureaucracy with little oversight. It operates using a mix of federal, state, local, and private centers, many of which are penal institutions. It has a history of abuse, and even when in conformity with its penal standards, it inflicts additional harm onto vulnerable people, especially asylum seekers and parents of minor children. It thus requires constant vigilance and concern. Our immigration policies and detention practices are deeply troubling, but until we elect to reform them, we have a special obligation to the vulnerable populations that we house in ICE detention.

INTRODUCTION

Francisco Castaneda came to the United States when he was ten years old, a refugee from the civil war in El Salvador. His mother died before she could apply for refugee status for the family, and Francisco ended up in ICE detention following his arrest for minor drug charges. Francisco repeatedly requested medical attention for a lesion

131

on his penis, but he was repeatedly denied care until the settlement of an ACLU lawsuit on his behalf. He subsequently died of penile cancer in 2008, at the age of thirty-five (Mooty 2010).

Victoria Arellano, a transgender woman from Mexico with AIDS, was detained in 2007. During detention, she was given her AIDS medication on a very random schedule. Despite repeated requests for help and symptoms ranging from nausea, vomiting blood, and fever, ICE denied her medical care until a week before her death. She died from pneumonia and meningitis at the age of twenty-three (Papst 2009).

These cases are truly horrifying, and given its secrecy and lack of accountability and oversight, it is not clear how many of the 121 deaths that have occurred to date in ICE detention are equally the result of grossly inadequate medical care (ICE Detainee Deaths). In what follows, I will describe the problem in more detail and argue that ICE has a moral obligation to offer adequate medical care to all its detainees.

GLOBAL BACKGROUND

There are approximately 191 million displaced persons in the world. Of that number, about seventeen million are designated by the UN High Commission on Refugees as refugees and stateless persons, with an additional sixteen million person internally displaced (UN High Commission on Refugees). In the United States there are approximately 11.2 million undocumented persons (Passel and Taylor 2010).

Just under fifty thousand of that number are asylum seekers (UN High Commission on Refugees). While undocumented persons do have some limited rights to health care in the United States, in practice their access to health care is extremely limited. *Plyler v. Doe* (1982) ruled that undocumented people were persons under the Fourteenth Amendment whose fundamental rights, including, presumably, some rights to health care, were thereby protected.

The 1986 Emergency Medical Treatment and Active Labor Act (EMTALA) mandates that all persons are entitled to receive emergency medical care until their condition is stabilized, but the 1996 Personal Responsibility and Work Opportunity Reconciliation Act (PRWORA) restricted most federal public benefits, including health care, for all classes of immigrants, legal and undocumented.

We could argue that all persons have a right to health care, but here I will make a more modest claim—that those undocumented persons who are held in immigration detention are entitled to appropriate health care. Since many medical conditions may be a natural consequence of the current ICE detention practices, this may turn out to be a far-ranging critique.

There are now over 1.1 million people overseen by ICE, with about thirty-three thousand detained in jails and federal detention centers around the country at any particular time (Schriro 2009). The average detention time is two months, but some are detained for much longer periods. Some detainees from the Mariel boatlift from

Cuba were detained for thirty years until the Supreme Court ordered their release (*Clark v. Martinez* 2005).

But the United States is not alone in detaining undocumented persons. This practice also occurs in Austria, Canada, Finland, Germany, Mexico, Netherlands, the United Kingdom, Japan, France, Italy, Greece, Spain, and Australia (Global Detention Project). While I think that a similar argument could be made for access to health care in all these countries, I will confine my remarks to immigration detention in the United States. Before I begin my argument, a bit of background is in order.

U.S. IMMIGRATION DETENTION POLICIES

The United States began detaining immigrants at Ellis Island in 1852, but this practice was largely discarded until the 1996 Illegal Immigration Reform and Immigrant Responsibility Act. Among its provisions are the following:

1. Most criminal offenses are grounds for mandatory, permanent deportation, and this provision applies even to offenses committed before the enactment of this legislation.
2. Mandatory detention is the norm for those in deportation proceedings.
3. The elimination of the right to federal review of the Immigration and Naturalization Service (INS) (The Homeland Security Act of 2002 replaced INS with Immigration and Customs Enforcement (ICE); United States Citizenship and Immigration Services; and Bureau of Customs and Border Protection) decisions.
4. Expedited removal procedures that allow INS (now ICE) employees broad discretion to deny admission, even to asylum seekers.
5. Evidence not available to immigrants or their lawyers can be used in deportation proceedings.

The 1996 Antiterrorism and Effective Death Penalty Act allows states to collaborate with Homeland Security in enforcing illegal immigration via 287(g) agreements. Florida was the first state to enter into a 287(g) agreement, which it did in 2002, and currently there are sixty-nine agencies in twenty-four states with 287(g) agreements (ICE Factsheet).

While ICE's emphasis on deporting immigrant "criminals" suggests that these are the only persons in ICE detention, this is far from the case. The categories of persons in ICE detention include asylum seekers; undocumented persons who are not asylum seekers, but who are not accused of any crime; undocumented persons who are accused of trivial offenses, including identity theft or felonious reentry; undocumented persons accused of serious offenses; and legal permanent residents who have committed a deportable offense. Until 2009, ICE also detained the children of undocumented adults, most of whom were American citizens. The practice of detaining "unaccompanied alien children" ended in 2003 with the transfer of these children to the Office of Refugee Resettlement.

ICE currently houses detainees in at least sixty-nine detention facilities (ICE Detention Reform). This is a constantly shifting number because ICE operates three different kinds of centers: Service Processing Centers (SPCs) that are run by ICE, Contract Detention Facilities (CDFs) that are run by private prison companies such as Corrections Corporation of America and GEO, and centers run under contract with state or local government correctional agencies.

Various concerns have been raised about these detention centers: They are often distant from the detainee's place of residence, making legal representation very difficult. In the prisons and jails that lease space to ICE, detainees are treated, in most respects, like prisoners, regardless of their status. Because correctional space is committed to other uses, detainees are transferred often and with little notice, making it difficult to find detainees. ICE recently included a detainee locator device on their website. Even when detainees can be located and are at a facility that allows the possibility of visitation, it is difficult and limited.

All detention centers require visitors to possess valid government-issued identification, and many family members of detained persons may not have such documents. Various other restrictions are put on visitation, with some centers mandating that all visits be noncontact and limited to thirty minutes (ICE Visitation).

CONCERNS ABOUT ICE HEALTH CARE

Finally, a number of very serious concerns have been raised about the lack of adequate health care in ICE detention facilities (Priest and Goldstein 2008, Keller 2003, Guzman 2009). Homer D. Venters, MD, an attending physician at the Bellevue/NYU Program for Survivors of Torture in New York City, said that "after adjusting for average length of detention, the data show that the mortality rate increased 29% between 2006 and 2007, from 27 to 34 per 100,000 detention-years" (AMA 2008).

First, though ICE adopted standards for the provision of health care in 2008, these standards were developed for penal institutions and are thus inappropriate for civil detention (Papst 2009). Second, there are no clear provisions for enforcing the standards and, thus, the number of serious complaints continues to rise. These range from suicide (Goldstein and Priest 2008) and lack of treatment for mental illness (Tillman 2009) to the denial of abortion services for a detainee who was raped (Walden 2009) to preventable deaths (Ferrell 2008). Concerns about the lack of translators and health care staff indifference and incompetence have also been raised (Mooty 2010).

ICE recently agreed to provide immigration detainees at two of its facilities with "constitutionally adequate levels of medical and mental health care" as part of an agreement to settle an American Civil Liberties Union lawsuit (*Woods v. Morton*). While this is clearly a step in the right direction, the limit of the agreement to two sites and ICE's history of intransigence on this issue suggest that continued vigilance and oversight is warranted. Kelsey Papst summarizes the reports of the ICE Inspector General for the years 2004 to 2006 and notes that despite the serious violations, as of 2008, ICE had not even responded to the report (Papst 2009).

I begin by distinguishing three categories of medical conditions, one of which imposes a different sort of moral obligation. The first is preexisting conditions, the second those that occur in detention but which have no causal connection to the conditions of detention, and the third are conditions that have a causal relationship to detention. All of the arguments I shall give for our obligation to provide adequate health care to detainees apply to all three categories of detainees, but the last category of detainees provides an especially compelling case. Here, we are obligated to mitigate the harm that is created by the detention practices that the United States chooses to employ.

Many detainees will enter detention with preexisting conditions. This is not surprising since this is a very vulnerable population. Most left their home countries for economic reasons, and their immigration status makes it very difficult to obtain care in the United States. The federal Emergency Medical Treatment and Active Labor Act (EMTALA) requires that hospitals treat and stabilize patients who present with emergencies, but at the same time there are no requirements to offer long-term or curative care.

In addition, the Personal Responsibility and Work Opportunity Reconciliation Act (PRWORA) restricts most federal public benefits, including medical care, for all classes of immigrants, legal and undocumented. Many hospitals are currently dealing with this conflict by repatriating undocumented patients, often without their fully informed consent (Johnson 2009, Bresa 2010, Babu and Wolpin 2010). It is reasonable to suppose that part of the reason why some people enter detention with preexisting conditions is because of the restrictions on access to health care that are enshrined in federal law.

The second category includes those that occur in detention but which have no causal connection to the conditions of detention. The final category is conditions that are either exacerbated or caused by the detention itself. Foremost among these are mental health problems.

MENTAL HEALTH ISSUES IN ICE DETENTION

The psychological effects of detention are profound and long lasting. Coffee et al. describe some of the mental health problems directly attributable to detention: isolation and fractured relationships, demoralization and depression, and changes in view of self (Coffey, Kaplan, Sampson, and Tucci 2010).

When the detainee is an asylum seeker, these problems are magnified through the lens of their previous mistreatment. Cutler cites problems in this population ranging from "anxiety to features of depressive illness, and features of post-traumatic stress to more serious conditions such as self-harm and suicide attempts" (Cutler 2005). These problems are especially serious for mothers. As one immigration attorney described it,

> It seems to me that there are so many unique issues with [detained] women. It's a higher psychological toll to be separated from their children. It gets to the point where you cannot even communicate with your client at all [because they are so distraught]. With men, there's definitely an impact, but with women it takes over their entire being. Anybody who works with women detainees who have been transferred away from children will tell you it's so much more emotionally taxing for them. (Rabin 2009)

While ICE claims to be continually upgrading its health care, as of May 2011, the only "reforms" they cite in the area of mental health are convening one workshop and a "full day mental health roundtable" (ICE Detention Reform).

COLLATERAL DAMAGE

The effect of ICE detention extends well beyond the detainee. Communities are undermined by the absence of contributing members. The fear of ICE detection encourages people to stay away from community activities and to endure abusive living and working conditions (Ray 2006, Kim 2009). The children of detained parents will often have the parent detained at a distant location, and in the worst case, the child will lose the parent through deportation.

If the child is among the approximately four million U.S.-born children with at least one noncitizen parent, and 79 percent of the children with undocumented parents were born in the United States (Passel and Taylor 2010), she may well face a devastating choice: to remain in the United States without the parent or move to a unfamiliar country, with prospects that are likely to be exceedingly poor (Rome 2010).

Since the experience of having one's parent detained in a prisonlike facility to which one has little access is very similar to the experience of having one's parent incarcerated for a criminal offense in a correctional institution, one would expect that long-term effects on children of parents detained by ICE would be roughly similar to those experienced by children of incarcerated parents. These consequences include severe and trauma-related stress; depression and difficulty forming attachments; difficulty sleeping and concentrating; withdrawing emotionally; cognitive delays; and difficulty developing trust, autonomy, initiative, productivity, and achieving identity (Miller 2006).

ARGUMENTS FOR OBLIGATION TO
DETAINEES: PUBLIC HEALTH

There are a number of arguments for the obligation to provide health services to detainees, and many of these arguments parallel the arguments offered in support of medical care for immigrants generally. The first is public health. Some of the detainees will later be released, and they may pose a threat to themselves or others if their health concerns are not addressed. One of the problems with this argument is that it does not go far enough. One could address this concern by offering services only to those that have a high probability of release into the United States, or to those who have a medical condition that would pose a public health hazard. Of course, defenders of this argument point out that one doesn't know who will constitute a public health hazard until they have been medically assessed. The CDC (2005) discussion of the prevalence of asymptomatic tuberculosis is instructive here.

JUSTICE

The question of justice most often comes up in bioethics in the context of the allocation of health care. The relevant issue for this chapter is whether and when persons are entitled to a minimum standard of health care. Rawls's principle of equal opportunity is often appealed to in this context (Rawls 1999). He argues that, in a fair bargaining situation, all persons would agree that everyone is entitled to equal opportunity. Meaningful equal opportunity requires, among other things, a right to at least a minimum standard of health care.

Defenders of a right to health care, such as Norman Daniels, argue that failure to respect this right is fundamentally unjust (Daniels 1998). This injustice is compounded when we note that people in ICE detention are unable to access health care on their own. As a result, even if one were persuaded that the right to health care is merely a negative right—one which requires only that others refrain from interfering with a person's act of securing health care—one would have to grant that the conditions of detention must either allow health care providers access to their detainee patients, or, if security requires limiting outside access, that health care be provided by ICE.

Critics might allege that a right to health care is something that society need only respect for its members and that persons in ICE detention are at best future members. But most defenders of the equal right to health care would base such a right on membership, not in any particular political community, but in the human community. Thus, the denial of health care violates a fundamental human right.

PROFESSIONAL RESPONSIBILITY

The third argument appeals to the professional responsibility of detention medical staff. They may be ICE employees or contractors, but I would argue that even in this conflict of dual loyalties, their professional responsibility is primarily as health care practitioners.

We can appeal here to four principles generally recognized in health care ethics: autonomy, justice, beneficence, and nonmaleficence. I think it is fairly obvious that denying appropriate health care to detainees runs afoul of some of these principles. Presumably, no rational person would choose to have his or her health issues ignored.

Beneficence points in the direction of offering care, and nonmaleficence deems cooperation of health care practitioners in detention practices that exacerbate health problems as professionally irresponsible. This provides another reason for thinking that the dual loyalty conflict must be settled in favor of the detainee patient.

STATE COERCION

The next argument is that state coercion is a sufficient condition for having certain basic rights. These rights include the right to participate in the government in some fashion. Michael Walzer argues that "the processes of self-determination through which a democratic state shapes its internal life, must be open, and equally open, to all those men and women who live within its territory, work in the local economy, and are subject to local law" (Walzer 1984). Following Henry Shue (1996), I would argue that this fundamental political right could not be meaningfully exercised unless one's basic subsistence rights are also provided for.

The Supreme Court made a similar argument in *Plyler v. Doe*, in which they claimed that undocumented children were persons under the Fourteenth Amendment and thus entitled to protection of their basic rights. One possible position is that no one is coerced into illegally migrating into the United States.

I have two responses here. The first is that there is indeed an element of coercion here, and I will return to this in the discussion of the U.S. role in causing migration. Second, once a person is in ICE detention, they are subject to substantial state coercion and thus should have some protections against the excessive use of state power. This leads into the next argument.

CRUEL AND UNUSUAL PUNISHMENT

The next argument applies specifically in the case of ICE detention. The Supreme Court has ruled that the denial of health care to incarcerated persons constitutes impermissible cruel and unusual punishment (*Brown v. Plata* 2011). As Justice Kennedy writes in *Plata*,

> As a consequence of their own actions, prisoners may be deprived of rights that are fundamental to liberty. Yet the law and the Constitution demand recognition of certain other rights. Prisoners retain the essence of human dignity inherent in all persons.

Respect for that dignity animates the Eighth Amendment prohibition against cruel and unusual punishment.

To incarcerate, society takes from prisoners the means to provide for their own needs. . . . A prison that deprives prisoners of basic sustenance, including adequate medical care, is incompatible with the concept of human dignity and has no place in civilized society.

It might be said that immigration detention is not identical to criminal incarceration and thus that *Plata* does not apply. However, in *Youngberg v. Romero* (1982), the Supreme Court held that persons who are involuntarily committed are entitled to better treatment than convicted criminals "whose conditions of confinement are designed to punish." Thus, I would argue that ICE detainees, who are subject to administrative and not criminal proceedings, are constitutionally entitled to adequate medical care.

DUE PROCESS

Detainees are detained during the processing of their various immigration pleas and while awaiting arrangements to be deported. During this process, they are constitutionally entitled to due process (*Demore v. Kim* 2003). Here we can appeal again to Shue's argument that basic political rights depend for their exercise on basic subsistence rights. It is very difficult and sometimes impossible to assert one's rights in any immigration process if one's basic health needs are not met.

FAMILY MEMBERSHIP

Family reunification has been a criterion for immigration since the Immigration Act of 1965. The underlying principle here is that strong family ties are important, both for individuals and for a flourishing national culture. This principle should apply to all families. The difficulty of reentering the United States has resulted in an undocumented population that is increasingly made up of families with minor children (Passel 2006). There are approximately four million U.S.-born children with at least one noncitizen parent, and 79 percent of the children with undocumented parents were born in the United States (Passel and Taylor 2010).

Given these statistics, it is reasonable to assume that a high percentage of people in ICE detention are the parents, siblings, or other relatives of U.S. citizens. This provides a general argument for loosening immigration restrictions on such persons. If such persons are morally entitled to consideration for entry on family grounds, presumably their treatment in detention should reflect their status as members, to some extent, of our society, and this status can ground the obligation to provide adequate health care to them.

COLLATERAL DAMAGE

If ICE detention imposes collateral damage on the innocent children of detainees, and if there is an acceptable alternative to detention, then we have a reason for supposing that we have an obligation to mitigate the harm. One simple way to do this is to move away from detention, at least for parents of minor children. There is good reason to think that alternatives to detention will not only mitigate some of the harms caused by detention but will also be effective and cost saving. A program run by the Vera Institute showed an appearance rate of over 90 percent for undocumented immigrants enrolled in its alternative nondetention program (Root 2000).

If the collateral damage undermines the detainee's ability to assert her rights in immigration proceedings, as it seems to do in the case of mothers, then we have an additional reason to adopt alternatives to detention. If this solution is not politically feasible, we are not thereby absolved of all obligations toward detainee parents. One way we can discharge some of our obligation is to offer them the appropriate health services to mitigate the harm that they are suffering in virtue of this collateral damage.

RECIPROCITY

James Dwyer (2004) argues, "Most undocumented workers do the jobs that citizens often eschew. They do difficult and disagreeable jobs at low wages . . . they have the worst jobs and work in the worst conditions," and that such work is a "social construction" that forms the basis of our obligation to provide health care.

I would add that, in addition to doing this work, undocumented workers pay taxes and receive few comparable benefits in return. They pay Social Security taxes under fake numbers that, according the Social Security Administration, add about $50 billion annually to the system (Porter 2005). In addition, they pay sales taxes, and some are homeowners who also pay property taxes. At the same time the 1996 Personal Responsibility and Work Opportunity Reconciliation Act prohibit them from collecting most public benefits.

THE U.S. ROLE IN CAUSING HEALTH PROBLEMS AND/OR IN CAUSING MIGRATION

Many theorists have argued that the political and economic policies of the global North are direct causes of migration. Thomas Pogge (2008) offers a global analysis and critique:

The existing global institutional order is neither natural nor God-given, but shaped and upheld by the more powerful governments and by other actors they control (such as the EU, NATO, UN, WTO, OECD, World Bank and IMF). At least the more privileged and influential citizens of the more powerful and approximately democratic countries bear then a collective responsibility for their governments' role in designing and imposing this global order and for their governments' failure to reform it toward greater human-rights fulfillment.

Whether or not we are convinced of such a global thesis, other theorists offer more local, empirically based accounts. David Bacon, for example, offers a detailed look at how U.S. policies created, and continue to create, tremendous pressures for Mexican illegal migration to the United States (Bacon 2008).

I will not debate this issue here, but if these theorists are correct, then we have reason to assert a negative duty to stop the policies that created the problem and a positive duty of reparation to mitigate the harm that we have caused.

Whether or not we are convinced that U.S. policies are causally implicated in undocumented immigration, there is no doubt that some detention practices are directly implicated in harm to detainees. The denial of care that results in unnecessary death or impaired function is a clear example.

The prisonlike detention conditions that detainees are subjected to, especially asylum seekers who are fleeing state torture, are a direct cause of subsequent mental health problems and exacerbations of such problems (Robjant, Robbins, and Senior 2009). In these cases, the only question is whether the duty of reparation should apply only to those directly wronged or to the larger class of detainees.

I would argue that since ICE makes no real attempt to sort out asylum seekers and other vulnerable people from other less vulnerable detainees, it has an affirmative duty to provide appropriate health care for all detainees.

ARGUMENTS AGAINST THE OBLIGATION TO DETAINEES: DETERRENCE

Brietta Clark discusses some of the standard objections to providing health care to undocumented immigrants in general, and these arguments apply to detainees as well (Clark 2008). First she discusses the deterrence argument that restricting such benefits would act as a deterrent to illegal immigration and that providing them would act as an incentive to such immigration. Her response to this argument is that it is employment, not health care, that is the primary motivator for illegal immigration.

Given the restrictions on health benefits for immigrants required by PRWORA, and the fact that by 2008, twenty-eight states had also restricted health care benefits for immigrants (Matthew 2010), it is very difficult to believe that undocumented immigrants come to the United States in search of publically subsidized health care.

LIMITED HEALTH CARE RESOURCES

The next argument Clark turns to is that we must restrict health care benefits because our health care resources are very limited. Her response is that health care is not an individual but a public good and that restricting it has overall bad consequences.

Presumably we might point to public health here. James Dwyer offers an additional response to this objection. He argues that we need not choose between health care for citizens and the undocumented. There are many other possible tradeoffs. Secondly, he points out that health care is a basic need and, as such, it is inappropriate to distribute it by appeal to a principle of desert.

DENIAL OF BENEFITS IS APPROPRIATE PUNISHMENT FOR LAW BREAKING

The final argument Clark considers is that benefit restrictions are justified as punishment for violations of the social contract. She has two responses here. The first is that not all excluded immigrants are undocumented—the five-year waiting period for Medicaid applies to legal immigrants as well.

This first response seems to exclude persons in ICE detention, but I would argue that it does not. Recall the categories of persons in ICE detention: asylum seekers; undocumented persons who are not asylum seekers, but who are not accused of any crime; undocumented persons who are accused of trivial offenses, including identity theft or felonious reentry; and undocumented persons accused of serious offenses and legal permanent residents (LPR) who have committed a deportable offense. Asylum seekers, in particular, are clearly not in violation of any social contract. Presenting oneself for asylum is within the rules of national and international law.

We can make a similar case for LPRs who are detained for committing a deportable offense. First, even if the offense occurred after the 1996 Illegal Immigration Reform and Immigrant Responsibility Act, I would argue that deportation is grossly disproportionate to most of the offenses that are currently classed as deportable offenses (DUI, for example). Second, the law allows for the deportation of LPRs for offenses that occurred in the past, even before the act became law.

The second response Clark gives is that while criminal sanctions might be seen as appropriate for violations of immigration law, this does not imply that denial of health care should be part of the punishment. Indeed, the Supreme Court has explicitly stated this position in *Plata*—denial of health care is a violation of the Eighth Amendment ban against cruel and unusual punishment.

RIGHT TO EXCLUDE AND RIGHT NOT TO TREAT

Some theorists have argued that legitimate states have a prima facie right to exclude immigrants from their territory (Wellman 2008). If undocumented persons have no right to be in the country, then it might seem to follow that they have no rights to benefits available to legitimate members of the state.

But I would argue that even if we accepted this position, such persons would still have a right against harm. Imagine that someone enters my property without my permission. Surely I would not be justified in shooting the intruder.

I would argue that the case is similar for detainees. The denial of needed medical services for someone who is otherwise unable to procure them by virtue of being detained is a harm, as is the unnecessary infliction of psychological distress on already vulnerable persons, such as asylum seekers. I think there is a much stronger case to be made for the obligation to provide health care for all, but the appeal to a right against harm suffices to show that persons who are detained by ICE have at least the right to be protected from the denial of medical services.

INSUFFICIENT RECIPROCITY

Some would argue that undocumented immigrants take more resources than they provide and thus are not entitled to services based on a principle of reciprocity. "They are taking our jobs" is one way this concern is raised. I think there is something right about this objection, but I don't think it accurately fixes the source of the problem. Richard Trumka, AFL-CIO president, states the problem succinctly: "Too many U.S. employers actually like the current state of the immigration system—a system where immigrants are both plentiful and undocumented—afraid and available. Too many employers like a system where our borders are closed and open at the same time—closed enough to turn immigrants into second-class citizens, open enough to ensure an endless supply of socially and legally powerless cheap labor."

In *Hoffman Plastics* (2002), the Supreme Court ruled that undocumented workers were not entitled to back pay, even if their various employment claims were sustained, since they were not legally available for work. This decision provides a perverse incentive to hire undocumented workers—no matter what you do to them they cannot be compensated with back pay in any lawsuit against you (Manning 2010). It is thus likely that having a class of exploitable workers does result in fewer jobs for American workers along with depressing wages in the unskilled sector. But the fault here is with employers and the Court, not with the undocumented workers.

A related objection is that immigrants don't pay enough in taxes to cover all the public benefits they use. This objection rests on an empirical claim about how much undocumented immigrants pay in taxes versus what they use in services. But even if we granted that the balance tilts in favor of the use of services, this is not the end of the story.

We can appeal to Dwyer's response to this objection. This objection sees society as a private business venture in which one benefits on the basis of what one invests, and, as Dwyer writes, "The business model is not an adequate model for thinking about voting, legal defense, library services, minimum wages, occupational safety and many other social benefits" (37).

EVEN IF THE UNITED STATES IS CAUSALLY IMPLICATED IN MIGRATION, THE BEST WAY TO FIX THE PROBLEM IS IN HOME COUNTRIES

I turn now to the final argument: That even if we accepted all the justifications for providing health care, and the causal role that wealthy countries play in creating migratory pressures, encouraging undocumented immigration is the wrong approach because it exacerbates the problem by encouraging the youngest, most productive workers to emigrate, leaving their home countries even worse off than they already are.

While I am convinced that a more comprehensive, global solution is ultimately in order, this simply does not absolve us of our obligation to those who are already within our borders, and especially those within our detention facilities.

CONCLUSION

ICE is a branch of a government agency in a democratic country, thus the citizens on whose behalf it allegedly operates have an obligation to ensure that it operates in conformity with the fundamental principles of justice on which this nation was founded.

ICE is a young and rapidly growing bureaucracy with little oversight. It operates using a mix of federal, state, local, and private centers, many of which are penal institutions. It has a history of serious abuse, and even when it operates in conformity with its penal standards, it inflicts additional harm onto vulnerable people, especially asylum seekers and parents of minor children. It thus requires our constant vigilance and concern.

Our immigration policies and detention practices are deeply troubling, but until we elect to reform them, we have a special obligation to the vulnerable populations that we house in ICE detention. Minimally, that includes being attentive to their medical needs.

REFERENCES

American Medical Association. 2008. "AMA Bulletin," *JAMA* 300 (2).

Babu, M. A., and J. B. Wolpin. 2010. Note and Comment: "Undocumented Immigrants, Healthcare Access, and Medical Repatriation after Serious Medical Illness." *American Health Lawyers Association, Journal of Health & Life Sciences Law* 3 (3): 83–101.

Bacon, D. 2008. *Illegal People: How Globalization Creates Migration and Criminalizes Immigrants.* Boston: Beacon Press.

Bresa, L. 2010. "Uninsured, Illegal, and in Need of Long-Term Care: The Repatriation of Undocumented Immigrants by U.S. Hospitals." *Seton Hall Law Review* 40 (4): 1663–96.

Brown v. Plata, 563 U.S. 678, 687 (2011).

Center for Disease Control (CDC). 2005. "Trends in Tuberculosis." http://www..gov/mmwr/preview/mmwrhtml/mm5511a3.htm.

Clark v. Martinez, 543 U.S. 371 (2005).

Clark, B. R. 2008. "The Immigrant Health Care Narrative and What It Tells Us about the U.S. Health Care System." *Loyola University Chicago School of Law, Beazley Institute for Health Law and Policy, Annals of Health Law* 17:229–78.

Coffey, G. J., I. Kaplan, R. C. Sampson, and M. M. Tucci. 2010. "The Meaning and Mental Health Consequences of Long-Term Immigration Detention for People Seeking Asylum." *Social Science & Medicine* 70 (12): 2070–79.

Cutler, S. 2005. "Fit to Be Detained? Challenging the Detention of Asylum Seekers and Migrants with Health Needs." Report by *BID (Bail for Immigration Detainees)*, based on the findings of a report by *Médecins Sans Frontières*.

Daniels, N. 1998. "Is There a Right to Health Care and, If So, What Does It Encompass?" In *A Companion to Bioethics*, edited by Helga Kuhse and Peter Singer, 316–25. Oxford: Blackwell.

Demore v. Kim, 538 U.S. 510, 553 (2003).

Dwyer, J. 2004. "Illegal Immigrants, Health Care, and Social Responsibility." *The Hastings Center Report* (January/February):35–40.

Ferrell, J. 2008, May 10. "Map: A Closer Look at 83 Deaths." *Washington Post*, http://www.washingtonpost.com/wp-srv/nation/specials/immigration/map.html.

Global Detention Project, http://www.globaldetentionproject.org/home.html.

Goldstein, A., and D. Priest. 2008, May 13. "Five Detainees Who Took Their Lives." *Washington Post*, http://www.washingtonpost.com/wp-dyn/content/article/2008/05/12/AR2008051202694.html.

Guzman, E. M. 2009. "Imprisonment, Deportation, and Family Separation: My American Nightmare." *Social Justice* 36 (2): 106–9.

Hoffman Plastics Compounds, Inc. v. NLRB 3, 535 U.S. 137 (2002).

Immigration and Customs Enforcement, ICE Detainee Deaths, http://www.ice.gov/doclib/foia/reports/detaineedeaths2003-present.pdf.

———. ICE Detention Reform, http://www.ice.gov/detention-reform/detention-reform.htm.

———. ICE Factsheet, http://www.ice.gov/news/library/factsheets/287g.html.

———. ICE Visitation, http://www.ice.gov/doclib/dro/facilities/pdf/etowaal.pdf.

Johnson, K. 2009. "Patients without Borders: Extralegal Deportation by Hospitals." *University of Cincinnati Law Review* 78 (Winter): 657–97.

Keller, A. S., MD et al. 2003. "The Impact of Detention on the Health of Asylum Seekers." *Journal of Ambulatory Care Management* 26 (4): 383–85.

Kim, K. 2009. "Civil Rights and the Low-Wage Worker: The Trafficked Worker as Private Attorney General: A Model for Enforcing the Civil Rights of Undocumented Workers." *The University of Chicago Legal Forum*: 247–310.

Manning, M. 2010. "A Mockery of the American Dream: How to Prevent Employers from Exploiting Immigration Status and Escaping Title VII Liability Post-*Hoffman*" (unpublished).

Matthew, D. B. 2010. "Race and Healthcare in America: The Social Psychology of Limiting Healthcare Benefits for Undocumented Immigrants—Moving beyond Race, Class, and Nativism." *Houston Journal of Health Law & Policy* 10 (Spring): 201–26.

Miller, K. M. 2006. "The Impact of Parental Incarceration on Children: An Emerging Need for Effective Interventions." *Child and Adolescent Social Work Journal* 23 (4): 472–86.

Mooty, B. M. 2010. "Solving the Medical Crisis for Immigration Detainees: Is the Proposed Detainee Basic Medical Care Act of 2008 the Answer?" *Law and Inequality: A Journal of Theory and Practice* 28:223–53.

Papst, K. E. 2009. "Protecting the Voiceless: Ensuring ICE's Compliance with Standards That Protect Immigration Detainees." *McGeorge Law Review* 40:261–89.

Passel, J. 2006. "The Size and Characteristics of the Unauthorized Migrant Population in the U.S.: Estimates based on the March 2005 Current Population Survey." Washington, DC: Pew Hispanic Center.

Passel, J., and P. Taylor. 2010. "Unauthorized Immigrants and Their U.S. Born Children." Washington, DC: Pew Hispanic Center.

Plyler v. Doe, 457 U.S. 202 (1982).

Pogge, T. 2008. *World Poverty and Human Rights*. Cambridge, UK: Polity Press.

Porter, E. 2005, April 5. "Illegal Immigrants Are Bolstering Social Security with Billions." *New York Times*. http://www.nytimes.com/2005/04/05/business/05immigration.html.

Priest, D., and A. Goldstein. 2008, May 11–14. "Careless Detention: System of Neglect." *Washington Post*. http://www.washingtonpost.com/wp-srv/nation/specials/immigration/cwc_d1p1.html.

Rabin, N. 2009. "Unseen Prisoners: Women in Immigration Detention Facilities in Arizona." *Georgetown Immigration Law Journal* 23 (Summer): 31–32.

Rawls, John A., *A Theory of Justice*, rev. ed. Cambridge, MA: Belknap, 1999.

Ray, M. 2006. "Undocumented Asian American Workers and State Wage Laws in the Aftermath of Hoffman Plastic Compounds." *Asian American Law Journal* 13:91–114.

Robjant, K., I. Robbins, and V. Senior. 2009. "Psychological Distress amongst Immigration Detainees: A Cross-Sectional Questionnaire Study." *British Journal of Clinical Psychology* 48:275–86.

Rome, S. H. 2010. "Promoting Family Integrity: The Child Citizen Protection Act and Its Implications for Public Child Welfare." *Journal of Public Child Welfare* 4 (3): 245–62.

Root, Oren, "The Appearance Assistance Program: An Alternative to Detention for Noncitizens in U.S. Immigration Removal Proceedings," http://www.vera.org/sites/default/files/resources/downloads/app_speech.pdf.

Saucedo, L. 2006. "The Employer Preference for the Subservient Worker and the Making of the Brown Collar Workplace." *Ohio State Law Journal* 67:964–6.

Schriro, D. 2009. "Immigration and Customs Enforcement: Rethinking Civil Detention and Supervision." *Arizona Attorney* 45:26–27.

Shue, H. 1996. *Basic Rights*. Princeton: Princeton University Press.

Tillman, L. 2009, February 19. "America's Immigration Gulags Overflowing with Mentally Ill Prisoners." *Brownsville Herald.* http://www.alternet.org/story/127451/.

Trumka, Richard. President, AFLCIO, Remarks at the City Club of Cleveland (June 18, 2010). http://www.aflcio.org/Press-Room/Speeches/Remarks-by-AFL-CIO-President-Richard-L.-Trumka-at-the-City-Club-of-Cleveland-Cleveland-Ohio.

UN High Commission on Refugees, http://www.unhcr.org/4cd91dc29.html.

Walden, A. 2009. "Abortion Rights for ICE Detainees: Evaluating Constitutional Challenges to Restrictions on the Right to Abortion for Women in ICE Detention." *University of San Francisco Law Review* 43:979–1012.

Walzer, M. 1984. *Spheres of Justice.* New York: Basic Books, 1984.

Wellman, C. H. 2008. "Immigration and Freedom of Association." *Ethics* 119:109–41.

Woods v. Morton. http://www.aclu.org/files/assets/2010-12-16-WoodsvMorton-Settlement Agreement.pdf.

Youngberg v. Romeo, 457 U.S. 307 (1982).

6

Global versus Local

The Use of Lethal Injection in China

Cher Weixia Chen

ABSTRACT

Lethal injection has not yet been commonly discussed in China. This chapter seeks to expand the existing literature by focusing on the most recent development of the death penalty in China—lethal injection. Lethal injection is something scholars have for the most part failed to examine. In this chapter I will look at its use from the perspectives of human rights and bioethics, both of which lethal injection by nature is intimately intertwined with. Two concerns will be given particular consideration: one, the participation of medical personnel in lethal injections and in the harvesting of organs from executed prisoners, and two, to offer some recommendations as to the need for guidelines.

INTRODUCTION

In the last two decades, China has accounted for a large portion of executions throughout the world. For example, in 2008, China carried out 1,718 out of 2,390 executions (72 percent) worldwide (Amnesty International 2008). China's death penalty system has always been seen as a violation of human rights. Its socialist government is said to use capital punishment to maintain its social order, to oppress its political opposition, and to curb the rising crime rate.

There is truth to these reports. However, Western media reports and academic research on the death penalty in China tend to be one-dimensional and oversimplified. They typically lack sufficient detail and overlook the complex nature of the issue. In addition, Western legal academics pay little attention to the most recent developments in China's practice of capital punishment.

Lethal injection has not yet been examined in China to the extent it has in the West. It merits a much more thorough analysis than it has received. In this chapter I will focus on the most recent development of the death penalty in China—and that is lethal injection. In particular, I will discuss its use from the perspectives of human rights and bioethics.

USE OF LETHAL INJECTIONS IN CHINA'S CAPITAL PUNISHMENT

In the twentieth century, lethal injection was included in the international human rights movement against methods of executions. This movement has been a restraining influence on China, which has been frequently cited as a violator of human rights because of its extensive use of the death penalty. It is the concern for a better global image that propelled China to research lethal injections as a preferable method for executions (Li 2008). This led to China adopting lethal injection in 1997. At that time, it was a relatively new method of execution. Its adoption was an effort to conform to the international human rights standards.

The use of lethal injections in China shares many elements with other countries while having some distinctive local peculiarities. A central comparison in this chapter will be with the United States. Given that the United States regularly uses lethal injection to execute convicts, its use will be addressed as a point of reference.

China's history is instructive. It previously used shooting as the sole legal method of execution, but it added lethal injection in 1997. A key contrast to shooting or other methods of execution is that lethal injection simulates a *medical procedure*. This has fundamentally transformed the practice.

From the violent nature of conventional executions, China introduced a method that potentially uses medical personnel on a regular basis. To undergo lethal injection, the inmate is typically put in an environment like an "operating" room. Medical or designated personnel are present to place a needle in the arm of the prisoner to induce sleep. The next step in the process is a drug-induced cardiac arrest, followed by the inmate's death (Maggio 2005: 48).

COMPARISON OF TECHNIQUES USED IN CHINA AND THE UNITED STATES

On the basis of research, China developed its own combination of drugs for lethal injections (Li 2008). The drug combination used in China is similar to those in the United States. It is composed of three ingredients: one is to cause loss of consciousness (pentothal), one is to paralyze the heart and suspend pulmonary activities (pavulon), and the third (potassium chloride) is to induce cardiac arrest (Yang 2008).

We should note, however, that there are differences between China and the United States with regard to the use of the death penalty. One major distinction is that lethal injection in China takes place in an "execution van" or "mobile execution chamber." In 1997 these execution vans were developed and used for the first time in Yunnan. They are windowless units. Amnesty International (2004) gives this report:

> The windowless execution chamber at the back contains a metal bed on which the prisoner is strapped down. Once a technician attaches the needle, a police officer presses a button and an automatic syringe injects the lethal drug into the prisoner's vein. The execution can be watched on a video monitor next to the driver's seat and can be recorded if required.

The Human Rights Committee has urged that "the death penalty . . . must be carried out in such a way as to cause the least possible physical and mental suffering" (ICCPR 1992: 6). It has been argued that lethal injection inflicts less physical and mental pain than its alternatives (Lifton and Mitchell 2000). In this sense, China's use of lethal injection is in conformity with the international human right standards. But the implementation of such international human rights standards concerning the method of execution is rather localized.

To some degree, the notion of an "execution van" is used by China to balance its international obligations and local realities. On the one hand, China sought to humanize its method of execution. Because of the influence of the global human rights movement, it adopted the method of lethal injection. On the other hand, the cost of building execution grounds for lethal injection could not be borne by local courts under the current circumstances. Thus, "execution vans" were developed in part to relieve the local courts of such financial burdens.

Though there is a concern among human rights activists that execution vans and their secrecy may cause the process to be less transparent, they are preferred over conventional execution grounds for at least three reasons. First, "execution vans" elicit much less resistance from the public than execution grounds. This is because most people do not want to be living close to an execution ground. It is deemed inauspicious in Chinese culture (Xu and Tang 2003: 33). Secondly, execution vans are windowless and, thus, do not involve a public spectacle. The vans prevent the widely condemned public executions rampant in the 1980s and 1990s (Amnesty International 2004). Evidently the move away from public displays has not been seen as problematic.

Finally, execution vans are more cost effective. They require less manpower and allow local courts to share and save on the cost. In light of the fact that execution grounds are expensive to build, the lower-priced execution vans have favor in financially stricken local courts ("Execution Van" 2009). Even so, execution vans pose a fiscal burden on local communities. As a result, some experts have called for a special fund to assist local courts in building execution vans (Yang 2008). For these reasons, execution vans are more suitable than the conventional execution grounds for the local settings in China and have, therefore, been encouraged.

LETHAL INJECTIONS AND HUMAN RIGHTS

Historically speaking, embracing the global human rights movement and adopting lethal injection signify a philosophical shift of the domestic criminal justice system in China. It is fair to say that the imperial law in China was primarily a prescription of punishments. For example, under the Code of Qing, there were 3,987 punishable offenses (Da Qing Hui Dian). By performing physical torture and mutilation, and very often in public, the state ensured that law was literally implicated into the body politic.

When convicts were decapitated, mutilated, or disemboweled, it was thought that justice was served. Lethal injection, in contrast, is viewed as painless (Pan and Wang 2008). It is intended to be more humane and to minimize the sufferings of both inmates and executioners (Zheng 2008). Not only have the policymakers valued the painless lethal injection, but the public also agreed that humane methods of execution are preferable. For this reason it was concluded that lethal injection should replace the traditional execution methods (Yuan 2009). From this standpoint, using painless lethal injection is a historical landmark in the evolution of the Chinese criminal justice system. This reason for this change was the rise of an international human rights movement.

China is seeking to expand the use of lethal injection on a nationwide basis. In 2008 there were about half of the 404 intermediate courts using lethal injection. One major obstacle to the expansive use of lethal injection is cost considerations. Consequently, in order to lower the cost and to expedite the reform, the Supreme People's Court took a bold step: It decided to provide the lethal cocktail used in the injection to the local courts for free (Bezlova 2008). The next step for China's death penalty is to legalize lethal injection so it becomes the only lawful method of execution. There are various reasons to recommend this reform. First, it results in less suffering. Compared to shooting and other methods of execution, lethal injection inflicts much less pain on convicts (LeGraw and Grodin 2002: 387). It is the method of execution least likely to constitute "cruel and unusual punishment."

Secondly, there are human rights' concerns. Lethal injection conforms to international human rights standards. As far as prisoners' rights, it is in accordance with inmate preferences. According to a Supreme Court poll, death row inmates overwhelmingly prefer lethal injection (Yang 2008). In this sense, to use lethal injection, a more humane method of execution favored by prisoners, is to respect prisoners' rights.

Thirdly, the invention of execution vans has effectively addressed local concerns throughout China. That is to say, they have provided a unique approach for China to implement global human rights standards within its own social context. For this reason, China should discontinue the use of shooting and establish lethal injection as the sole method of execution.

Lastly, by making lethal injections the only form of capital punishment, discrimination and corruption among officials will be reduced. Public opinion polls indicate a concern about the fair use of lethal injections. Several media reports indicate that lethal injection has become the "privilege" of wealthy convicts, while others receive shooting instead (Bezlova 2008). Some experts argue that this phenomenon is not because of corruption but an "economic" reason instead. Since the use of lethal injection proves to be too costly for many less developed areas, it is plausible that corrupt officials allow lethal injection more often for wealthy criminals than for those who are more disadvantaged.

Nonetheless, a consistent and detailed implementation guideline that explicitly prescribes who receives lethal injection and how it should be carried out is imperative (Yang 2008, Bezlova 2008). This is not simply a matter of honoring the last wish of the convicts but an issue of fairness and integrity of the criminal justice system as a whole.

LETHAL INJECTIONS AND BIOETHICS

In general, the use of lethal injection is a positive step forward in China's reform of its death penalty system. Its "humane" feature identifies with the spirit of the international human rights standards. Nevertheless, the "medical" nature of lethal injection demands that any discussion of its use should involve bioethics.

In China the implementation of lethal injection has raised several bioethical concerns with some distinctive local features. Currently there are two key bioethical issues that need to be attended to, other than the question of the moral permissibility of the death penalty in the first place. Once that question is put to rest, two issues come to the fore. These are the role of the medical profession and the harvesting of organs from executed prisoners. Let us look at both of these concerns.

The Role of Medical Professionals

One source of the controversy surrounding lethal injection is the involvement of medical professionals. Before 1997, China only used shooting as the legal method of execution. No other medical personnel other than forensic officers took part in the process. But to carry out lethal injection, medical knowledge is essential. As a result, medical professionals or personnel with medical training have to take part in the implementation of lethal injection. Whether such involvement violates medical ethics is subject to debate (Amnesty International 1994: 8).

In the United States, the medical profession has expressed mixed views on participating in the process of lethal injection (Maggio 2005: 48). One argument is that it violates the Hippocratic Oath of "first do no harm." However, there is no agreement yet as to what exactly constitutes "participation" in an execution, even though physicians, nurses, and other medically trained personnel "play a vital role" in lethal injection, at least in the United States (LeGraw and Grodin 2002: 384). Participation of medical professionals in lethal injection is considered to be morally impermissible by some scholars. They are accused of using their medical knowledge to assist in state-sanctioned killing—"judicial homicide." Furthermore, it is argued that they facilitate the process and glorify the death penalty by taking part. One concern is that this then shields capital punishment from legal challenge (LeGraw and Grodin 2002: 386).

Some scholars in China have argued that "do no harm" is a relative concept. It does not necessarily entail humanitarianism. Under certain circumstances, only relative humanitarianism can be achieved (Zhou 1997: 26). Generally speaking, the role of medical professionals in the process of lethal injection has yet to become as much a source of debate in China as in the United States. One way to solve the ethical dilemma for the medical profession is to abolish the death penalty so that lethal injection will not be needed. After all, the death penalty itself has long been challenged as a violation of human rights.

There has been a worldwide movement toward the end of capital punishment (Schabas 2002). Such international trends have pressured the Chinese government to compromise (Cohen 1987: 532). While acknowledging the international trend toward the abolition of the death penalty, it is crucial to be aware of the important role that local culture can play.

Overall, the death penalty law in China is headed in the right direction; namely, toward conforming to international human rights law. With ongoing reform, China will abolish the death penalty all together (*China Daily* 2005). Until then, it appears that "killing fewer and killing carefully" will be the new policy. If so, this will be a step closer to the ultimate abolition of capital punishment and is more applicable to the social reality of China (Stetler 2008: 27).

It helps to look at the issue in a historical context. The use of capital punishment constituting "cruel and unusual punishment" is a fairly new and modern concept. There had been general acceptance of the necessity of harsh punishments for thousands of years in China (Moore 2001: 731; Zhang 2008: 166). Drastic change might be counterproductive. Nonetheless, among Chinese policymakers and academics is an increasing willingness to reconsider the use of the death penalty. There is also an increasing eagerness to reform their death penalty system.

We can see a dramatic rhetoric change in examining the discussion on the death penalty among the Chinese policymakers since the economic reform took place in 1978. This change indicates less and less stress on the local context over time. In 1987, Gao Mingxuan, a prominent legal scholar and official, claimed that the death penalty was indispensable in China "to protect the fundamental interests of the state and people, to safeguard our socialist construction and to secure and promote the development of productive forces" (Fitzpatrick and Miller 1993: 278; Wyman 1997: 561).

In 1993, a top Chinese official asserted at the World Conference on Human Rights that "countries at different development stages or with different historical traditions and cultural backgrounds . . . have different understanding and practice of human rights" (Schabas 2002; Wyman 1997: 561). But in 2008, Xiao Yang, the former chief justice of the Supreme People's Court, reported to the National People's Congress. He stated that executions in China were now limited to an "extremely small number of extremely serious and extremely vile criminals posing a grievous threat to society" (Bodeen 2008). Evidently there is a growing interest in the issue of the death penalty among Chinese authorities. They are more receptive to the global trend of an abolitionist movement and have adjusted their local policies accordingly. It seems that the death penalty in China will continue to be reformed and seems likely that it will be abolished in the future.

The debates on the death penalty among Chinese legal scholars have shifted the focus from the justification of its use to how to eventually abolish it (Sun 2009: 106). With the global abolitionist movement in mind, fewer Chinese legal scholars believe in the permanent necessity of capital punishment in China. More and more agree that it is just a matter of when and how to abolish it. They have proposed a strategy for the gradual abolition of the death penalty in an attempt to maintain a balance between the international trend and the local reality (Wei 2008: 57).

To a large extent, a gradual abolition is a workable and realistic proposal. It could be dangerous to become abolitionist overnight, especially if that country is known for its overuse of the death penalty (Sharoni 2001: 284). "Killing fewer and killing carefully," as a transitional policy toward the ultimate abolition of capital punishment in China, should be allowed. Until China abolishes the death penalty, lethal injection is a relatively humane method of execution to use. Thus, as long as lethal injection is used in capital punishment, the ethical dilemma for the medical profession remains.

China has found an uncommon way to moderately solve this ethical dilemma by sheltering the entire medical profession, including physicians and nurses, from the process. In China local prison officers are trained to carry out lethal injection and forensic officers are present only to pronounce the death of prisoners.

It was the ethical concern mentioned above that has led to such practice (Zhuang 2005: 24). Essentially this practice minimizes the involvement of medical personnel and to a certain extent frees them from the ethical predicament. Undoubtedly it will require strict protocols to avoid any botched executions. But at least the medical profession can somewhat be exempted from the ethical dilemma that their American colleagues face with lethal injections. However, even though according to the current practice in China the medical profession does not have to participate directly in the process of actual lethal injection, other issues arise. They still have to be involved in the process, such as training prisoner officers and developing a safe formula for drugs to be used in lethal injection. The latter two activities may or may not constitute "participation in execution."

According to the American Medical Association (AMA) definition, to train prisoner officers to carry out lethal injection is "an action which would assist, supervise, or contribute to the ability of another individual to directly cause the death of the condemned." To develop a safe drug formula to be used in lethal injection could also constitute "participation in execution" (AMA Code of Medical Ethics, Opinion

2.06). In this sense, the current practice in China has not completely excused the medical profession from the ethical dilemma.

ETHICAL DILEMMAS IN HARVESTING ORGANS

In addition to the ethical predicament of the medical profession, harvesting organs of death row inmates is another major bioethical issue associated with lethal injection. Both shooting and lethal injection offer the opportunity to harvest organs of prisoners, as these two methods of execution allow most organs to remain intact.

There has been an outcry that China practices harvesting prisoners' organs without their consent (Brown 1996: 1073–74). Human rights activists worried that the use of lethal injection and execution vans makes the body undamaged and therefore might promote the actual harvesting of organs of prisoners in China (Bezlova 2008).

The issue of harvesting organs of prisoners is multifaceted. First, death row inmates should be allowed the opportunity to *donate* their organs. When an organ is transplanted, the donor may perceive that his/her life has been continued in the recipient (Shen 1997: 102). This act of altruism is the ethical foundation for organ transplants (Guan and Li 2001: 8). As members of the society, death row inmates should be granted organ donation if they explicitly express that wish. Conversely, death row inmates should have the right to refuse to donate their organs. Because the practice of harvesting prisoners' organs without their consent has occurred in China, this side of the arguments should be emphasized to prevent any injustice.

Second, if prisoners do not give consent, harvesting their organs is morally wrong and should be illegal. The percentage of the Chinese favoring organ transplants is around 70 percent, but the donation rate is much lower (Wang, Su, and Liu 2002: 21). Such discrepancy reflects the impact of the traditional culture.

According to Confucianism, our bodies are received from our parents and donation is the most unfilial act. Many people still think that to keep a dead body intact is a respectful act and hope they can have an unbroken body after death (Xie, Huang, and Liu 2000: 39). This is to say that a significant number of Chinese people culturally oppose the idea of donating their organs. Thus, to lure or force death row inmates to donate their organs, or to harvest their organs without their consent, is considered repugnant by those holding this point of view.

Third, harvesting organs requires medical knowledge. One way to thwart illegal harvesting is to have a strict ethical code prohibiting medical professionals from engaging in the illegal harvesting of organs of executed prisoners (Brown 1996: 1073–74). In response to such concern, the Ministry of Health in China issued a ban on the sale of organs ("Execution Van" 2009). In addition, the People's Supreme Court issued an order stipulating that, only with the consent of death row inmates or their families, can their organs be harvested (Liu 2006). The effect of these orders remains to be seen.

ETHICAL GUIDELINES TO ADDRESS THE TWO ISSUES

In order to address those two bioethical dilemmas—that of medical personnel participating in lethal injections or harvesting executed prisoners' organs—a detailed implementation guideline on lethal injection is imperative. This guideline ought to be based on widely accepted principles of bioethics, such as those proposed by Beauchamp and Childress (Beauchamp and Childress 2008). Their transformative four principles are those of autonomy, nonmaleficence, beneficence, and justice. All are strongly relevant to bioethics in China. For example, their theory of "autonomy" could be useful to look at the meaning of consent with respect to condemned prisoners donating their organs. How to apply these theories to the specific policies is challenging, but they seem very fruitful.

China has incorporated international standards into their major national bioethics regulations that explicitly refer to the international bioethics documents such as the Declaration of Helsinki (WMA 2004). Nevertheless, the principal concern is that these regulations lack specifics, a problem that the new guideline on lethal injection should overcome (Hennig 2006). A guideline with specifics will also help prevent the occurrence of botched lethal injections, as happened in the United States. In particular, the administering of the drugs in the United States has been found problematic. The botched executions of Raymond Landry, Stephen McCoy, and Billy Wayne White all raised the question on how to improve the safety of administering lethal injection and to minimize the pain inflicted on prisoners (Maggio 2005: 48).

So far in China no such cases have been reported. Nevertheless, China could learn from what has occurred in the United States. The People's Supreme Court of China issued the Notice on Using Lethal Injection in Executions in 2001 to standardize the procedures (Liu 2006). But the Notice itself lacks details and lags behind in addressing some critical issues, such as the role of the medical profession and the use of organ transplants.

It is worth mentioning that the psychological impact on executioners has been duly noticed in China. In Chinese culture, it is normally considered inauspicious to administer an execution. Because of such a heavy psychological burden, some prisoner officers were reluctant to carry out lethal injections (He and Li 2008: 77). How to seek professional psychologists' aid for those involved in lethal injections should also be included in the guidelines (Yang 2008). If lethal injection is to be effectively applied in China, there needs to be the satisfactory implementation of global human rights and bioethical norms, as well as the cultural considerations noted above.

CONCLUSION

To sum up, the use of lethal injections represents a progressive development of the death penalty in China. It is an attempt to balance China's international obligations with its own social and cultural realities. The practice of lethal injections in China indicates that, when abstract international human rights and bioethical norms are implemented in local contexts, there exists a degree of variation. Such variation is inevitable and ought to be tolerated. The use of execution vans is a case in point. As the Universal Declaration on Bioethics and Human Rights justly puts, "the importance of cultural diversity and pluralism should be given due regard" (UNESCO 2005, art. 12).

Lethal injection requires a continuous reform to ensure its safe and fair use. Such reform should consider local details while incorporating the global standards. Practical application of global norms necessitates deep knowledge of local conditions. Neglecting local conditions and cultural factors that influence values and perceptions could be disastrous.

Two major related bioethics challenges including the role of the medical profession and organ harvesting of condemned prisoners call for legislative and judiciary action. A detailed implementation guideline of lethal injection based on the local specifics should be developed to adequately address these challenges. It is not easy to find a balance between global norms and local reality, especially when the global norms are new to the local culture. But it is not impossible.

REFERENCES

American Medical Association. n.d. Code of Medical Ethics, Opinion 2.06. http://www.ama-assn.org/ama/pub/physician-resources/medical-ethics/code-medical-ethics/opinion206.shtml.

Amnesty International. 2004. "Undermining Global Security: The European Union's Arms Exports." http://www.amnesty.org/en/library/info/ACT30/003/2004.

Amnesty International. 2008. "Abolish the Death Penalty." http://www.amnesty.org/en/death-penalty.

Beauchamp, T. L., and J. F. Childress. 2008. *Principles of Biomedical Ethics*, 6th ed. New York: Oxford University Press.

Bezlova, A. 2008, June 16. "China: Will the People Choose the Death Penalty?" http://ipsnews.net/news.asp?idnews=42810.

Bodeen, C. 2008, March 1. "China Hails Reform of Death Penalty." http://www.usatoday.com/news/world/2008-03-10-975780323_x.htm.

Brown, K. M. 1996. "Execution for Profit? A Constitutional Analysis of China's Practice of Harvesting Executed Prisoners' Organs." *Seton Hall Constitutional Law Journal* 6:1029–82.

China Daily. 2005. "China Questions Death Penalty." http://www.chinadaily.com.cn/english/doc/2005-01/27/content_412758.htm.

Cohen, R. 1987. "People's Republic of China: The Human Rights Exception." *Human Rights Quarterly* 9 (4).

Da Qing Hui Dian (Collected Institutes of the Great Qing Dynasty), 54:1a–b.

Execution Van. 2009. Wikipedia. http://en.wikipedia.org/wiki/Execution_van.

Fitzpatrick, J., and A. Miller. 1993. "International Standards on the Death Penalty: Shifting Discourse." *Brooklyn Journal of International Law* 19:273–366.

Guan, W., and K. Li. 2001. "Kaizhan huoti qiguan yizhi de lunli xue sikao." *Yixue yu Zhexue* (*Medicine and Philosophy*) 22–26:8.

He, C., and J. Li. 2008. "Kaowen zhushe sixing de sanda nanyan zhiyin." *Fazhi Yanjiu* (*Legal Research*) 10:75–79.

Hennig, W. 2006. "Bioethics in China." http://www.nature.com/embor/journal/v7/n9/full/7400794.html.

ICCPR. 1992. General Comment 20, U.N. HRC, 44th Session, U.N. Doc ccpr/c/21/Add.3.

LeGraw, J. M., and M. A. Grodin. 2002. "Health Professionals and Lethal Injection Execution in the United States." *Human Rights Quarterly* 24 (2): 382–423.

Li, J. 2008. "Zhushe sixing." http://news.hexun.com/2008-11-03/110795102.html.

Lifton, R., and G. Mitchell. 2000. *Who Owns Death? Capital Punishment, the American Conscience, and the End of the Death Penalty.* New York: William Morrow.

Liu, X. 2006. "Zhejiang jiuyue yiri qi zhushe daiti qiangjue zhixing sixing." *Legal Daily.* http://news.sina.com.cn/c/2006-06-25/150410248870.shtml.

Maggio, E. J., Esq. 2005. "A Violent Roman Tradition." *National Italian American Bar Association Law Journal* 13(35): 35–49.

Moore, B., Jr. 2001. "Cruel and Unusual Punishment in the Roman Empire and Dynastic China." *International Journal of Politics, Culture, and Society* 14 (4): 729–72.

Pan, X., and X. Wang. 2008, April 10. "Zuihou yiqiang-zhongguo jiasu puji zhushe sixing." *Nanfang Zhoumo* (*Southern Weekend*): A03.

Schabas, W. A. 2002. *The Abolition of the Death Penalty in International Law*, 3rd edition. Cambridge: Cambridge University Press.

Sharoni, M. M. 2001. "A Journey of Two Countries: A Comparative Study of the Death Penalty in Israel and South Africa." *Hastings International Comparative Law Review* 24 (2).

Shen, M. 1997. "Shengsi JuShan, Rendao Biyi. Shanghai Shehui Kexue Yuan Xueshu Jikan." *Academic Seasonal Journal of Shanghai Academy of Social Science* 2.

Stetler, R. 2008. "Killing Fewer, and Killing Carefully: Death Penalty Defense in China on the Eve of the Beijing Olympics." *Champion* 32 (22): 27.

Sun, W. 2009. "Sixing cunzai de beilun yu feizhi de genben dongle. Huadong Zhengfa Daxue Xuebao." *Journal of The East China University of Political Science and Law* 2:106–12.

Wang, H., B. Su, and J. Liu. 2002. "Guanyu Woguo Qiguan Yizhi de Youguan Falv he Lunli Wenti. Zhongguo Yixue Lunli Xue." *Chinese Medical Ethics* 4:21.

UNESCO. 2005. Universal Declaration on Bioethics and Human Rights. http://portal.unesco.org/en/ev.php-URL_ID=31058&URL_DO=DO_TOPIC&URL_SECTION=201.html.

Wei, Y. 2008. "Qiu xinglong he 96ming sixingfan tongjian. Nanfang Renwu Zhoukan." *Southern People Weekly* 12:57–59.

WMA. 2004. "*Declaration of Helsinki: Ethical Principles for Medical Research Involving Human Subjects.*" Ferney-le-Voltaire, France: World Medical Association.

Wyman, J. H. 1997. "Vengeance Is Whose?: The Death Penalty and Cultural Relativism in International Law." *Journal of Transnational Law and Policy* 6:543–67.

Xie, M., C. Huang, and X. Liu. 2000. "Guanyu Woguo Qiguan Yizhi yu Qiguan Juanxian de Sikao. Zhongguo Yixue Lunli Xue." *Chinese Medical Ethics* 6:39.

Xu, R., and J. Tang. 2003. "Yunnan tuiguang zhushe sixing: guannian zuai." *Xinwen Zhoukan* (*News Weekly*) 9:32–33.

Yang, X. 2008, January 3. "Expert: China Is Fit for Lethal Injections." http://www.china.org.cn/english/GS-e/237842.htm.

Yuan, B. 2009. "Woguo minzong sixing jinben guannian shizheng fenxi." *Xingfa Luncong (Criminal Law Review)* 1:36.

Zhang, Y. 2008. "Woguo sixing zhidu xianzhuang zhi fansi yu chonggou." *Fazhi yu Shehui (Legal Systems and Society)* 8:166.

Zheng, J. 2008. "Zhushe sixing de rendao zhuyi tanxi." *Sheke Zongheng (Social Sciences Review)* 4:263.

Zhou, C. 1997. "Yixue lunli shengsi guan de kunjiong yu chongjian." *Jingzhou Shizuan Xuebao (Academic Journal of Jingzhou Normative College)* 4:26.

Zhuang, Xujun. 2005. "Qianxi woguo zhushe sixing zhifu." *Xinan Keji Daxue Xuebao (Journal of Southwest University of Science and Technology)* 22:24.

7

Ethics, Human Rights, and Sexual/Reproductive Health in Africa

Exploratory Sociocultural Considerations

Godfrey B. Tangwa

ABSTRACT

In this chapter I consider, from a very broad perspective, the evolving relationship between ethics and human rights in the particular domain of sexual and reproductive health within the context of Africa. Human rights theory can be seen as an offspring of ethics or morality, which is one of the overarching values of all human societies, communities, or cultures. Human beings develop a culture marked by a common worldview—the sharing of common ideas, beliefs, values, customs, traditions, and practices. Cultures differ widely in practical details, but all are concerned with ethics (morality) and rationality, which can be called the universals of all cultures. As a derivative of ethics, human rights are a powerful heuristic device that emerged at a particular historical epoch as an effective tool for canvassing ethical conduct and facilitating behavior change. Cultural ideas, values, and practices are usually very resistant to change, particularly in the sexual/reproductive domain where open and frank discussion and debate are not usual, let alone encouraged. Considering the intersections and interplay between ethics and human rights, I discuss sexual/reproductive health in its traditional cultural and evolving forms, and I highlight the complex nature of the interplay between culture, ethics, and human rights and suggest how this might evolve in the present context and situation of Africa.

INTRODUCTION

Since "human reproduction is the means by which each society perpetuates itself and its traditions,"[1] the importance of reproduction for all human societies is self-evident, as no society could possibly want to go out of existence. All human societies also cherish their culture, customs, and traditions as things of value and of the very last importance. Human cultures, with their different customs, traditions, and practices, are also remarkably diverse, differing each from the others in many practical details.

If we define culture as "a way of life of a group of people, underpinned by adaptation to a common environment, similar ways of thinking and acting and doing, similar attitudes and expectations, similar ideas, beliefs and practices, etc.,"[2] then culture is intrinsically *relative* to the society or people for which it has application. But human cultures, diverse as they may be, do have in common that they are all *human* cultures, held together or underpinned by reason or rationality and morality (ethics). Rationality and morality can be called the *universals of cultures*, and it is on their account that human culture in general is possible. They are of the very essence or definition of being human or having a culture, and no human culture seems possible without them. Human rights are a subset or derivative of ethics/morality, a powerful heuristic device or tool for canvassing ethical conduct and facilitating behavior change in the modern world.

And since "reproductive health implies that people are able to have a satisfying and safe sex life, the capability to reproduce, and the freedom to decide if, when, and how often to do so,"[3] the potential importance of human rights for reproductive health, a domain in which social, cultural, and religious values strongly shape and condition attitudes, is both obvious and rather critical for many particular contexts. Similarly, law is also a derivative or subset of ethics/morality with the notable advantage of being more robust and efficacious in its coercive and behavior-changing effects, but restricted to particular or specific politico-geographical areas of jurisdiction.

The idea of "international law" or of "international human rights law" is today still basically a prescriptive ideal whose limitations are set by the idea of "national sovereignty." Nevertheless, following World War II and the Holocaust that marked it, the resulting shock on the conscience of the whole world, the formation of the United Nations against war and its attendant atrocities, the crafting of the Universal Declaration of Human Rights (UDHR) in 1948,[4] followed in 1966 by the International Covenant on Civil and Political Rights[5] and the International Covenant on Economic, Social and Cultural Rights,[6] a solid foundation and groundwork has been laid for the flourishing of human rights and international law all over the globe.

In Africa, two recent events increased awareness of the importance and connections between ethics and human rights, including sexual and reproductive rights: the Truth and Reconciliation Commission[7] that followed the collapse of the apartheid system in South Africa and the HIV/AIDS pandemic.[8, 9, 10, 11, 12, 13] Particularly in South Africa, advocacy and public debate resulted in the provision of appropriate legal underpinnings for the modern imperatives of ethics and human rights, particularly in the sexual and reproductive domains. Other parts of Africa lag behind in that respect, but the impetus of globalization will surely rouse them from their lethargic slumber.

In modern societies, particularly in the industrialized Western world, good conduct and responsible behavior are assured by the interplay between ethics, human rights, and law. In traditional societies, particularly in Africa, good conduct and responsible behavior were assured by the interplay between ethics, customs, and taboos. Many of the mores, customs, and taboos of such societies were aimed at regulating sexual behavior and reproductive conduct. The concepts of human rights and positive laws were not evident in an explicit manner in traditional societies although their essence was incorporated in ethics, customs, and taboos. The idea of "customary law" as it existed in many African countries in the colonial era is a concept that basically looked back at traditional society and tried to deduce its laws from its mores, customs, traditions, and taboos. In considering the intersections and interplay between ethics, human rights, and sexual/reproductive health in Africa, therefore, it is important to consider the traditional state of affairs in its stable or evolving forms and how the modern concept of human rights and the prescriptive ideals of international law might effect a smooth and acceptable mutation.

In what follows, I will sketch a loose framework from the point of view of African culture, within which this interplay might function. I start by discussing the place of human reproduction within African cultures; next, I discuss the ideas of reproductive health and sexual health; then I discuss a paradigm case of a system of traditional African marriage as an illustrative background context in which to conceptualize the reproductive and sexual problems of the traditional setting; and finally, I discuss the interplay between human rights and reproductive and sexual health, while recognizing the complex interplay between culture, ethics, and human rights in the contemporary situation of Africa.

HUMAN REPRODUCTION AND AFRICAN CULTURES

As a matter of fact, all human societies and cultures in all historical epochs have been deeply concerned, if not obsessed, with reproduction and allied processes; a concern/obsession reflected in laws, religious dogmas/injunctions, customs, traditions, taboos, and practices. And while human reproduction and human sexuality have been a concern and a value in all human cultures, this is even more so the case in African cultures, noted for their great love of procreation, large families, and the practice of polygamous forms of marriage. Children are so highly valued in African cultures that procreation is the express and main purpose of marriage and its absence the main cause of divorce or conversion of monogamy into polygamy, while childlessness for whatever reason is a highly undesirable state of being for both men and women.[14] This state of affairs has resulted in the ambivalence of many Africans to modern biotechnological methods of assisted reproduction. On the one hand, the great need for offspring attracts to these methods and, on the other, there is the technophobia of nonindustrialized cultures and mistrust of the artificial and the demystified arising from the background of traditional religion and worldview.

The idea of "reproductive health" and of "sexual health" as a minor consequential corollary was present in African traditional cultures and was assured by means of customs and taboos. Such, for instance, were practices whereby a pregnant woman left the husband's lineage and returned to her own lineage until she had safely delivered and weaned her baby; the prescription or proscription of the intake of certain foods during pregnancy; the consumption of various substances by men to enhance potency and erectile staying power; the prohibition of sex with a menstruating woman; the tabooing of incest or of sex with minors, and more. Rightly or wrongly, these prescriptions and proscriptions were believed to be either enhancing or subversive of sexual and/or reproductive health.

In this situation, sexual health was considered important for the married or, in any case, procreating adult, but not for the unmarried young for whom sexual activity was not only proscribed but often severely repressed. This was more so for young girls for whom virginity at marriage was a highly cherished value. No other category of patient consults the modern physician or the traditional healer more than the barren woman and the impotent man,[15] but the reasons for this have less to do with a desire to enjoy sex as an independent value and more to do with a desire to maintain potency for parenthood.

The same underlying reason is partly responsible for the frequent refusal of many African patients to accept surgical removal of any organs closely connected with procreation (even if on account of advanced age or other such reason they now serve merely a symbolic function), such as breasts or testes, even under threat of death; the other part being the value attached to intactness of limbs and other bodily members in life or in death.

The idea of "sexual health" as a separate and independent value, therefore, is not evident in traditional African cultures. And yet, it is plausible to claim that sex was meant by nature for its own sake and not merely as a tool for reproduction and that, in the cause of evolution, it had probably taken time for humans to realize that there was a direct, causal link between the sexual act, assured by instinctive impulses, and the event of pregnancy resulting in birth. It is easy to imagine that under a strong religious or magical worldview humans could attribute pregnancy and childbirth to supernatural forces, until observation of mating among domestic animals and its evident consequences pricked their skeptical consciences regarding mating among humans.

In any case, the actual situation of things is that many different and complex factors—increasing acceptance of singlehood as a respectable mood of existence, delayed marriage, pressures on family size, earlier emancipation of young people of both genders from strict parental control, and more—have contributed to make sex without its procreative component the only option for an increasing number of people. This state of affairs makes it easier than heretofore to canvas sexual activity as an independent value and a human right. Such developments and the fact that the customs and traditional practices of Africa have been severely subverted, for good or for ill, by the contact with Western cultures, religions, and education, and are slowly receding into the past, makes modern legislation and other supporting structures for reproductive and sexual health an urgent necessity.

Such legislation needs to be fully aware of and sensitive to traditional attitudes and practices so as to facilitate a smooth transition to a modern setting and to salvage what is of enduring value in them, so as not to throw away the baby, as it were, with the bathwater. It is also necessary to avoid imposing the ideologies or idiosyncratic practices of one culture on another without sufficient justification. Cultural borrowing is inevitable and is justifiable only where what is borrowed is demonstrably both rational and ethical.

REPRODUCTIVE HEALTH

The World Health Organization (WHO) has popularized the understanding of health as "a state of complete physical, mental, and social well-being and not merely the absence of disease or infirmity."[16] Along the same conceptual path, reproductive and sexual health can be understood as a state of complete physical, mental, and social well-being in the domain of reproduction and sexual activity. Such a definition is evidently an ideal standard, necessary as the target of aspirations and practical projects; in practice it is hardly achievable for all members of any society or human community. The actual overall state of health of any individual at any given point in time will always be less than complete or perfect. In fact, at the individual level, even if such a state of complete or perfect mental, physical, and social well-being were achieved, one could hardly know for certain that it had been achieved; human ambitions and aspirations will, understandably, always stay ahead of the status quo or what is actually achievable because human beings are by nature aspiring but limited beings.

Be that as it may, while reproductive health has been a perennial concern from time immemorial in all societies and cultures, it is only in recent times that it has received the focal attention of medical researchers and research funders. Programs and projects and associations now abound, which are making a great impact globally on reproductive health. Furthermore, assisted reproduction technologies (ARTs) and assisted conception are making reproduction not only possible for those for whom it would otherwise have been impossible but also safer and healthier than in the past.

Except for very sophisticated methods, like ICSI (cytoplasmic sperm injection) and EF (embryo freezing), nearly all the other ARTs are already available in Africa,[17] although in terms of demand there is a clear preference for artificial insemination using a husband's sperm (AIH) rather than other possible options. But economic factors will likely ensure increasing resort to the other methods of ART. Economic determinism is already leading to both a delay in the assumption of the burdens of parenthood and a reduction in family size for many Africans. Delayed parenthood will come with difficulties in achieving conception normally or naturally, making resorting to ARTs inevitable.

SEXUAL HEALTH

As mentioned above, the idea of sexual health as a separate and independent value was almost completely absent in traditional African societies. But even in Western societies, where for a long time sexual health has been accepted as an integral part of reproductive health, it is only recently that sexual health has emerged as a clearly separate and independent value.

Many factors are responsible for the increasing importance of sexuality as a separate and independent concern, irrespective of reproduction. These include, besides those already enumerated, such phenomena as voluntarily childless marriage, much earlier discovery or introduction to sexuality, increasing rates of sexually transmitted infections particularly of HIV/AIDS, increasing recognition or acceptance of homosexuality, the impact of biotechnologies on reproduction, and more. The WHO has already announced[18] the imminent publication of a number of very important studies focusing exclusively on sexual health, such as: *Defining Sexual Health: Report of a Technical Consultation on Sexual Health*; K. Wood and P. Aggleton, *A Conceptual Framework for Sexual Health Programming*; and K. de Koning, S. Hawkes, A. Martin Hilber, M. Waelkens, M. Colombini, A. van der Kwaak, and H. Ormel, *Integrating Sexual Health Interventions into Reproductive Health Programmes: Experiences from Developing Countries*. Rebecca Cook, Bernard Dickens, and Mahmoud Fathalla have characterized sexual health as including "the ability to enjoy mutually fulfilling sexual relationships, freedom from sexual abuse, coercion, or harassment, safety from sexually transmitted diseases, and success in achieving or in preventing pregnancy."[19]

In the context of Africa, where traditional ways of thinking, attitudes, habits, and practices still hold sway, this understanding of sexual health in its comprehensiveness involves a call to a different way of looking at things and developing new attitudes, habits, and practices, inasmuch as the idea of sexual pleasure within the traditional worldview was simply a welcome by-product of a process aimed at fecundation in which the idea of preventing pregnancy would have been self-contradictory. Even the idea of fertility regulation in that context boiled down to child spacing, and the person seeking permanent sterilization would have been looked upon as indeed "odd" if not downright evil.

It is against such a background also that the various forms of marriage in Africa, especially family-arranged marriages, can properly be understood. In some cases the bride and groom could be meeting for the first time on their wedding night. In arranging a marriage, the family was always less concerned about the physical beauty or sexual attractiveness (which admittedly are in the eye of the beholder) of the marriage partner and more concerned about such other qualities as good family background, general physical and mental health, reliability, honesty, hard work, and, above all, the likelihood of being fertile.

In that setting it was extremely difficult to find convincing reasons for, say, refusal of a potential spouse on grounds connected with mere personal preference/choice or for divorce of any marriage, which had been blessed with at least an offspring. A woman who had borne offspring with the husband knew very well that her place in the patrilineage was more secure than that of her husband, who could always be reminded that the woman was not his wife alone but the wife of the entire lineage.

This situation, as sketched above, is in a state of rapid mutation and change, under the powerful influences of contact with Western culture and Western religions, the emergence of sundry epidemics connected with sexuality, the phenomenon of globalization, increased migration, the information revolution, and more. Under the impact of these phenomena, it is evident that the traditional African family and traditional African marriage, ideas, attitudes, and practices related to sexuality and procreation can no longer be wholly sustained. Nowadays, sexual debut is occurring much earlier than in the traditional setting, and increased urbanization and the HIV/AIDS epidemic have violently jolted traditional attitudes and ways of thinking. Change is inevitable and almost complete on many issues at the ideational level, but it is still to impact completely on attitudes and practices.

For example, many Africans today readily accept the idea of individual choice as a consequence of individual autonomy of, say, a marriage partner, but this still has to be reconciled and harmonized with attitudes and practices that emphasize community and group values over individual ones. Nor is it a matter of "either/or" in the exclusive sense. The two sets of values (which summarily can be described as "communal" and "individual") are reconcilable and harmonizeable, although the result to be expected will surely be heavily shaped and colored by context and perspective.

Nearly all traditional African communities affirm by varying degrees and conceptual appellations the philosophy of *Ubuntu*,[20, 21] which in actual fact is a balance between individual autonomy and communal values; establishing a dialectic relationship between them by means of which alone each finds meaning. John Mbiti has popularized this philosophy with the epigram: "I am because we are; and since we are, therefore I am."

TRADITIONAL MARRIAGE AMONG THE NSO' AS A PARADIGMATIC EXAMPLE

Marriage is a particularly important area in which traditional African customs, laws, and ethics seem to coalesce perfectly. Marriage, of course, is a cultural universal, in the sense that even though marriageless societies have been advocated (in Plato's *Republic*, for example), no actual culture has ever succeeded in doing without it. But the form and shape marriage takes is culture bound, a cultural particular. In Western cultures, marriage is generally understood as a legal union between two individuals to the exclusion of all others, 'til death or legal divorce do they part. In traditional African cultures marriage is understood mainly in (extended) familial terms as the inclusion rather than exclusion of many others, as marriage typically turns two hitherto indifferent lineages into significant others of each other.

In my natal culture, that of the Nso' of the Western grasslands of Cameroon, as elsewhere in traditional Africa, both monogamy and polygamy were practiced within a plastically flexible framework that tried to balance both freedom and rigidity.[22] This plastic flexibility when transported to the modern setting without the supporting traditional structures is liable to result in the type of promiscuity and sexual license characteristic of many present-day urban towns and cities of Africa. Traditional marriage in Nso' was plastically indissoluble, but it was not required that one signed a contract or took a vow to maintain the chosen marital status for life because it could change without such change having been wished or foreseen.

But to be married at all was to assume sexual responsibility. A married person was not expected to engage in casual or opportunistic sex, which was tantamount to wasting a precious, procreative treasure. If a married man proved sexually insatiable and medication failed to help, the wife would be the first person to initiate the search for a co-wife or co-wives for him. If a married woman proved sexually insatiable the situation was much more complex, but two frequent results were either separation, or she could seek sexual satisfaction outside the home with the covert approval of the husband—but, in any case, any children she bore traditionally belonged to the husband, as long as there had been no divorce.

Among the Nso' both polygamous and monogamous marriages exist, although polygamy is preponderantly for kings (*afon*), great councillors of the kingdom (*vibai*), and lineage/compound heads (*atarla*), while the vast majority of ordinary people are monogamists. Among the titled categories, polygamy is not a matter of choice. As soon as you are selected and installed into any of these positions, you automatically inherit all the wives of your predecessor in position before adding to that harem your own wife or wives and any new ones you might acquire in the course of time. For ordinary citizens there were, before the recent introduction of "civil status marriage," three main roads to a recognized valid marriage (monogamous or polygamous) in traditional Nso': *vidjin* (orthodox marriage), *kincem* or *nceemi* (unorthodox marriage), and *villem* (wife inheritance).[23]

In orthodox marriage, the first or only daughter of a woman who had also married in orthodox fashion is always given out in marriage by her maternal grandfather (*taryiy*) and all the other daughters by their paternal lineage head (*tarla'* or *fai*). A father arranged the marriage of the first wife of each of his sons as well as the marriage of each of all the first or only daughters of all his daughters. A peculiarity of Nso' marriage, vis-à-vis marriage among other African peoples, is that there is no bride-price/wealth or dowry. Ceremonial gifts are, however, exchanged at prescribed times with the proviso that the total value of marriage gifts received on behalf of a girl should not exceed the total value of the gifts that were given on behalf of her mother.

A lot of time and attention are, however, devoted to checking the familial background of the prospective spouses to make sure that there is no blood relationship between them and that there exists no old and unsettled grudge, quarrel, or feud between the two family lineages. The prospect of marriage is also an occasion and an incentive for the ritual settlement of persisting differences, grudges, and problems between families, lineages, and communities. But once the marriage ceremonies and rituals have been performed, the two families/lineages now become "in-laws" (*a sëjuu*), committed to coming to each other's assistance in times of need, such as tilling, harvesting, building, birth, marriage, installation, death, and more.

In unorthodox marriage, a man takes unto himself a wife and a woman a husband without the above formalities of orthodox marriage; they simply "move in together."

Though recognized and tolerated, this form of marriage was not at all encouraged. Children begotten of such marriages belong, by Nso' custom and tradition, to the parents of the woman, the man being considered in this situation as a mere "he-goat" (*kibev*), having no claim whatsoever over his own biological offspring.

Furthermore, female children begotten through this form of marriage cannot marry in orthodox fashion but must also marry, if at all, in unorthodox fashion. They miss all the colorful rituals and ceremonies of orthodox marriage. This was a great disincentive and constraining factor for this form of marriage. However, many of such marriages, if they proved stable, happy, and successful, could, retrospectively, be orthodoxified by performing all the requirements of orthodox marriage—some, obviously, merely symbolically.

In *villem* (wife inheritance) a man inherits the widow of his father, son, or brother as his wife. When the occasion arises, it is usually the lineage head, in consultation with the women and elders of the compound, who checks for possible impediments and who decides who is to inherit whom. This form of marriage served as a sort of insurance and security for married women and had the consequence of reinforcing polygamy among ordinary citizens by converting initial monogamists into polygamists, whether or not they were enthusiastic about such conversion. This form of marriage did not necessarily or always have a sexual dimension. Sometimes the inherited wife or wives might have already attained menopause, in which case sexual relations were not expected. Other factors that tended to promote polygamy (or polygyny to be more exact) in this setting were power, wealth, and popularity. If a man was wealthy, powerful, or socially popular, families and lineages tried to associate with him by offering him one of their daughters in marriage.

What would it take to modernize a marriage system such as that sketched above? No matter how modernization may be conceived, ethics, human rights, and law, in that order of priority, need to be implicated. Clearly, unethical practices can never be justified anywhere or at any time. Ethically controversial or ethically neutral practices are highly recommendable or disrecommendable to the extent that they cohere or fail to cohere with human rights principles. The law should ideally come in only when the ethics and human rights issues have been clearly and unequivocally settled.

An additional reason for this is the thought that in all societies, as the ancient Greek philosopher Thrasymachus (c. 400 BC) is reputed to have remarked, the law tends always to protect the interest of the strong and powerful in the society. An antidote to this tendency is provided by human rights principles and discourse, which, nevertheless, need to strive to avoid the above Thrasymachian pitfall of laws.

This is the time to ensure that what is of enduring value in the traditional system should not be thrown away with what must change. Empirical research on a myriad of issues in this domain to determine the current state of affairs is strongly indicated. What, for instance, is the rate of singlehood among mature adults in the various African communities? What is the actual rate of polygamous marriages? What is the current family size average? What is the rate of homosexuality, if it exists? What is the rate of celibacy among unmarried, mature men and women? What is the frequency of sexual encounters among different categories of men and women in given communities, and other issues?

One way of helping along justifiable change, however, would be the linkage of desirable changes with the concept and principles of human rights, a highly heuristic device liable to assist rapid change in behaviors and practices but also liable to be used covertly by powerful and influential cultures in proselytizing and propagating their own values.

HUMAN RIGHTS AND REPRODUCTIVE/SEXUAL HEALTH

The idea of human rights may be a purely heuristic device, but, in practice, it is a quite powerful means of effecting positive changes in systems otherwise highly recalcitrant to change. Human rights have such a strong appeal around the globe that their profession constitutes the highest form of political correctness in the contemporary world, while their violation draws the automatic condemnation of all and sundry. Human rights are, of course, not provable and cannot be philosophically justified without either logical circularity or reference to the most general assumptions, postulates, or axioms of ethical principles. As Mann et al. have rightly stated:

> Modern human rights is a civilizational achievement, a historic effort to identify and agree upon what governments should not do to people and what they should assure to all. Human rights are non-provable statements that derive their legitimacy from having been developed, voted upon and adopted by the nations of the world and having been incorporated into the domain of international law; they do not achieve their status from divine inspiration or religion.[24]

But even though human rights are not directly derivable from religious doctrines, they are quite compatible with religious worldviews. The *Universal Declaration of Human Rights*,[25] the touchstone document for human rights discourses, is, of course, a purely secular document aimed at providing protections in the public domain particularly. Its focus is on societal-level conditions and determinants of well-being, including health and related issues and concerns. There is no religion or culture for which human well-being and the preconditions of its attainment are not a central concern. Without belaboring the issue, putative human rights can be recognized by applying the test of reasonableness. What is unreasonable cannot be a human right.

In public health the central concern is that of ensuring the conditions in which citizens can live healthy lives, avoiding preventable disease, disability, and premature death. Intensive international travel and communication, coupled with the emergence of some highly infectious diseases, give public health concerns in our day a global and urgent dimension. In present-day Africa, there are arguably more infectious and epidemic diseases than have ever been seen in the past. Public health is the particular responsibility of civil authorities and governments. For that reason, human rights concerns in public health focus primarily on governmental actions/

inactions and how they impact on human health, human well-being, and other rights enshrined in international human rights law.

Public health targets populations rather than individuals and in this way has clear affinities with traditional African attitudes that prioritized communal over individual values. The concept of human rights provides an important imperative for monitoring governmental responsibility and accountability relative to fundamental rights affecting human health.

Violations of human rights, such as unjustified discrimination, torture, and other forms of physical and psychological abuse, impact directly on health and well-being. These considerations, relevant and applicable to all countries, are critical for African countries in their present situation, where traditional ways of life and governance have been displaced, with as yet nothing definite and firm enough to replace them, and where civil war, poverty, disease, dictatorship and make-believe democracy are the order of the day.

PUBLIC HEALTH AND HUMAN RIGHTS ARE NATURAL ALLIES[26]

Public health goals and human rights norms when combined complement each other and lead to more effective and sustained health policies and programs. As already mentioned, human rights are nonprovable, but they do not derive their legitimacy solely from the fact of "having been developed, voted upon and adopted by the nations of the world and having been incorporated into the domain of international law."[27]

Certainly human rights have been greatly empowered by such procedures and acts that ensure that they will be respected and not violated with impunity. But such empowerment notwithstanding, whatever can be canvassed as a human right can also independently be established and justified, using only common sense and the most general of moral principles, although the justification of morality itself remains irremediably problematic and the cause of interminable controversies, as there is no antidote to extreme moral skepticism or amoralism. Legislation also tends to put issues in a straitjacket, whereas the very rapid evolution of our thinking and attitudes in an age of information revolution and globalization calls for constant reappraisal and revision of our accepted ideas, attitudes, and practices.

The delivery of health care, particularly in reproductive and sexual health, is fraught with quandaries and dilemmas for both the provider and the receiver in which the generally accepted fundamental bioethical principles of autonomy, beneficence, nonmaleficence, and justice are either in conflict or need delicate balancing. Dealing with adolescents, HIV-positive people, polygamists, homosexuals, prostitutes, wives of physically abusive men, husbands of verbally abusive women, and more, for example, pose peculiar ethical problems in each case.

Take, for instance, the principle of autonomy, which imposes on health workers or care providers the duty of respect for persons and their privacy or confidentiality. But there will be circumstances in which breaching confidentiality may seem ethically correct to protect the health of the public at large or even to protect the well-being and future interest of the very person whose confidentiality is being breached. An adolescent, for instance, seeking, say an abortion or permanent sterilization, creates a situation in which many ethical dilemmas must be faced by both herself and her health care provider. In such a case, can her health-seeking behavior be helped without very careful counseling or without the knowledge and consent of the parents? Such and many other similar ethical dilemmas in the African context concern basic issues that need to be carefully thought through in the prospect or process of using legislation grounded on ethics and human rights to effect changes in the traditional systems of Africa.

CONCLUSION

In a world fast becoming a veritable global village, thanks to the technological and informational revolutions, no culture will be able to remain an island unto itself. The local and the global are fast fusing into one. Disciplines are equally collapsing into an interdisciplinary general pool. In this situation, human health and particularly reproductive and sexual health, ethics and human rights are fruitfully contending with each other.

African culture and social life have no choice but to join in the dance. Africa needs to listen carefully to the global drum beats of reproductive and sexual health, ethics and human rights, but it needs to dance its own dance with its feet firmly planted on the solid ground of its own culture, social life, historical experience, and worldview.

NOTES

1. Rebecca J. Cook, Bernard M. Dickens, and Mahmoud F. Fathalla, *Reproductive Health and Human Rights: Integrating Medicine, Ethics, and Law* (Oxford: Clarendon Press, 2003), 3.

2. Godfrey B. Tangwa, "Morality and Culture: Are Ethics Culture-Dependent?" in *Bioethics in a Small World*, edited by F. Thiele and R. E. Ashcroft (Berlin/Heidelberg: Springer Verlag, 2005).

3. Ibid., 5.

4. http://www.ohchr.org/en/udhr/pages/introduction.aspx.

5. http://www.ohchr.org/en/professionalinterest/pages/ccpr.aspx.

6. http://www.ohchr.org/EN/ProfessionalInterest/Pages/CESCR.aspx.

7. http://www.justice.gov.za/trc/.

8. L. London, L. Rubenstein, and L. Baldwin-Ragaven, "The Problem of Dual Loyalty and Role Conflict in Public Health," in *Rights-Based Approaches to Public Health*, 119–41, edited by E. Beracochea, C. Weinstein, and D. Evans (New York: Springer, 2010), chapter 7.

9. L. London, A. Kagee, K. Moodley, and L. Swartz, "Ethics, Human Rights and HIV Vaccine Trials in Low Income Contexts," *Journal of Medical Ethics* 28 (2012): 286–93.

10. L. Baldwin-Ragaven, J. de Gruchy, and L. London, *An Ambulance of the Wrong Colour: Health Professionals, Human Rights and Ethics in South Africa* (Cape Town: University of Cape Town Press, 1999).

11. L. London, "Human Rights, Environmental Justice, and the Health of Farm Workers in South Africa," *International Journal of Occupational and Environmental Health* 9 (2003): 59–68.

12. L. London, "Dual Loyalties and the Ethical and Human Rights Obligations of Occupational Health Professionals," *American Journal of Industrial Medicine* 47 (2005): 322–32.

13. L. London, and G. McCarthy, "Teaching Medical Students on the Ethical Dimensions of Human Rights: Meeting the Challenge in South Africa," *Journal of Medical Ethics* 24 (4) (1998): 257–62.

14. Godfrey B. Tangwa, "ART and African Sociocultural Practices: Worldview, Belief and Value Systems with Particular Reference to Francophone Africa," in *Current Practices and Controversies in Assisted Reproduction*, edited by Effy Vayena, Patrick J. Rowe, and P. David Griffin (Geneva: World Health Organization, 2002).

15. Ibid., 56.

16. Preamble to the Constitution of the World Health Organization as adopted by the International Health Conference, New York, June 19–22, 1946; signed on July 22, 1946, by the representatives of sixty-one States (Official Records of the World Health Organization, no. 2, 100) and entered into force on April 7, 1948.

17. Osato F. Giwa-Osagie, "ART in Developing Countries with Particular Reference to Sub-Saharan Africa," ibid., 23.

18. See *Progress in Reproductive Health Research* 67:1.

19. *Reproductive Health and Human Rights: Integrating Medicine, Ethics, and Law* (Oxford: Clarendon Press, 2003), 8.

20. John S. Mbiti, *African Religions and Philosophy* (New York: Doubleday, 1970).

21. Mogobe B. Ramose, *African Philosophy through Ubuntu* (Harare, Zimbabwe: Mond Books, 1999).

22. For a good description of such plasticity and flexibility in the marriage laws and customs of another African peoples, see Ulrike Wanitzek, "Between Continuity and Change: The Marriage Laws of the Bulsa of Northern Ghana," in *Commission on Folk Law and Pluralism, Papers of the Commission's Xth International Congress*, University of Ghana, Legon, Ghana, 1995.

23. For a more detailed description of these and other aspects of Nso' traditional marriage, see L. S. Fonka, "Nso Marriage Customs" and W. Banboye, *Methods of Wife Acquisition*, a Nso' History Society Production, Nooremac Press 6, Abiodun Street Mushin, Lagos, Nigeria (undated but circa 1958).

24. Jonathan M. Mann, Sofia Gruskin, Michael A. Grodin, and George J. Annas, eds., *Health and Human Rights* (New York/London: Routledge, 1999), 2.

25. http://www.un.org/en/documents/udhr/.

26. Stephanie Nixon and Lisa Forman, "Exploring Synergies between Human Rights and Public Health Ethics: A Whole Greater Than the Sum of Its Parts," *New England Journal of Medicine* 339 (24) (1998): 1778–81.

27. Ibid.

Discussion Topics: Part II

Wanda Teays

1. John-Stewart Gordon argues that a global bioethics should be able to consider both universal moral claims *and* cultural differences so that it enriches bioethical discourses. He further suggests that a global bioethics should appeal to a universal standard using human rights and the notion of human dignity to solve cross-cultural bioethical problems.
   Answer the following:
   a. How might his idea of using human rights and human dignity as an over-arching principle be a good starting point for a global bioethics?
   b. Can you see how a human rights model can apply to the different areas of bioethics? Share two or three ideas.
2. What should we do when there are human rights violations that are not recognized or addressed by the government or ruling parties of a particular country? Can you think of examples to illustrate your suggestions?
3. In setting out a historical perspective on human rights, Robert Baker asserts that

   > Pandemics leap from continent to continent, companies peddle their cures around the world, biomedical experiments sponsored in the developed world are conducted in the developing world, and, in all corners of the globe, the new biology foments culture shock. Bioethical issues do not stop for border crossings. Thus, we need global bioethics. But the principlism that has served American bioethics so well is too parochial to play on an international stage, and so to meet the challenges of global bioethics, we need to turn to the more cosmopolitan concept of human rights.

   Answer the following:
   a. State four or five examples of biomedical issues that "do not stop for border crossings"—that is, issues that are fundamentally international.

    b. What do you think should be included or excluded from a concept of human rights so it can apply on the international level?

    c. Do you agree with Baker that American bioethics is too parochial to serve as a model for a global bioethics?

4. Nurses as well as doctors have participated in force-feeding of detainees. As practiced, it has been described as brutal and painful, and even if without discomfort, it violates an informed consent right of refusal under patient autonomy.

Answer the following:

Besides the public stands against the participation of its members, is there something more professional organizations should be doing?

5. On its website on September 15, 2013, Amnesty International praised the Canadian government for apologizing to Canadian citizen Maher Arar. This was for Arar's torture while a victim of mistaken identity as a terrorism suspect in the war on terror. Amnesty International called for the United States to apologize as well. This has yet to happen.

Answer the following:

    a. What should professional organizations (the AMA, WMA, etc.) do by way of a response when physician-members enable or assist in torture or "harsh interrogation"?

    b. Given medical personnel were likely participants in Arar's torture, should the WMA or the AMA also be asked to issue an apology?

6. Disability rights as human rights: According to the United Nations' Statement on Human Rights, "Persons with disabilities are still often 'invisible' in society, either segregated or simply ignored as passive objects of charity. They are denied their rights to be included in the general school system, to be employed, to live independently in the community, to move freely, to vote, to participate in sport and cultural activities, to enjoy social protection, to live in an accessible built and technological environment, to access justice, to enjoy freedom to choose medical treatments and to enter freely into legal commitments such as buying and selling property" (See http://www.ohchr.org/EN/Issues/Disability/Pages/DisabilityIndex.aspx).

Answer the following:

    a. Share your thoughts about how more attention could be brought to bear on the sorts of "invisibility" as set out in the quote above.

    b. What needs to shift in terms of attitudes and resources in order to make an appreciable change for a person with disabilities?

7. Given the significant numbers of hearing-impaired people, should movie theaters and TV and cable channels be required to provide subtitles for the hearing impaired? Set out your recommendations—picture that you are an advocate for the hearing impaired.

8. Discuss the ethical issues in medical personnel participating in coercive force-feeding by hunger strikers in prisons (e.g., those in Pelican Bay, California, in 2013) or by detainees (e.g., those held at Guantanamo Bay, Cuba, in 2013). When a hunger striker may be close to death, is life-saving intervention via force-feeding morally acceptable?

9. ICE has new rules on solitary confinement intended to limit its use. Read the following comments about enforcement of those limits and share your responses and ideas regarding how to ensure compliance.

"Solitary confinement in both immigration detention and the criminal justice system is cruel, expensive, and ineffective," said Ruthie Epstein [of the American Civil Liberties Union (ACLU)]. . . . "If strictly enforced throughout the ICE detention system—including at county jails and contract facilities—ICE's new policy could represent significant progress in curtailing this inhumane practice."

Half of ICE detainees are placed in county jails, she explains, adding it will be a challenge to ensure the new practices are followed not just in county jails but privately contracted facilities (See Sandra Lilly, "New ICE Directive Limiting Solitary Confinement a Good Step, but Issue Is Compliance, Say Rights Groups," *NBC Latino*, September 6, 2013).

10. What should be done about the use of long-term solitary confinement in prisons? Look, for example, at the case of Herman Wallace, who was in solitary for forty-one years—convicted of killing a prison guard—he maintained that he was innocent. (See E. Woo, "Herman Wallace Dies at 71; Ex-Inmate Held in Solitary for 41 Years," *The Los Angeles Times*, October 8, 2013).

11. Do you think scientists should use data obtained from experiments that are now seen as immoral, unjust, or exploitative—for example, the Nazi hypothermia studies, the Tuskegee syphilis studies, the Guatemalan studies, the human radiation studies, and so on? Share your thoughts about using information obtained by means that violate human rights.

12. Should children be allowed to be human subjects in nontherapeutic experimentation? Are there societal or medical benefits that would justify use of children?

13. When the EPA (Environmental Protection Agency) planned a two-year environmental study using infants and children up to three years old, they offered the families $970, children's clothes, and a camcorder in exchange for using pesticides in their homes. State your major concerns and then respond to this argument for using children in pesticide studies:

Linda S. Sheldon, acting administrator for the human exposure and atmospheric sciences division of the EPA's Office of Research and Development, said the agency would educate families participating in the study and inform them if their children's urine showed risky levels of pesticides. She said it was crucial for the agency to study small children because so little is known about how their bodies absorb harmful chemicals (See Juliet Eilperin, "Study of Pesticides and Children Stirs Protests," *The Washington Post*, October 30, 2004).

14. There are other questions about the use of human subjects. In a May 9, 2005, press release, the Public Employees for Environmental Responsibility (PEER)

raised concerns about government oversight of human experimentation by the Environmental Protection Agency (EPA):

Under its new policy, EPA would accept all human chemical dosing studies "unless there is clear evidence that the conduct of these studies was fundamentally unethical . . . or was significantly deficient relative to the ethical standards prevailing at the time the study was conducted." Since industry is not required to disclose the conditions under which experiments were conducted, it is not clear how the EPA will ever learn of "fundamentally unethical" practices. Moreover, the EPA is unwilling to define what ethical lapses would disqualify an industry submission from being used for regulatory purposes.

Answer the following:

    a. Do you think PEER's concerns about monitoring "fundamentally unethical" practices are justified? How much transparency should we expect?

    b. From the point of view of industry, some degree of animal and/or human testing is advisable before its use by the public. What are reasonable standards to expect—or require?

15. What sort of policy restrictions should be placed on pharmaceutical companies or other parties doing clinical studies in African nations such as Nigeria, in light of the death of children-subjects in Pfizer's Trovan meningitis studies in 1996? Donald G. McNeil Jr. points out:

The deaths and injuries of children during the Trovan trial, along with the dispute over the cause, first gained broad attention in 2000, when *The [Washington] Post* published a series of articles that raised major questions about drug testing overseas. The articles touched off demonstrations in Nigeria.

The distrust of Western medicine that the dispute engendered was one of several factors that led many families in northern Nigeria to refuse to let their children be vaccinated against polio. (Other factors were rumors that the polio vaccine contained the AIDS virus or represented a Western plot to sterilize Muslim girls.) Northern Nigeria is still one of the world's last remaining epicenters of polio.

Trovan was introduced in 1998 and became a lucrative product for Pfizer, but it was later withdrawn in Europe and restricted in the United States after the drug was blamed for cases of fatal liver damage (See "Nigerians Receive First Payments for Children Who Died in 1996 Meningitis Drug Trial," *The New York Times*, August 11, 2011).

16. When a country has practices such as capital punishment that are seen as morally objectionable in the wider global community, how could professional groups like the AMA, the WMA, and the ANA play a role in effecting change? Amnesty International objects to lethal injections in capital punish-

ment and raises concerns on its website about the involvement of medical personnel. They state:

Lethal injection was designed to prevent many of the disturbing images associated with other forms of execution. However, lethal injection increases the risk that medical personnel will be involved in killing for the state, in breach of long-standing principles of medical ethics.

Virtually all codes of professional ethics that consider the death penalty oppose health professional participation. Despite this, health professionals are required by law in many death penalty states to assist executions and in some cases have carried out the killings (See "Anything But Humane," *Amnesty International*, http://www.amnestyusa.org/our-work/issues/death-penalty/lethal-injection).

Answer the following:
a. Set out an argument opposing the use of medical professionals in lethal injection in the death penalty.
b. Set out an argument supporting the use of medical professionals in lethal injections in death penalty cases.

17. In her chapter on lethal injections in China, Cher Weixia Chen argues,

In China the implementation of lethal injection has raised several bioethical concerns with some distinctive local features. Currently there are two key bioethical issues that need to be attended to, other than the question of the moral permissibility of the death penalty in the first place. Once that question is put to rest, two issues come to the fore. These are the role of medical professionals and the harvesting of organs from executed prisoners.

Answer the following:
a. What do *you* think should be the role of medical personnel when it comes to harvesting organs from condemned prisoners?
b. State *one* argument for and *one* argument against harvesting organs from executed prisoners.

III

CULTURE

Introduction to Part III: Culture

Alison Dundes Renteln

Many of the most significant bioethics issues are of concern across the globe. Because of cultural variation, communities respond differently to these challenges. Toward the end of the twentieth century, researchers investigating matters of health and human rights called "Western" conceptions of normative standards into question (Airhihenbuwa 1995). In the twenty-first century this scholarship has increasingly reflected a wider range of issues considered part of bioethics as well as diverse societal approaches to them (Alora and Lumitao 2001). With more frequent migration, medical professionals are confronted more than ever before with unfamiliar moral and cultural conflicts. In part III, the authors wrestle with specific bioethics issues that put these types of conflicts in stark relief.

The contributors analyze specific bioethics questions, such as when, if ever, physicians are obligated to tell patients their precise diagnoses, differing notions of what constitutes a family, surgical procedures sometimes regarded as mutilation, sex-selective abortion, and research ethics on vulnerable communities—both the transnational implications of conducting clinical trials in Africa and the impact on indigenous people when they are subjects in experiments.

These chapters delve into policy debates in particular contexts, so that we may contemplate whether any ethical principles are truly universal. This is, admittedly, a controversial enterprise. The authors' willingness to acknowledge how communities differ in their approach to concrete health issues, in an effort to document agreement on normative principles, should help make possible a truly global bioethics.

Part III begins with an essay concerning the interpretation of truth-telling. When an individual is diagnosed with a health problem, it is generally understood that medical professionals must inform either the patient or the family of the patient. The question of what type of "truth-telling" is ethically required is central to Ilhan Ilkiliç's chapter. The presumption that a patient must be notified about his or her condition appears not to be shared worldwide. His analysis affords insight into possible interpretations of bioethics principles potentially applicable to this difficult matter. Although some might disagree that patient autonomy could be interpreted so as not to require being informed, others seek to incorporate a presumption against being told into the concept of patient autonomy.

Another fundamental bioethics issue concerns the appropriate use of reproductive technology. We need only look at the fertility market. It is international in scope—from Southern California's high-tech fertility centers to India's low-cost in vitro fertilization and surrogacy tourism. What is permitted *prior* to conception, much less afterward, has generated numerous moral and cultural conflicts. A major concern is the boundary of personal autonomy, particularly when others are asked to play a role in the exercise of the "right" of procreative liberty. That the market includes those who sell their own gametes to those who gestate the genetic children of others is at least part of the reason this merits our scrutiny. Moreover, both reproductive autonomy and patient autonomy at the end of life bring the issue of self-determination to center stage.

What duties do others have in ensuring personal autonomy is upheld? Can I ask you—or pay you—to give birth to my genetic child? Can I ask you to take my life when I want to die? What are the limits of self-determination when others are part of the equation? And what do we do when those others have moral qualms about carrying out my wishes? The ethical concerns go beyond what we do to our own bodies to how others are used to accomplish our ends.

The next chapter is by Maya Sabatello, in which she examines family rights from an international human rights perspective. In looking at the intersection between law, gendered identities, culture, and science, she analyzes how courts have responded to various problems about family relations as well as personal autonomy. She shows how the concept of "family" has been transformed by such scientific developments as IVF, in vitro genetic manipulation, sex selection, and the use of surrogate mothers. These changes have led to debates about access and the cultural construction of "family"—such as whether these procedures should be open to gay and transgendered people. Sabatello makes the case that the social and cultural barriers must be addressed from a human rights perspective that can then be used to help resolve the complexities that arise.

In my chapter, I offer a cross-cultural interpretation of controversial surgical procedures. This chapter exposes the tacit assumptions about classifying medical procedures properly considered enhancements and others regarded as mutilation. Many bioethics controversies hinge on the question of what types of cutting are permissible, according to ethical principles such as nonmalificence. I show that it can be problematic to ascertain which procedures are harms in pluralistic societies. While I support a presumption against surgery for children, with a few possible exceptions, it is unclear what limits should be imposed on adults who voluntarily choose to undergo surgery. As there are culturally varying notions of aesthetics, this is a vexed question. Underlying some of these debates is the serious matter of whether the state can legislate morality, and if so, whose moral code should be applied. I conclude by arguing that the ethical aspects of surgical practice deserve far greater consideration in bioethics.

Following the analytic chapters come four cases. The first is concerned with the use of reproductive technology to abort female fetuses. This practice, widespread in India and elsewhere, has drastically affected the ratio of males to females, resulting in even greater violence against women. One of the leading authorities on this subject, Vibhuti Patel, delves into the reasons behind the perpetuation of this custom in the context of South Asia. She questions whether women exercise "choice" here. Her essay underscores the need to determine the limits of reproductive autonomy. Mary Anne Warren's *Gendercide* (1985) put a name to the systematic elimination of females, and Patel shows us that, over twenty-five years later, the concern is no less pressing. It results in skewed sex ratios, as male infants grow into men who then face the societal repercussions of this abhorrent practice.

As we have seen throughout this volume, the perspective taken can make all the difference. This is the case both in the framing of the problems themselves and the very concepts that are used, and it is demonstrated in the next chapter with Cecilia Wee's discussion of active and passive euthanasia from the perspective of Confucianism. Her explication helps us see how morality, culture, and religion intersect on such matters as these. She points out key differences between Confucian and Western notions around acts of omission and acts of commission—and the impact this has on the attitude toward killing versus letting die.

In particular, the distinction drawn between active and passive euthanasia, between "killing versus letting die"—which is such a point of contention in the Western debate—has little force in Confucianism. Her examination helps us see how much assumptions and values can affect the way in which bioethical issues and decision making are framed. The definition of the problem shapes the search for a solution. Distinctions perceived as crucial in one worldview may be of minimal significance in another and, thus, have a transformative effect on policies and societal norms.

Wee contends that in a role-based morality as found in Confucianism, the distinction between acting and omitting to act may be largely irrelevant to moral decision making. Consequently, active euthanasia (acts of commission) and passive euthanasia (acts of omission) are no longer seen as polar opposites. The result is that, in Confucian societies, end-of-life decision making contrasts with that of the West and other societies that do not rest on a role-based morality.

In the last two cases the scholars focus on the risk of exploitation posed by clinical research on vulnerable communities, including persons with disabilities, children, married women, and prisoners. Peter F. Omonzejele examines the trend toward clinical trials on new drugs in West African communities when the side effects and long-term consequences of treatment are unknown. He highlights the potential for devastating harm, although where research does not occur, there may be virtually no access to medication. Here the reader is exposed to various definitions of vulnerability, including its formulation in the policies of the Council for International Organizations of Medical Sciences (CIOMS). Ultimately the question turns on informed consent, particularly when it is difficult to obtain, as with individuals with mental and intellectual disabilities.

In the last chapter in part III, Marlene Brant Castellano analyzes research ethics as it relates to indigenous groups. Her study of Aboriginal people in Canada advances the argument that they should have the right to participate in setting standards for research that affects the well-being of their communities. This sovereignty argument reveals the unequal bargaining power of government and the medical establishment vis-à-vis indigenous groups. Castellano favors the empowerment of First Nations and other disadvantaged groups through the formulation of ethical principles that reflect their worldview and customary law.

All the chapters in this section highlight conflicts over specific medical or health issues. Insofar as different parts of the world have their own distinctive value systems, their perceptions of what is ethical conduct vary. The chapters here document illustrations of these. Some of the authors do acknowledge that culture-based arguments might be construed so as to preclude the possibility of moral criticism, that is, Ilkiliç.

They also refer to scholarship that expresses skepticism about the relevance of the concept of culture and question its utility because of colonialism (e.g., Ahmad 1996). However, cultural relativism can be construed as a descriptive theory that permits moral criticism (Renteln 1988, 1990). Most of the contributors are motivated by a desire to show the need for a more nuanced approach to bioethics issues that is not limited by a presumption of universality.

Should there exist a global consensus on specific principles, then that would pave the way for a cross-cultural universal code. These chapters should generate greater discussion of specific principles in transnational and transcultural perspectives. Thus, the analysis of moral and cultural conflicts may ultimately help identify shared values linked to cross-cultural universals.

REFERENCES

Ahmad, Waqar. 1996. "The Trouble with Culture." In *Researching Cultural Differences in Health*, edited by David Kelleher and Sheila Hillier, 190–219. London: Routledge.

Airhihenbuwa, Collins O. 1995. *Health and Culture: Beyond the Western Paradigm*. Thousand Oaks: Sage Publications.

Alora, Angeles Tan, and Josephine M. Lumitao, eds. 2001. *Beyond a Western Bioethics: Voices from the Developing World*. Washington, DC: Georgetown University Press.

Benatar, S. R. 2002. "Reflections and Recommendations on Research Ethics in Developing Countries." *Social Science & Medicine* 54 (7): 1131–41.

Callahan, Daniel. 2009. "The Contested Terrain of American Bioethics." *ESKA/Journal International de Bioethique* 20 (4): 25–33.

Durante, Chris. 2009. "Bioethics in a Pluralistic Society: Bioethical Methodology in Lieu of Moral Diversity." *Medical Health Care and Philosophy* 12:35–47.

Hellsten, Sirkku K. 2008. "Global Bioethics: Utopia or Reality?" *Developing World Bioethics* 8 (2): 70–81.

Marshall, Patricia A. 2005. "Human Rights, Cultural Pluralism, and International Health Research." *Theoretical Medicine and Bioethics* 26 (6): 529–57.

Renteln, Alison Dundes. 1988. "Relativism and the Search for Human Rights." *American Anthropologist* 90:56–72.

———. 1990. *International Human Rights: Universalism Versus Relativism*. Newbury Park, CA: Sage; reissued in 2013 by Quid Pro Books.

Ryan, Maura A. 2004. "Beyond a Western Bioethics?" *Theological Studies* 65:158–77.

1

Culture and Ethical Aspects of Truth-Telling in a Value Pluralistic Society[1]

Ilhan Ilkiliç

ABSTRACT

Advances in medical science and technology offer us not only new diagnostic measures and possibilities but also allow us to make better prognoses in terminal disease stages. As a consequence, physicians can work out more precise diagnoses, enabling them to inform their patients about the expected future course of their condition. Under these circumstances, truth-telling as a classical issue of medical ethics remains a highly charged problem. The concept of truth-telling has become controversial in multicultural societies because of the differences in attitude toward this practice based on diverse cultural value systems and preferences. The demographic changes effected by migrant groups especially in western European countries mean that truth-telling will be an ever more common problem in everyday medical practice, posing serious challenges for health care professionals. This chapter describes some arguments pertinent to this issue and discusses a real case history recorded at a German hospital. Telling the truth about a diagnosis in an intercultural setting and the participation of family members in the decision-making process in a multicultural society are identified as the key ethical points of this case. It also discusses some metaethical issues, such as the universal applicability of the ethical principle of "respect for autonomy" with regard to truth-telling. Some practical suggestions for everyday medical practice in a multicultural society are developed, and in the conclusion, some ethical theses are proposed.

INTRODUCTION

Rapid developments in medicine enable us not only to produce better diagnoses but also to make more accurate predictions about the future development of illnesses. As

185

a result of these developments, unfavorable diagnoses such as malignant cancer are made more frequently and in dire prognoses are to be communicated to patients. Thus, the standard question of medical ethics concerning the morally correct way of handling the disclosure of unfavorable diagnoses and prognoses persists. It is even more complicated given the existence of different values among patients and caregivers. Ethical questions in medical practice have increased as a consequence of pluralistic value systems and demographic changes associated with new migrants in western European countries.

The first part of this chapter discusses arguments in the context of the communication of an unfavorable diagnosis and prognosis. The second part provides a concrete case in an intercultural setting recorded in a German hospital, involving a patient and his family coming from a Muslim country. The central problems included the demand of family members to be involved in the decision-making process, identifying the appropriate mode of communication, and the general search for an ethically acceptable way of dealing with a patient from a foreign culture. Because the patient and his family were Muslims, I consider Islamic principles relevant to truth-telling. The third part discusses two ethical approaches associated with possible options for action in such a conflict situation and evaluates them. Finally, I offer practical recommendations for dealing with such conflicts in a pluralistic society in an ethically appropriate way.

PART ONE: ARGUMENTS IN THE CONTEXT OF COMMUNICATING AN UNFAVORABLE DIAGNOSIS AND PROGNOSIS

In industrial countries, well into the 1960s the disclosure of an unfavorable diagnosis and dire prognosis to patients was considered to contravene the Hippocratic principle of "doing no damage" (*nil nocere*). Empirical studies from the early 1960s made in the United States show that 90 percent of doctors were against informing their patients of a diagnosis of cancer (Oken 1961). Physicians, on their own, chose to withhold information from patients ostensibly to save them from fear and desperation, so as not to weaken their powers of recovery (Van de Loo 2000).

This attitude changed somewhat in the 1970s when the self-determination and responsibility of the patient in the relationship between doctor and patient were deemed more important (Steinhart 2002). In another study from the United States conducted in 1977, only 2 percent of American doctors spoke out against informing a patient of an unfavorable diagnosis and prognosis (Novack, Plumer et al. 1979). Eventually, informing the patient about the diagnosis, therapy options, and prognosis became an integral part of a doctor's responsibilities (Brown 1995). The historical analysis of this development, in particular in the European and Western world, indicates that the moral assessment of this practice is closely tied to the value placed on the autonomy of the patient (Faden and Beauchamp 1986, Tuckett 2004, Surbone 2006).

Truthfulness in conversations with a patient is crucial for establishing a relationship of trust between patient and doctor. It represents the indispensable basis for any ethically acceptable medical intervention, and it cannot be established without honesty on the part of the doctor. This implies being informed of any illness, even if it is difficult or impossible to cure (Jameton 1995, Van de Loo 2000, Salomon 2003).

In addition to the issue of truthfulness, there are other substantial arguments in favor of communicating a negative prognosis (Sullivan, Menapace et al. 2001). Rapid developments in biomedicine have created new diagnostic and therapeutic measures allowing for better treatments and sometimes even healing diseases previously considered incurable. There are also increasingly more options for treating an illness with various impacts on a patient's quality of life. For this reason, being informed enables patients to weigh their options, according to their values and preferences, thereby being involved in determining their own futures (Jameton 1995).

Receiving information about a serious illness allows the patient to contemplate the serious side effects of, say, chemotherapy, on an adequate informational basis—one cannot expect a patient left with the impression that he or she has only a harmless illness to agree to a therapy with serious side effects (Salomon 2003). The patient can only evaluate such a therapy appropriately if he or she is in a position to perceive the benefits offered and to decide about them on the basis of the required information. Only if the danger of a disease becomes more evident is one prepared to undergo a long and unpleasant therapy. Communicating the gravity of a condition can thus support patient compliance.

Besides the ethical arguments, there are also legal norms that determine the framework for medical decision making and action. In the German legal system, every medical intervention for diagnostic and therapeutic purposes is seen as a potential personal injury and can only be legitimated by gaining the patient's informed consent (Walter 2000). The validity of such consent presupposes the patient's ability to understand the planned intervention and thus his or her being appropriately informed by the doctor. It follows from these premises that the doctor is obligated, in all but a few exceptional cases, to communicate unfavorable diagnoses to the patient. These legal regulations and the guidelines of professional institutions in Germany are based on specific ethical norms, including the concepts of human well-being and human dignity. A contravention of these regulations and guidelines leads to sanctions or criminal proceedings (Ulsenheimer 2008).

Despite these arguments, one can imagine situations in which withholding an unfavorable diagnosis would be legitimate and even ethically desirable. The central paradigm "respect for the autonomous decision of the patient" implies not only the right to know but also the right not to know (Macklin 1999: 100; Chadwick 1997). Consequently, withholding medical information could be ethically allowed if the patient wants to make use of his or her negative rights and refuses to receive relevant information.

In addition, withholding information can also be ethically justified if the information to be communicated would harm the patient seriously without benefiting him or her in any way. In this case, it is the doctor, not the patient, who decides, because of the professional scientific expertise and experience with the procedure. A perceived risk of suicide or a serious depression after being informed of the diagnosis can legitimate such medical decisions. For good reason, this procedure requires a very sensitive investigation of the situation and a critical approach to the case on the part of the doctor in charge (Brody 1997).

Withholding an unfavorable diagnosis, however, does bring up numerous ethical problems. Regardless of whether this withholding of information has been requested by the patient or contemplated by the doctor, it must not lead to refusing therapy, as a patient might refuse to hear the true diagnosis ("right not to know") but nevertheless wants an appropriate therapy. But this poses a problem: How can necessary chemotherapy with its serious side effects be carried out legitimately without the patient suspecting a cancer diagnosis? In a case like this, one wonders if it is reasonable to expect a desirable degree of compliance at all.

The communication of such information is also *lege artis* of central importance. A quiet place without time pressure or the presence of others is certainly more appropriate for the communication of a negative diagnosis and prognosis than a crowded ward (Pilchmaier 1999, Salomon 2003). It is desirable to create suitable circumstances for answering patients' various questions. The use of easy-to-understand language and an appropriate tone of voice are bound to have a positive effect on the communication. Providing for professional psychological counseling of the patient following the conversation is equally important.

PART TWO: TRUTH-TELLING IN AN INTERCULTURAL CONTEXT

In a multicultural society characterized by the existence of different cultures and value systems, truth-telling gives rise to several ethical questions. First, it may be difficult for the physician to understand how the values of a patient from another culture (or family members' attempts to influence the doctor's procedure in communicating an unfavorable diagnosis and prognosis) can cause ethical conflicts. Legal regulations, codes of conduct established by professional institutions, and procedural conventions can limit the options for dealing with actual problems. As an example, let us consider some ethical problems that arose in an actual case in a German hospital. My colleagues, Dr. Abdullah Takim and Dr. Rainer Brömer, informed me about this case:

A twenty-three-year-old Turkish man was diagnosed with malignant cancer. Several cycles of chemotherapy achieved no success in treatment. The patient's state of health deteriorated progressively, making his imminent death more and more likely. The patient was transferred to a palliative ward. Both the patient and his parents had only rudimentary knowledge of the German language, which did not allow for an adequate communication with the medical team. With the help of an interpreter, who was a member of their wider family, the doctor in charge informed the parents about their son's hopeless situation; the son was also partly involved in this talk.

A nurse of Turkish descent happened to overhear the conversation and later informed the doctors that the interpreter had not passed on to the patient the information about his expected imminent death, probably on the request of his parents. The doctors considered this a clear contravention of the patient's "right to know." With the help of a different interpreter, they arranged another conversation with the patient during which he was informed of the possibility that he might soon die. Two days later the patient passed away. The parents later accused the doctors of being responsible for their son's death: they had contributed to the worsening of his condition and thus hastened his demise.

There is a conflict of opinion here between the patient's parents and the medical team regarding disclosure to the patient of an unfavorable diagnosis and prognosis. In this ethical conflict, the medical team believes that the patient should decide if he wants to receive the full information about his condition. The balance between the *right to know* and the *right not to know* should be made by the patient himself, out of a respect for the patient's autonomous decision making. Among the other norms, autonomy is accorded the highest priority in the medical team's decision-making process. As an adult and autonomous human being, the patient should decide through an individual evaluation of his various options. Withholding requisite information would mean disenfranchising the patient and violating his right of self-determination.

The starting point for the parents' decision and attitude is, however, a different one. Their approach may be described as caring and consequentialist. In their decision-making process, patient autonomy does not play a central role. For the parents, the issue is primarily whether the disclosure of the dire prognosis will affect their son's well-being. They expect that the medical team's course of action will upset their son and thus weaken his regenerative powers. This approach is regarded as harmful in preference to one of withholding the diagnosis and prognosis. In this case, the patient died two days after receiving the information. His parents therefore felt that their decision was vindicated and accused the medical team of having acted wrongly.

Communication and Dealing with the Family

Communication difficulties often play a decisive role in the processes leading up to clinical-ethical conflicts in medical practice. Linguistic and cultural barriers in an intercultural setting increase those difficulties, further complicating the conflict (Ilkilic 2002 and 2007, Hancock, Clayton et al. 2007). Since the solution of such conflicts initially requires the clarification of the conflict parties' different interests, overcoming these barriers is of central importance (Krakauer, Crenner et al. 2002; Valente 2004; Volker 2005).

In an intercultural context, a linguistic understanding of the patient's wishes and preferences is necessary, but it is often not sufficient to guarantee an ethically appropriate way of dealing with a given problem. Rather, the significance and sometimes the background of these wishes in a given culture should be clarified in writing as well as verbally (Kagawa-Singer and Blackhall 2001). Only then can one hope for an appropriate ethical evaluation of goods.

In the case described above, it is striking to observe that no conversation took place between the two conflicting parties after the patient's death—that is, the medical team and the parents. Neither party really knew why the other acted the way it did, nor did they grasp the different sets of values brought to bear on the decision making. The medical team probably saw in the family's position a clear violation of the patient's autonomy and self-determination and considered it to be ethically unacceptable. The family members, on the other hand, believed that the patient must be protected at all costs from the damage that his being informed about his unfavorable diagnosis would presumably cause. They did not understand why the medical team would want to harm him in such a way.

In this case, it would have been sensible for the responsible doctor to take the initiative in a conversation with the parents. Such a conversation could have provided both parties more information about the backgrounds of the other's position, opening a broader access to the culturally alien motivation, possibly enabling a reflective attitude to their own positions. A better understanding of one another based on such a conversation, even though it cannot guarantee consensus in such cases, seems to be an indispensable instrument—particularly in an intercultural setting.

In such a conversation, the family members could have informed the medical team from their own cultural perspective about the normative meaning of withholding an unfavorable diagnosis and prognosis to be understood, in their culture, as a moral imperative based on the conviction that the communication of such information directly harms the affected person and is therefore to be avoided. Disclosure would also destroy the hope of healing, which would create, according to this anthropology, an unacceptable situation. In addition, this knowledge would be a burden for the patient and thus decrease his quality of life. Not to know about one's imminent death is considered beneficial for the patient's well-being and is therefore a desirable condition.

On the other hand, the medical team could have informed the family about the legal constraints of which they probably were unaware. This information would have given the family a better idea of the range of options for decision making and action available to the medical team and thus perhaps created a basis for understanding the chosen action. In addition, ethical arguments and their backgrounds could have been presented, including the conviction that a person as a self-determined and thus responsible being has a right to make decisions about his current state. This presupposes, further, the doctor's responsibility to provide information about the medical conditions of this state (Van de Loo 2000: 284).

In medical ethical terms, the communication of an unfavorable diagnosis and dire prognosis is not to be viewed as direct harm. Such harm arises only through the perception and reflection of the affected person. From this understanding, the wishes and preferences of the family members cannot be allowed to guide the attitude of the doctors—unless they can provide information about the presumed will of the patient. However, this aspect is irrelevant in this case, since the patient himself was competent to express his own opinion and make his own decisions. Even though it is not to be expected that this comprehensive exchange of views will lead directly to consensus, it would contribute significantly to preventing an escalation.

The Actions of the Medical Team

The German Medical Association (*Bundesärztekammer*) prescribes in its guidelines for medical treatment of the terminally ill that the information given to a dying person about his or her condition and treatment options must be truthful. This information and the way it is delivered "must however take account of the dying person's situation and present fears" (*Bundesärztekammer* 2004: 1).

The doctor in charge may withhold information about the hopeless situation of his or her patient if she is convinced that this would clearly and unequivocally cause damage to the patient. He or she should withhold an unfavorable diagnosis (1) if the patient himself explicitly asks the doctor to do so, (2) if the doctor is convinced that such information would lead to a suicide attempt, and (3) if this information would cause serious psychological disturbance. Family members may only be informed about such a diagnosis with the permission of the patient (*Bundesärztekammer* 2004: 1).

These principles are firmly based on the respect for the patient's personal rights, particularly the right of self-determination. Medical treatment therefore requires a patient to be informed before having to consent to any intervention (*Bundesärztekammer* 2007). The patient needs to be given information not only about the therapy to be carried out but also about the critical reasons for the specific therapeutic measures chosen. In our example, the reasons for stopping conventional cancer therapy and shifting to palliative care should be explained to the patient, requiring him or her to be informed of the dire prognosis.

The position of the family members in the decision-making process, scarcely attended to by the medical team, can also be traced back to the patient-centered attitude described here. This attitude is based on an anthropocentric, individualistic concept of the human being. The procedure adopted by the medical team also implies a cultural invariance claim as if in no culture the family had normative significance for decision making unless explicitly desired by the patient. It should be noted that just this attitude led to the escalation of the conflict.

Medical guidelines and legal regulations allow medical practice to be performed more simply and, in the course of time, lead to a certain routine. This routine is based on well-considered ethical arguments; it is, however, easily interrupted as soon as culturally conditioned ethical problems arise. The way the medical team acted may be viewed as a conventional attitude based on the ethical norms and legal regulations described above. It remains to be considered, though, whether there could be further pragmatic reasons for this attitude.

One reason for the behavior of the medical team could be "wanting to stay on the right side of the law." Following the parents' wishes without the assent of the patient could have legal consequences. Legal sanctions now increasingly play a major role in the decisions and actions of doctors, especially those with less professional experience. Critical discussions and concerns debated among academics and the public produce headlines such as "the making of medicine into law" or "the dictatorship of legal constraints" (Ulsenheimer 2008).

A further reason can be a lack of time for a detailed conversation with family members or with the patient (Hancock, Clayton et al. 2007). Time pressure has long been a phenomenon in everyday medical practice, and it may present a barrier to an ethically appropriate delivery of medical care. One example is the decrease in time devoted to informing patients or discussing treatment options in detail. Despite this situation, it is necessary to find an appropriate context for longer conversations not only with the patient but also with family members. "Time pressure must play no role," says the training brochure for further education that is published by the German Medical Association (*Bundesärztekammer* 1998: 114).

An additional problem can arise from a lack of *intercultural competence*. Intercultural competence means the ability to both discern and analyze the basic elements of an intercultural conflict and integrate them into the medical/ethical decision-making process (Ilkilic 2008). In the absence of this competence, the reality of cultural components in a conflict might initially be overlooked. In this case, the integration of culture-specific values and connected wishes into the decision-making process is prevented.

It is also difficult to clarify the normative significance of culture-specific attitudes and preferences for practice. One cannot, of course, expect such a difficult achievement from a medical team; nevertheless, there should be some sensitivity to the cultural phenomena in everyday life. In complex cases in which the team faces a challenge for which it feels unprepared, outside experts can be called upon and the clinical ethics committee or clinical ethics consultants can be involved (Paul 2008).

Establishing the Will of the Patient

Finding out the patient's actual will to be informed of an unfavorable diagnosis and prognosis and the parents' attitude(s) is of central importance. In an intercultural setting of this kind, it is difficult for the doctor to "take account of [the patient's] present fears" (*Bundesärztekammer* 2004: 1). It is conceivable that a conversation with family members might be able to clarify the patient's attitude to being informed about an unfavorable diagnosis and prognosis. It is more likely that an appropriate approach could be found on this basis. This attempt requires, however, a certain degree of caution.

There is no reason to expect from the outset that the family members will communicate this information perfectly. Given a conflict of interests, the patient's real attitude may be concealed or misrepresented. Here a relationship of trust between the family members and the medical teams is necessary. In certain circumstances this information could be checked against statements made by acquaintances or friends of the patient. However, this may be impossible because of the lack of time or personnel.

Finding out the will of the patient directly by means of a conversation between the patient and his doctor may be difficult because of the linguistic and cultural barriers. The presence of an interpreter creates another barrier to a direct conversation. Sensitive nuances and subtle formulations can be lost in translation. Similarly, the doctor will be unable to interpret certain gestures and expressions of the patient's body language, firstly because she might not know the meaning of the patient's movements in his cultural context and secondly because the content transmitted by emphasis is easily lost in the interpreter's rendition. Thus, access to the patient's will is filtered through multiple layers of mediation. These difficulties can be minimized by use of interpreters specifically trained for such situations.

In any case, gaining an adequate understanding of the patient's preferences requires an optimized strategy. The difficulty in choosing such a strategy consists, among other things, in the alien appearance of the patient's culture. For this reason, a preliminary conversation can be helpful to allow access to the patient's personality. In a conversation of this kind, one can discuss the patient's current knowledge of his or her condition and possibly also ask about any expectations regarding treatment options or the course of the medical condition. The significance and value of his family can also be addressed in this conversation. One can even ask directly whether a direct involvement of family members in the decision-making process would be in accordance with his wishes.

The information and impressions gained in the initial conversation can be helpful for determining the strategy for the second talk. They can also help to eliminate strategies found to be inappropriate. Sensitivity and caution should accompany the doctor's actions in these conversations. "The question about the truth about the seriousness of the illness is therefore ultimately a question about the appropriate truth" (*Bundesärztekammer* 1998: 114).

Family and Truth-Telling

Withholding an unfavorable diagnosis or prognosis on the request of family members is not a rare occurrence in some countries in the world. Such a practice is often encountered outside the "Western world," in particular in Asian and South American countries, but also in the Near East and in Muslim countries (Berger 1998, Mobeireek et al. 2008). The medical ethicist Yali Chong from the Peking University Health Care Center emphasizes the importance of the family in decisions about informing a patient of his condition. He even speaks of the model of a family-patient-doctor in the Chinese-Confucian culture (Cong 2004).

Here, the seriousness of the illness also determines the influence of the family on the procedure to be adopted. "If the illness is very easy to cure, the family member will directly disclose all the information to the patient, or allow the patient to do so. Otherwise, the family member offers only partial information or lies to the patient" (Cong 2004: 152). Jotkowitz and his colleagues argue similarly on this topic and speak of a similar reserve with respect to informing a patient fully about a bad diagnosis and prognosis in the Jewish tradition (Jotkowitz, Glick et al. 2006).

In Turkey, family members' desire to be involved in determining medical treatment is also strong if the illness is incurable and terminal (Ozdogan et al. 2006, Aksoy 2005). It is common for family members to express to the doctor their wish that the patient not be informed of a bad diagnosis, often before the diagnosis has even been made. It is also not rare for the doctor, in the case of an unfavorable diagnosis, to discuss the further procedure with family members first. The attitude of the parents in the case described above can be viewed as a typical instance of such cases.

It would certainly be wrong to see this attitude as a merely cultural attitude without any moral foundations. Two forms of argumentation can be constructed from the perspective of the Turkish-Islamic culture that is rarely made explicit in practice. The first one assumes that informing patients about an incurable disease or imminent death would upset them and thus cause a psychological burden. This action is to be viewed as unequivocally harmful and hence to be avoided.

Here, the classical medical-ethical principle of avoiding harm comes to the fore. This form of argumentation is not foreign to western European medical ethics and also not insignificant in common practice. The important difference consists in the normative interpretation of the individual assessment of this practice. In the Turkish-Islamic culture, this principle of doing no harm is initially independent of an individual attitude. Family members are involved in the decision-making process on this basis. The central importance accorded to the family in social life generally makes this involvement easier. Even from an individualist perspective, this action is not *eo ipso* to be seen as detrimental to the patient's well-being. Whether this action is harmful can only be decided on the basis of the patient's own attitude to this practice.

The attitude of the family members in the above-mentioned case can also be justified by Islamic belief. In Islamic thought, the time of death is set by God and remains hidden from human beings (Quran Sura 56:60). Humans can speculate about it with the means at their disposal, but they cannot predict this moment with absolute certainty. A predictive statement about end of life is viewed critically from this religious perspective. "One is ultimately not God" is the reaction to such statements. It is worth noting that such reactions more frequently follow negative prognoses. Such an assertion is also seen as an open attack on the theological concept of hope.

To take away the hope of healing would contradict the implicit attributes of God in Islamic belief, since this attitude would deny God's omnipotence. This theological foundation would also make the family's attitude in the situation described above plausible, from the perspective of their religious beliefs, even if it was not made explicit at the time.

PART THREE: UNIVERSALISTIC AND PARTICULARISTIC APPROACHES TO TRUTH-TELLING

When it comes to medical-ethical conflicts in an intercultural setting, such as those discussed and analyzed above, the conceptualization of the cultural phenomena, their ethical analyses evaluation, and their integration into the decision-making process take on central importance. As the example has shown, cultural phenomena are often given little attention in the procedure followed by the medical team.

At this point, it is important to ask whether the approach adopted in this conflict is the only ethically legitimate course of action, or if a different procedure might provide a better way of dealing with the conflict. In other words, is an anthropocentric, individualistic ethical approach based on human dignity, personal rights, and the right to self-determination able to take account of cultural phenomena and to integrate them into the decision-making process? The latter question is directly connected with the ethical assessment of culturally specific values. This and similar questions have already been addressed by medical ethicists in discussions about the universality of the principle of respect for patient autonomy. In what follows, two basic positions on the topic of truth-telling will be examined.

American bioethicist Ruth Macklin argues that established fundamental ethical principles could adequately address cultural phenomena in medical care and integrate them into the decision-making process in an appropriate way. She distinguishes between the principles of "respect for the person" and "respect for autonomy" and subordinates the latter principle to the former (Macklin 1998). Autonomy, a self-evident consequence of the principle of respect for the person, does not in her opinion exclude withholding an unfavorable diagnosis and taking family members' choices into account during the decision-making process.

Provided the patient agrees, family members can contribute to the health care team's deliberations. In the same way, the patient's wish not to be informed about an unfavorable diagnosis can be honored by the physician (Macklin 1998: 7). Note that this approach claims universal validity and is thought capable of resolving conflicts in an intercultural physician-patient relationship.

Chinese medical ethicist Ruiping Fan denies the universally binding character of "Western bioethical principles" and questions their "abstract content" that would offer a basis for the moral evaluation of medical practices in all cultures (Fan 1997). He argues his position, taking the principle of autonomy as an example and discussing two forms of determination that can be derived from it—namely, self-determination and determination by the family.

In his opinion, the Western principle of autonomy leads to self-determination where the starting point is individual free will and the subjective determinability of moral goods. Determination by the family can be derived, on the other hand, from the East Asian principle of autonomy. This form of determination claims an objective understanding of moral goods and emphasizes the value of harmonious dependency within the family. These two concepts of autonomy cannot, according to Fan, be equated with each other, as they imply different moral actions.

Fan illustrates these theoretical discussions with instances of truth-telling in the case of an unfavorable diagnosis and prognosis. From the Chinese or Confucian perspective, withholding a diagnosis and prognosis can be ethically justified. First, the family members should be informed, and subsequently the further procedure should be decided upon in consultation with the family. If the family decides to withhold information from the patient, the doctor should respect this decision

(Fan and Li 2004). According to Fan and Li's particularistic approach, this procedure rests on the following conditions:

1. the physician finds evidence of manifest mutual concern of the family members for the patient
2. the family's wishes are not egregiously in discord with the physician's professional judgment regarding the medical best interests of the patient

If either or both of the two necessary conditions are not met, the physician should communicate directly with the patient (Fan and Li 2004: 189).

CRITICAL DISCUSSION OF UNIVERSALISTIC AND PARTICULARISTIC APPROACHES

A major concern of the universalistic approaches argued by Macklin and others is the prevention of harm, which can reach the degree of a violation of human rights. For this reason, every medical action must first be examined to assess if it represents a violation of human rights. In a second step, the intervention should be evaluated from the patient perspective. Only then can it be ethically legitimated in medical practice.

This approach presupposes a hierarchy among ethical principles, according to which patient autonomy is most important (Macklin 1998). To argue for the universal application of this approach assumes the validity of this hierarchy among ethical principles. Yet as long as such a hierarchy in the form just described is not accepted in a given culture, this approach cannot be applied ("unbridgeable moral gap between Western individualism and non-Western communalism"; Baker 1998: 212).

A further deficiency of the universalistic approach is its inability to ethically assess culturally dependent moral phenomena such as family autonomy. It is not able to ascribe a normative value to such phenomena. This approach is always dependent from the individualistic understanding of the human being. Therefore, this ascription of ethical value thus has a *hypothetical* character and not an a priori one.

If one applies the entire approach to our case study, the attitude of the medical team can be ethically legitimated on its basis. The medical team deliberately ignored the wishes of the family and instead turned to the patient himself. The reason given was the patient's autonomy. As long as the patient does not assent, no normative value can be ascribed to the wishes of the family. It is obvious that just this ignorance of the cultural phenomena led to the escalation of the conflict.

In addition, this approach presupposes a responsible, adult, and informed patient with whom one can communicate perfectly without linguistic or cultural barriers. A further difficulty comes in when the patient is not able to express himself, as is the case, for example, with an incompetent or comatose patient, infant, or fetus.

Despite these difficulties, this approach possesses an important strength for a multicultural society, the constituent groups of which are by no means homogenous. It is ethically unjustifiable to decide about the treatment given to a patient merely on the basis of his (perceived) membership in a religious or ethnic group. An indiscriminate application of the knowledge gained about the patient's culture or the extrapolation from previous individual experiences can turn out to be mistaken in a current case. For this reason, it is always important to uncover the individual patient's attitude to a specific practice.

The normatively relativist or particularistic approach promises a better account of cultural phenomena in making ethical judgments than a universalistic one. Particularists can derive moral maxims for actions from culturally specific phenomena. Because the moral judgments within a culture are affected by other cultural phenomena, they receive as such a normative value—without being examined according to fundamental ethical principles. Thus, withholding an unfavorable diagnosis, for example, is morally right if this practice is morally accepted within a certain culture. This position is clearly supported especially by cultural anthropology.

Unfortunately, this approach implies a *culturalistic fallacy.* I understand under the culturalistic fallacy that the ethical justification of a moral practice or attitude is only through its existence in a certain group. According to this attitude, a reflection upon or criticism of a culture's moral practice is impossible.

A comprehensive application of this approach is not only problematic because of the culturalistic fallacy but also because of its prerequisite moral homogeneity within a given ethnic group. In the age of globalization a profound change in values is taking place, even in societies considered closed to the outside world, so that disparate values emerge within each culture. If the members of a certain culture live in another country, the influence of the dominant values in the host country would be strong and thus support the heterogeneity of values within this ethnic group.

If one applies this approach to our case study, the relatives' wish attains normative value and can under certain circumstances be acted on. If the patient's expectations agree with those of the family, this approach is better able to take account of the cultural phenomena. If the patient does not agree with the family's wishes, however, the patient could then be restrained in his decisions, even disenfranchised. An insoluble problem is also presented by the juridical justification of the medical team's actions. Withholding medical information without the patient's assent can have legal as well as moral repercussions for the doctor.

CONCLUSION

The disclosure of an unfavorable diagnosis and dire prognosis to a patient, communicating essential (and existential) information to the person most immediately concerned, has historically been a controversial topic. Today, it has lost nothing of its controversial status. On the contrary, we encounter this question in medical practice much more frequently and with a growing complexity. Truth-telling in the intercultural setting of a value-pluralistic society requires a better-founded and more comprehensive discussion of the problem than has hitherto taken place.

From the comprehensive discussion and analysis presented above, the following conclusions on a practical and theoretical level can be developed:

- An ethically appropriate way of handling the disclosure of an unfavorable diagnosis and infaust prognosis in an intercultural setting requires first of all culturally sensitive and successful communication, especially in case of a conflict of preferences and interests, in order for the conflict parties to reach a mutual understanding of their values and of the specific reasons for their attitude. Translation by relatives or hospital staff has often proven counterproductive and ethically problematic, hence communication should be mediated by professional interpreters trained for medical practice.
- An ethically legitimate resolution of such conflicts often requires intercultural competence, to be understood as the ability to recognize and analyze the goods at stake in an intercultural conflict and to integrate them into medical-ethical decision making. The availability of such competence cannot, however, be taken as a given. It should be imparted during medical studies and supported in professional life by means of further training. Intercultural competence must also be recognized as an important competence for members of ethics committees in a value pluralistic society.
- The decisions and actions of doctors must be taken within the limits of the law and conforming to the regulations of professional institutions. These regulations should be laid down in such a way as to leave sufficient space for taking account of cultural phenomena. Equally, in a culturally determined medical-ethical conflict it should be investigated whether a procedure diverging from the conventional practice is possible. For reasons presented above, it often happens that options that are in principle available for medical decision making are not pursued. With a culturally sensitive attitude and intercultural competence, additional options can be better integrated into medical decision making.
- The ethical problems that arise in applying the universalistic and particularistic approaches were discussed in detail above. A rigid application of any of these approaches appears to be problematic in many respects. Instead, an integrative procedure should be followed. This procedure entails taking account of the ethical goods at issue in the conflict from the perspective of the conflict parties. This does not mean prioritizing either patient autonomy or family autonomy, but rather contextualizing these forms of autonomy sensitively in concrete terms.

Only then can both the wholesale application of patient autonomy often found in conventional practice and the overruling of the individual patient's wishes based on his presumed belonging to a certain culture be prevented. This process of argumentation and reflection, however, presents a challenge for the medical team, which should therefore in complex situations have access to expertise from a competence center or to ethical consultancy by a clinical ethics committee or clinical ethics consultant.

ACKNOWLEDGMENT

The author would like to thank Dr. Rainer Brömer for his important comments and critical perusal of this manuscript.

NOTE

1. This paper has developed out of the project Medical Ethical Decisions at the End of Life in Intercultural Setting, supported by Johannes Gutenberg University Mainz (Förderlinie der Stufe I).

REFERENCES

Aksoy, S. 2005. "End-of-Life Decisions Making in Turkey." In *End-of-Life Decision Making: A Cross-National Study*, edited by R. H. Blank and J. C. Merrick, 183–95 (Cambridge: MIT Press).

Baker, R. 1998. "A Theory of International Bioethics: Multiculturalism, Postmodernism, and the Bankruptcy of Fundamentalism." *Kennedy Institute of Ethics Journal* 8 (3): 201–31.

Berger, J. T. 1998. "Culture and Ethnicity in Clinical Care." *Archives of Internal Medicine* 158 (19): 2085–90.

Brody, H. 1997. "The Physician-Patient Relationship." In *Medical Ethics*, 2nd edition, edited by R. W. Veatch, 75–101. Boston: Jones and Bartlett Publishers.

Brown, K. H. 1995. "Information Disclosure." In *Encyclopedia of Bioethics*, edited by W. Reich, 1221–24. New York: Free Press.

Bundesärztekammer. 1998. *Gesundheit im Alter. Texte und Materialien der Bundesärztekammer zur Fortbildung und Weiterbildung*, Köln.

———. 2004. "Grundsätze der Bundesärztekammer zur ärztlichen Sterbebegleitung." *Deutsches Ärzteblatt* 19:1–2.

———. 2007. *Berufsordnung für die deutschen Ärztinnen und Ärzte*.

Chadwick, R. 1997. "Das Recht auf Wissen und das Recht auf Nichtwissen aus philosophischer Sicht." In *Perspektiven der Humangenetik*, edited by F. W. Silvia Petermann and Michael Quante, 195–207. Paderborn: Ferdinand Schöningh.

Cong, Y. 2004. "Doctor-Family-Patient Relationship: The Chinese Paradigm of Informed Consent." *Journal of Medical Philosophy* 29 (2): 149–78.

Faden, R. R., and T. L. Beauchamp. 1986. *A History and Theory of Informed Consent*. New York: Oxford University Press.

Fan, R. 1997. "Self-Determination vs. Family-Determination: Two Incommensurable Principles of Autonomy: A Report from East Asia." *Bioethics* 11 (3–4): 309–22.

Fan, R., and B. Li. 2004. "Truth Telling in Medicine: The Confucian View." *Journal of Medicine and Philosophy* 29 (2): 179–93.

Hancock, K., et al. 2007. "Truth-Telling in Discussing Prognosis in Advanced Life-Limiting Illnesses: A Systematic Review." *Palliative Medicine* 21 (6): 507–17.

Ilkilic, I. 2002. *Der muslimische Patient. Medizinethische Aspekte des muslimischen Krankheitsverständnisses in einer wertpluralen Gesellschaft*, Diss., Münster London: Lit.

———. 2007. "Medizinethische Aspekte im Umgang mit muslimischen Patienten." *Deutsche Medizinische Wochenschrift* 132 (30): 1587–90.

———. 2008. "Kulturelle Aspekte bei ethischen Entscheidungen am Lebensende und interkulturelle Kompetenz." *Bundesgesundheitsblatt Gesundheitsforschung Gesundheitsschutz* 51 (8): 857–64.

Jameton, A. 1995. "Information Disclosure: Ethical Issues." In *Encyclopedia of Bioethics*, edited by W. Reich, 1225–1332. New York: Free Press.

Jotkowitz, A., et al. 2006. "Truth-Telling in a Culturally Diverse World." *Cancer Investigation* 24 (8): 786–89.

Kagawa-Singer, M., and L. J. Blackhall. 2001. "Negotiating Cross-Cultural Issues at the End of Life: 'You Got to Go Where He Lives.'" *JAMA* 286 (23): 2993–3001.

Krakauer, E. L., et al. 2002. "Barriers to Optimum End-of-Life Care for Minority Patients." *Journal of the American Geriatric Society* 50 (1): 182–90.

Macklin, R. 1998. "Ethical Relativism in a Multicultural Society." *Kennedy Institute of Ethics Journal* 8 (1): 1–22.

———. 1999. *Against Relativism. Cultural Diversity and the Search for Ethical Universals in Medicine*. New York: Oxford University Press.

Mobeireek, A. F., et al. 2008. "Information Disclosure and Decision-Making: The Middle East versus the Far East and the West." *Journal of Medical Ethics* 34 (4): 225–29.

Novack, D. H., et al. 1979. "Changes in Physicians' Attitudes toward Telling the Cancer Patient." *Journal of the American Medical Association* 241 (9): 897–900.

Oken, D. 1961. "What to Tell Cancer Patients: A Study of Medical Attitudes." *Journal of the American Medical Association* 175:1120–28.

Ozdogan, M., et al. 2006. "Factors Related to Truth-Telling Practice of Physicians Treating Patients with Cancer in Turkey." *Journal of Palliative Medicine* 9 (5): 1114–19.

Paul, N. W. 2008. "Klinische Ethikberatung: Therapieziele, Patientenwille und Entscheidungsprobleme in der modernen Medizin." In *Grenzsituationen in der Intensivmedizin*, edited by T. Junginger, 208–17. Berlin: Springer.

Pichlmaier, H. 1999. "Wahrheit und Wahrhaftigkeit am Krankenbett." *Deutsches Ärzteblatt* 96 (9): 536–37.

Salomon, F. 2003. "Wahrheit vermitteln am Krankenbett." *Deutsche Medizinische Wochenschrift* 128 (23): 1307–10.

Steinhart, B. 2002. "Patient Autonomy: Evolution of the Doctor-Patient Relationship." *Haemophilia* 8 (3): 441–46.

Sullivan, R. J., et al. 2001. "Truth-Telling and Patient Diagnoses." *Journal of Medical Ethics* 27 (3): 192–97.

Surbone, A. 2006. "Telling the Truth to Patients with Cancer: What Is the Truth?" *Lancet Oncology* 7 (11): 944–50.

Tuckett, A. G. 2004. "Truth-Telling in Clinical Practice and the Arguments For and Against: A Review of the Literature." *Nursing Ethics* 11 (5): 500–13.

Ulsenheimer, K. 2008. *Arztstrafrecht in der Praxis*. Heidelberg: C. F. Müller.

Valente, S. M. 2004. "End of Life and Ethnicity." *Journal for Nurses in Staff Development* 20 (6): 285–93.

Van De Loo, J. 2000. "Aufklärung/Aufklärungspflicht." In *Lexikon der Bioethik*, edited by W. Korff, 284–87. Gütersloh: Gütersloher Verlagshaus.

Volker, D. L. 2005. "Control and End-of-Life Care: Does Ethnicity Matter?" *American Journal of Hospice Palliative Medicine* 22 (6): 442–46.

Walter, U. 2000. "Aufklärung/Aufklärungspflicht. Rechtlich." In *Lexikon der Bioethik*, edited by W. Korff, 287–8. Gütersloh: Gütersloher Verlagshaus, S.

2

Controlled Parenthood

Bioethics and the Notion of the Family

Maya Sabatello

ABSTRACT

The chapter examines the issue of family rights in the scientific era from an international human rights perspective. It looks at the intersection between law, gendered identities, culture, and science, and it analyzes how courts have responded to the quandaries arising in the context of family relations. I argue that the complexities are not only the result of the challenges such questions pose to the moral and cultural construct of the family institution but also, in particular, the gaps between scientific developments and society, and between science as culture and the conceptualization of human rights. Here, it is argued, while scientific progress may play a significant role in the advancement of individuals' family rights, in reality, cultural and morally based barriers hamper such development. The chapter thus provides an innovative, international human rights approach to resolve such dilemmas.

INTRODUCTION

Scientific developments in the past decades have changed the landscape of the family. IVF procedures, surrogacy agreements, gamete donors, and others have enabled the creation of families in circumstances that wouldn't have been possible otherwise. Genetic manipulations have also made it possible to create particular family compositions—disability-free, with a selected sex or other chosen genetic makeup. Even though some celebrate these reproductive technologies (Robertson 1996, 2007–2008), they pose ethical challenges to the family institution "as we know it." Can parental reproductive choice ever be too much? Should gay couples or transgender individuals be eligible for IVF procedures? What are the limits of using such technologies?

Most scholarship focuses on parental reproductive freedom, pressures on women, and the market that has subsequently developed. Less has been written about children who are the product of such technologies. Examining family rights from an international perspective, this chapter looks at the intersection between law, culture, and science. I argue that in addition to the moral and cultural construct of the family institution, the challenges lie in the gaps between scientific developments and society, as in the variance between adults and children's familial perspectives and interests. I therefore propose a child-centered approach to resolve such bioethical dilemmas.

THE TWO REVOLUTIONS AND THE FAMILY

Scientific technologies have created two major revolutions in the family context. First is the development of assisted reproductive technologies (ART). From in vitro fertilization (IVF)[1] to intracytoplasmic sperm injection (ICSI)[2]; from the gametes' harvesting from the dead to using frozen, fertilized embryos; from sperm and egg donation to embryo donation and to partial or full surrogacy;[3] and from ooplasm transfer, creating a child with three genetic parents,[4] to a womb's implantation (Caplan et al. 2007), and to the creation of human sperm that would ostensibly allow a woman to get pregnant without a man (Walsh 2009),[5] the estimation is that "for almost 95% of [infertility] cases today, [there is] an answer" (Wahrman 2005–2006: 128).

The second revolution occurred with the progress in the study of human genetics. The development of preimplementation genetic diagnosis (PGD) has enabled the identification of some gene carriers for major disorders (e.g., cystic fibrosis, Tay Sachs) and of genetic propensity to developing major disorders later in life (e.g., heart disease, cancer, Alzheimer's). It has also enabled the determination of inherited disabilities, the sex of a fetus, and of other genetic traits (Jones 1992–1993). Although improvement of one's genetic endowment and cloning are currently prohibited,[6] these options may be possible in the near future.

The combined effect of these revolutions is tremendous. First, the demographic patterns of reproduction have changed, encouraging nontraditional families: births by older and even postmenopausal women, single mothers, and same-sex couples (Daar 2008: 32–33; Shapiro 2005–2006: 608). Through ART, lesbian couples can be both biologically linked to the child: one partner provides the egg (genetic mother), the other serves as the gestating mother. Individuals may also parent children long after their death if their gametes were properly harvested (Dwyer 1999–2000, Katz 2006). Parenthood, therefore, now exists in many forms.

Childhood is also increasingly experienced in familial pluralism—from traditional mother and father to single parent to same-sex couples and to orphanhood by parental or others' choice. Furthermore, the genetic commonality among siblings within a family may vary significantly—from similar genetic parents, to about two-thirds in ooplasm transfer, to 50 percent in sperm or egg donation, to no genetic link at all (full gametes donation). Moreover, genetic siblings may be scattered across the globe.

Second, ART creates a complex web of procreation, which today potentially includes many partners. Doctors are vital players, holding the power to decide whom they will treat.[7] It is possible that religious and other cultural considerations, for example, of same-sex couples or of single parenthood, influence their decision (Appel 2006: 20–21). Gametes donors and surrogate mothers may also be critical actors. The lack of such services in some countries has led to "fertility (or reproductive) tourism," whereby the gametes and reproductive services are bought and sold across borders (Smerdon 2008: 22; Storrow 2005–2006: 203).

Additionally, as a growing number of states changed their regulations to identifiable donors, prospective parents turn to other countries where anonymity is allowed (Van den Akker 2006: 95). Consequently, a child born through ART may have five or more individuals playing a significant role in the reproductive process.[8]

Finally, the demography of ART children has changed, with a rise in multiple births (twins, triplets, and more). The birth of twins following fertility treatment is especially common,[9] particularly when the private market controls the use of such technologies (as in the United States). The high costs paid from personal resources often leads prospective parents to opt for multiple births, regardless of risks (Robertson 2009: 28).[10]

Simultaneously, the development of genetic diagnosis and manipulation have led to far more genetic screening for fetuses with disabilities, particularly among ART users, as women of older age, multiple births, and arguably, the technologies themselves have been linked to increased birth defects, genetic disorders, and other ailments (Skloot 2009; Carbone 2007–2008: 1764).[11] Preimplantation genetic diagnosis (PGD) has been increasingly used also for other reasons, however—such as sex selection and "matching tissue siblings" (Aulisio et al. 2001: 408), and it gave rise to parental requests for other traits that the future child will have—for example, height, hair color, athletic potential (Davis 2009: 25–26). What are, then, the parental rights, obligations, and duties toward the child? And where are the ART children in this discourse?

A RIGHT TO (ASSISTED) FOUND A FAMILY?

Most scholarly work on ART has focused on the legal, philosophical, and political aspects of parental decision to found a family—and perhaps intuitively so. Indeed, an array of international treaties acknowledge the family as the "natural and fundamental group unit of society," entitling it to protection by society and state. International human rights instruments also explicitly recognize the right to found a family, to enjoy the rights and responsibilities as parents, and the right to "decide freely and responsibly on the number and spacing of their children."[12]

The Children's Convention holds the family as the chief actor in the child's well-being and development. Articles 7 and 8 of the Convention explicitly stipulate that a child has "a right, . . . as far as possible, to know and be cared for by his or her parents"; and that states "undertake to respect the right of the child to preserve his or her identity, including . . . family relations." These articles are unique, and I will return to them later. For now, these family-rights provisions raise two sets of questions. First, are these rights translated into one's right to use ART? Is parental selection of an offspring's characteristics part of one's reproductive freedom? As will be examined, both questions have been highly controversial. The second set pertains to ART children, and whether such technologies are in line with children's bioethical, familial, and other rights.

ART AND THE RIGHT TO FOUND A FAMILY

Some recent developments suggest that ART may be included within the universal right to found a family. The estimation is that 10 to 20 percent of couples in the Western/developed world experience infertility (Goodwin 2005–2006: 16). Infertility is further prevalent with late childbearing, particularly when race is factored in,[13] among economically and socially less privileged groups, and in developing countries, where poverty, the lack of proper health services, and other environmental hazards result in infertility.[14] There are also male factors causing barrenness (Goodwin 2005–2006: 20) and the emotional/psychological costs of infertility. Health insurance programs increasingly acknowledge infertility as a medical condition and cover some costs associated with ART (Daar 2008: 30–31; Lauritzen 1990: 43).

Another argument centers on what some term social infertility. Included here are individuals who can reproduce in "the traditional way," yet that for various social and other reasons cannot—or do not want—to do so. Gay couples, for example, may be physically fertile yet need reproductive assistance, as they are not engaged in heterosexual relations. Persons with disabilities are often excluded from reproductive services, assuming that their disability (whatever it is) prevents them from functioning as parents (Degener 2001). Transgender individuals are another example: Some state's laws condition eligibility for sex-reassignment surgery and for the change of legal documents on infertility, forcing such individuals to discard otherwise naturally healthy reproductive organs, along with their hope for genetic offspring (Eisfeld 2008: 21; Norton 2006: 189–90).

The rubric of social infertility includes single-parent families, particularly single women without a partner who depend on reproductive technologies to procreate (Daar 2008: 31–32). Many of these women delayed childbirth as part of the Western "new middle class morality" that emphasizes higher education, professionalization, and financial independence prior to childbirth, and a sense of entitlement to reproductive technologies (Carbone 2007–2008: 1762). Thus, excluding all those who suffer from physical and social infertility from the scope of the right to found a family and to procreate would compromise the rights granted under international law.

Some have taken the scope of one's reproductive freedom in the ART context beyond infertility. Considering the financial, social, emotional, and other burdens associated with raising that child, it is argued that parental decision about their commitment should be respected (Robertson 1996, Hull 2006). Accordingly, one's right to reproductive freedom should include one's choice of how to procreate, under what circumstances to do so (economically disadvantaged, multiples pregnancy, posthumous conception, etc.), and also a choice regarding the screening against inherited disability, selection of an offspring's sex, and other genetic characteristics (Robertson 1996), including, potentially, a "savior sibling" (Robertson et al. 2002).

Not all support this proposition, however. Opponents raise liberal-based objections, including concerns about the child's commodification and the potential loss of the child's status as a subject with inherent moral value as a human being (Davis 1997: 12). Religious authorities have raised concerns about the moral adequacy of "playing God" in the holy act of human creation (Wahrman 2005–2006: 130), the status of pre-embryos and embryos (Cohen 2006), and the child's religious identity (Schenker 2003: 257).[15]

The accuracy of this proposition is questionable on legal grounds. State laws often reflect religious, cultural, and other historical considerations, making it impossible to discern a universal standard of reproductive services (Robertson 2004–2005, Ravitsky 2004, Zahraa and Shafie 2006). Relevant international bodies have interpreted the right to found a family only conservatively, focusing on gender equality in the family without suggesting any positive duties on states to assist those seeking to procreate (Harris-Short 2004: 339–40). Indeed, such qualification may be in place: The costs associated with ART[16] may be beyond the reach—and the reasonable expectation—that states, particularly impoverished ones, have an obligation to fulfill.

European treaties on biomedicine and human rights seem to support this conclusion as well. Sex selection and genetic modifications for nonheredity-related diseases are prohibited (Articles 13, 14 of the Convention), and although screening for disabilities has gained legal acceptance (Articles 12, 13, 18), there is a strong disability rights movement that has fervently challenged it (Pfeiffer 1999, Shakespeare 2006).

Courts provide inconsistent and often contradictory answers. For instance, in a frozen embryo conflict,[17] the ECHR found the right *not* to procreate prevails over the right to procreate, although the implications were that the woman has lost all possibilities of becoming a genetic mother (*Evans v. UK* 2006).[18] This decision follows American state courts (Waldman 2003–2004) but opposes the Israeli Supreme Court decision of *Nachmani v. Nachmani* (1996).

In another case, and in contrast to some U.S. cases (Beatie 2008),[19] the ECHR rejected an application of a couple consisting of a woman and a woman-to-male transgender that the latter be recognized as the legal father of a child conceived via IVF with an anonymous donor. This was so although both the sex-change operation and the IVF procedure were covered by the national health insurance and despite the father's written informed consent and formal commitment, before the IVF, that he would serve as such (*X, Y, Z v. UK* 1997).

Conversely, the ECHR accepted the petition of a couple, the man serving a life sentence in prison, that the authorities' refusal to allow them to use ART violated their right to family and privacy (*Dickson v. UK* 2007). Yet again in another recent decision, the Grand Chamber of the ECHR rejected the applicants' argument that the governmental policy prohibiting the use of gamete donation of ova or sperm for IVF constitutes discrimination and violates their rights to family and private life. Reversing the ECHR's ruling of April 2010, this decision was issued although the requested procedure would have been the only way for the applicants to conceive children.

Drawing all-inclusive answers is thus impossible, but the sense that, although the Court recognizes reproductive freedom and autonomy, value-laden, sociocultural considerations are behind the rulings. They elucidate how the interests, perspectives, and ultimately (family) rights of ART children have been ignored.

CHILDREN BORN OF ART: EXISTING APPROACHES

Internationally, about three million babies were born following the use of ART so far, and two hundred thousand babies are born each year to women using IVF (Daar 2008: 29–30). Thus, although parents and medical professionals clearly hold a decision-making power, a discussion on children born of ART is in order. What sort of interests or rights, then, does a future child or the child born of ART have?

Literature about ART and the genetic selection of offspring has only recently tackled the issue from a child-centered perspective. This is a result of social pressure: Infertility is often viewed as shameful, and using ART, particularly donated gametes, frequently remains a secret from the closest family—including from the child born as a result (Van den Akker 2006: 96). Existing scholastic work, on the other hand, generally takes one of the two following approaches. The first relies on the concepts of "the child's welfare" and "best interests" as enshrined in the Children's Convention. Some legal frameworks and soft law regulations have adopted these standards as well, requiring doctors to evaluate whether prospective parents are "able to provide adequate child-rearing" before the provision of fertility services (Robertson 2009: 27).

The second approach, advanced by children's rights advocates, suggests that the main concern should be the protection of "the child's right to an open future" (Feinberg 1980: 125–27). The doctrine suggests that children have some protectable "rights-in-trust" for the child to exercise later in adulthood, and that policies should maximize the child's possible life choices (Davis 2001: 24).

In practice, these approaches often led to similar bioethical conclusions. Selection for a disability-free offspring should be respected, whereas sex-selection and parental choosing of other genetic characteristics are to be avoided (Davis 2009). Consideration of the child's interests has also led some to determine that untraditional family structures, particularly homosexuals and posthumous conceptions, would not provide a sufficiently stable physical, emotional, and financial environment for the child's maximum development and growth (Fasoulioties and Schenker 1995: 27; Katz 2006).

Although these approaches are commonly used, their application is limited in that they are vague and fail to see the many cultural constructions of a child's welfare, best interests, and also what would the child's "right to on open future" entail. Which disabilities are substantial enough to undermine the child's interest and give rise to a duty to avoid? Considering that nature itself allows for a continuum of physiological sex, can selection for a girl or for a boy be against the child's interest? And as courts around the world have recognized instances in which children's donation of organs is in their best interests (Aulisio et al. 2001: 409–10), is parental selection for a "savior sibling," where the future child has tissue composition that could be used to treat a sibling with a fatal disease, necessarily wrong? Or, where should the line be drawn (only umbilical cord, blood quotas, bone marrow, kidney)? As it becomes clear, these approaches are inherently open for the subjective judgment, indeed, the sociocultural preferences, of the decision maker.

The context of children is further complex. First, the biomedical decisions are made by adults (parents, doctors, courts, etc.) on their behalf. Children are not—and in the ART context, also clearly cannot be—regarded as the patients, and besides, their young age often excludes them from giving an informed consent on their own. They are, however, the most direct product of the reproductive decisions taken. Second, the calculation of factors to consider in regard to a proposed infertility treatment, on the one hand, and the (future) child's interests, on the other hand, is oftentimes too simplistic.

Often, the child's (future) welfare and best interests are merely positioned in opposition to the parental reproductive freedom and autonomy. However, such balancing is impossible considering the different nature of these two values (Davis 2001: 23). It is also too individual oriented, failing to view the family's interests as a whole (Dwyer and Vig 1995: 9; Lindemann and Lindemann Nelson 2008: 20). Subsequently, it also fails to consider the (future) child's own voice.

How should ART dilemmas be resolved from a child-centered perspective, then? To state the obvious, no one bright-rule for all cases can be stipulated, and decisions should be made on a case-by-case basis. Exploring all the possible ART scenarios, however, is also too broad. The remainder of this chapter thus merely aims to draw attention to some of the factors that, from a child-centered perspective, are most important to consider. As it will be revealed, the discussion on ART children has been heavily based on adults' perspectives regarding disabilities, gender roles, the genetic tie, and ultimately, about what constitutes "proper" families, but very little on children's own views.

CHILDREN'S BIOETHICS AND THE FAMILY IN THE NEW SCIENTIFIC ERA

Elsewhere, I suggested an alternative dual model to examine children's bioethical rights (Sabatello 2009: 189–95). The first path examines the medical/health implications of the medical intervention on the (future) child; the second path explores the identity implications of such a procedure; and the balancing of these two determines the result. The combination of these two paths, I argued, provides the space to capture the web of relations in which biomedical decisions are made and the contextual interdependency in which the (future) child (and in fact, all individuals) will exercise her rights.[20]

Furthermore, as children do not have traditional autonomy, conceptualized as "freedom from others," it was suggested that, first, children's autonomy is understood as "autonomy in relations" or "autonomy with others," that is, that their autonomy is inherently intertwined with their relationships with others; and second, that from a child's perspective, this autonomy is translated into identity.

Identity embodies the "entire fabric around [one's] knot," including family, ancestors, and successors, other webs of relationships, and one's sense of belonging (Panikkar 1982: 90–91), and thus it provides children the (only) space in which they exercise any given interests or rights (Bilsky 1998: 144–5).[21] Coming to examine the bioethical dilemmas arising from the two ART revolutions from a child-centered perspective, I now turn to discuss both paths.

MEDICAL/HEALTH PATH

In the ART context, two main issues arise under the medical/health path. First, there is a risk of disabilities and genetic defects, which is arguably higher (see above); and second, there is the sense that the selection of desired characteristics is almost offhand for individuals and couples who resort to IVF and PGD for physical or social infertility as they are already in a position in which only a few of the created embryos will be selected and implanted in the womb. The question is therefore: When is the selection of genetic characteristics *medically* justified?

Clearly, not all ART-related conception stories raise direct concerns under this path. Posthumous conception, sex selection, or choosing an offspring with a matching tissue, for example, do not pose a medical/health dilemma on their own, or, at least, not much beyond traditional reproduction: they can all occur naturally. The most prevalent claim raised in this regard is about parental responsibility—possibly also moral duty—to screen against disabilities.[22] As the argument goes, the ART context requires the application of a concept of *wronging*, of treating one unjustly or injuriously, and hence it also justifies interference with others' interests and rights (Kahn 1991a).

Although disability-related concerns may be valid, the discussion has been greatly occupied by some misconceptions about disability that may unjustly tilt toward a disability-free resolution. Most significantly are the habitual equation between disability and (bad) health, although in most types of disabilities no such connection can be made[23]; the usual connotation between disability and suffering, even a life of misery (Kahn 1991a: 303–6), although in practice, for most persons with disabilities the impairment is merely a part of everyday life that ontologically is "unimportant" (Watson 2002: 518, 524); and finally, the conventional supposition that disability (and in fact, also the "suffering" or even the "intolerable suffering" associated with it) is an objective medical condition that is well known and agreed upon.

In reality, there is no cross-cultural definition of "disability," and the term can only be defined by the norms of normalcy and the expected roles and tasks within each given cultural group (Renteln 2003: 59). These have also been reinforced in research with children. The disability was often not viewed as "different" or "abnormal," and also when they observed differences, they did not attribute to it the negative connotation as adults (Stalker and Connors 2004, 224–25; Deal 2003: 899).

As with other ART-related conception stories (sex selection, posthumous conception, etc.), relying on the health and disease-related rationales as general justification for genetic interventions to eradicate disabilities is incorrect. The typical reaction to disability does not correspond to the individual's experience of persons with disabilities—including children—of their own impairment (Reeve 2002: 495, 504), and furthermore, a determination of any consensual objective criteria to distinguish between "easy" and "severe" disabilities, or of which types give rise to parental and others' biomedical duty to avoid, is impossible.

Thus, from the future child's perspective, once ART were used, the most basic—and possibly, only—medical/health consideration is whether or not she would survive.[24] Accordingly, parental reproductive choice that significantly raises the likelihood of death should be rejected. Aside from degenerate disabilities, the only ART scenario that squarely falls within this rubric is parental intentional decision of multifetal pregnancy (beyond triplet). Indeed, in contrast to the handful of astonishing stories of sextuplets, octuplets, and more, many other multiple-birth children do not survive (Fasouliotis and Schenker 1995: 31).

I would also limit savior-sibling scenarios under this path. While donation of tissue from the umbilical cord poses no health implications to the donor child, donations that require medical intervention that substantially raise the likelihood of complications (particularly nonrenewable organs) should be prohibited. The determination is, of course, more complex, as between these two extremes the degrees and types of medical risks greatly vary for different organs or tissue. This, however, is also where broader family considerations, most pertinent the donor child's own perception of her (future) familial relations, come into play, necessitating, along with the other ART-related scenarios, the examination of their compatibility with the identity path as well.

IDENTITY PATH

Identity considerations are increasingly recognized as integral to the resolution of bioethical dilemmas. Indeed, also the European Conventions on Biomedicine and Human Rights state as their goal the protection of "dignity and identity of all human beings."[25] The disentanglement between identity and bioethics is especially evident in ART children as using such technologies may create mixtures of familial environments and may have significant implications on their status within their community.[26] What sort of identity considerations does a child perspective entail? The examination focuses on two main points that, in my view, require reconsideration.

First is the connection between genetic characteristics and identity. Too often, opponents of offspring's genetic selection justify their stance, at least partially, in the presumed (negative) impact it would have on the child's identity. In the context of disabilities, the assumptions have been that there is a "disabled identity" that is inherently based on one's impairment (Watson 2002: 513) and that it is substantially different from an "abled identity" and for the worst.

Selecting for a girl (for nondisability-related reasons) has been opposed, also in cases of "family balancing," on the ground that it would fixate gender roles and impose a stereotyped gendered identity on the child (Davis 2001: 100–1). Similarly, "savior-siblings" critics have argued that it would force a "donor identity" on the child characterized by anxiety, a lesser sense of worth, and living in the shadow of the ill sibling, regardless of his or her other characteristics and interests (Goodwin 2006–2007: 364, 371).

While these concerns cannot be rejected on the spot, their flaw is that they give too much weight to one or more biological factors in the construction of the child's identity. Although one's genetic combination certainly determines some aspects—for example, appearance and certain personal traits—there are multiple other factors such as family relations, peers, and a given sociocultural environment that play an even greater role in the formation of the child's (and adult's) identity (Hur and Bouchard 1995: 341). Identities are also not fixed, and they are always in the process of changing, greatly depending on one's social interaction (Persson 1995: 22).

Opponents of genetic selection do not necessarily ignore this, as they raise concerns that the procedure would "de-emphasize important parts of parental responsibility," particularly the sense of relatedness, warmth, and love (McGee 1997: 17–18), or that parents would be more frustrated, intolerant, and possibly also detached from the child if disappointed with the actual outcome (Davis 2009: 26–27). Such suggestions seem a sweeping generalization, however, and they also show the double standard in the relationship between genetics and identity.

There is no evidence that parents of children with disabilities detach themselves more than is prevalent in the general population, and that sex selection may be for reasons that significantly differ from a parental desire to entrench specific gender roles in the child.[27] Also in savior-sibling cases there is no reason to assume that parents who love one child enough to have another will care any less about the savior child once born (Aulisio 2001: 415). Indeed, no evidence was found that negative psychological impact would necessarily occur, and furthermore, although the dynamic among the family members may certainly be more complex, it has been suggested that such donation among siblings may strengthen the familial bonds and the child's own sense of value within the family (Lotz 2009: 296).

Focusing on narrow genetic characteristics as the determinants of one's identity to prohibit parental selection is thus misguided, as it unjustly essentializes something that cannot be essentialized. Moreover, by doing so, it strengthens the stereotypes that are associated with it: disability-free—yes; sex-selection and savior sibling—no; although ultimately in all these instances the real issues at stake are not genetics but the sociocultural norms.

Such essentialism of identity also ignores the child's voice. Studies with children with disabilities have shown fluidity and pluralism of identities, also within groups of disabilities, depending on their social and familial relationships as well as ethnic, religious, and cultural backgrounds (Sabatello 2009: 215–20). The process of identity formation resembles among children regardless of disability, sex, and other factors— that is, it is formed by both processes of inclusion and exclusion and by means of comparing others to them (Stalker and Connors 2004: 224).

Furthermore, children's sexual and other identity-related development has much to do with the activities they are allowed or disallowed to perform (Kelle 2001), and no differences were found between children who are raised by traditional, single parent, or same-sex families in this regard (Fasouliotis and Schenker 1995: 28). In fact, studies have consistently shown that in terms of family relations, parenting qualities, and social and emotional development, ART children are better off than their naturally conceived children (Golombok et al. 1995; Papaligoura and Trevarthen 2001).

Put differently, a child—any child—has no preference (or say) on her own as to whether being of one sex rather than the other, disabled rather than abled-body, matching or not matching tissue sibling, and so forth, is preferable over the other. For the child, this is the reality into which he or she is being born—that's the only reality he or she knows. Indeed, this is the unique—and nevertheless only one piece of—the life story that each of us has as part of our identity.

Secondly, the importance attributed to the genetic tie needs reconsideration. This issue has been acutely debated in regard to the anonymity of donor gametes, suggesting that donor offspring suffer negative consequences of poor self-perception, feelings of being different in the family in which she is raised, and generally, that she would have identity crises—or in an analogy to an adoptee: confusion regarding her family descent ("genealogical bewilderment") if not provided with at least some identifying information about her genetic origin (Roberts 1995: 217; Van den Akker 2006: 96; McWhinnie 2001: 814).

The narrative of children's rights has often been used, with children's rights advocates commonly reiterating Articles 7 and 8 of the Children's Convention, insisting that ART children have a right to know their conception story and their genetic origin (e.g., Frith 2001). As Van den Akker blatantly argued, "If the best interests of the child are considered, clearly non-disclosing parents are not considering the child's rights, but their own" (Van den Akker 2006: 96).[28]

True, the drafters of the aforementioned articles had biological origins in mind, and some states (e.g., the UK, Austria, Switzerland) have also interpreted them in this manner (Frith 2001: 821, Blyth and Frith 2009). A few points need stressing, however. First, the significance of the genetic link to the notion of the family is not equally relevant across cultures and communities—also within Western states. Among African Americans, for example, informal adoption and a network of women caring for children not genetically linked to them is prevalent, and the notion of the family, brotherhood, and sisterhood is based on a political—not genetic—agenda (Roberts 1995: 232).

In fact, also in Western and U.S. legal structure, the bond between biological parenthood (particularly fatherhood) and parental-child psychological attachment was never a "natural given" but a social construct (Roberts 1995, Waldman 2003–2004). This disconnection between the genetic tie and the family is especially apparent in the "new family": studies consistently show that gametes donors, mainly sperm donors, are unconcerned with the offspring their sperm/egg creates, have no sense of attachment to it, do not want to meet them in the future, and that their motivation for donating is overwhelmingly financial (Waldman 2003–2004: 1049–52).[29] Considering the characteristics of gamete donors, notably following the trend to nonanonymity (older men, often married, some reported mild psychopathology and alcohol abuse) (Van den Akker 2006: 94), the genetic father may be far from what the child has had in mind.

By insisting on the child's right to know her genetic origins, there is therefore a risk of exposing her to the experience of abandonment akin to an adoptee, and indeed, it can create a possible identity crisis. Second, it is not clear that the genetic link is as important to the children themselves. Instances in which donor offspring expressed anger, frustration, and other behavior more likely happened in traumatic circumstances (e.g., during divorce battles), or when the offspring were already adults (Van den Akker 2006: 96; McWhinnie 2001: 812).

This does not necessarily reinforce the importance of the genetic tie, however—first, as the anger may have occurred when the expected familial trust failed (rather than the lack of knowledge about genetic origins per se),[30] and second, as it is possible that by the time of disclosure, these adults were already fully acculturated into the traditional notion of the family as necessitating a genetic link.

On the other hand, research with ART children has shown no harmful consequences of nondisclosure (Van den Akker 2006: 96). Indeed, considering that most donor offspring do not know about their story of conception, it is improbable to assume otherwise. Moreover, studies with young children who were told about the donors have shown inconclusive results. Four-year-olds in The Netherlands who were born to heterosexual couples reacted neutrally to the subject or did not show any reaction, although they were the ones who raised the question about how they were born (Leeb-Lundberg et al. 2006: 79); and among children ages seven to seventeen raised by lesbian couples in Belgium, about half preferred donor anonymity, 27 percent were interested in meeting the donor (mostly boys), and the rest were satisfied with nonidentifying information.

Differences were also found between siblings raised in one family (including siblings from the same donor), leading the researchers to conclude that the importance of learning about the genetic origin is individual (Vanfraussen et al. 2001: 2021). Finally, these results also make sense from a sociological perspective.

Research with children on kinship has consistently shown that children include in their definition of "my family" household members, pets, a range of relatives, and individuals from other households (Mason and Tipper 2008: 441, 453–56). Thus, the insistence on the child's right to know her genetic origin seems more in the adults' interest based on the importance of the genetic link rather than of the child's own voice. Indeed, it is also for this reason that the decision of the ECHR in the *X*,

Y and Z case rejecting the request of the woman-to-man transgender/social father to be registered as the legal father is all the more appalling. Without even asking for the (then) six-year-old child's opinion, the Court merely adopted an adult's perspective, reasoning its decision on her *possible* interest in finding out one day who her biological father was.

This survey is not intended to undermine the efforts of children's rights advocates to create appropriate mechanisms for disclosing donor offspring's genetic origin. Certainly, disclosure may be of interest to some children, and open communication between parents and their ART children is preferable. Instead, the issue at stake here is the exaggerated importance we attribute to the genetic link in the determination of one's familial and other identity. So where does that leave the notion of the family in the scientific era?

BIOETHICS, CHILDREN, AND THE NEW FAMILY

New scientific developments in the context of reproduction have shaken up some deeply rooted sociocultural notions about the family's structure, and further, about what family is. The examination of the consequent bioethical dilemmas has been overwhelmingly subjugated by adults' discourse. The leading themes have been parental reproductive freedom, autonomy, and privacy in family life, often translated into the bioethical requirement of informed consent; the market forces; and the ever-increasing control of doctors in the act of procreation. While intuitive, and certainly important, constructing the discussion in this way has also meant that only little room has been left for the examination of the interests—and particularly views—of children born of ART.

Scholarly work on ART children has only recently begun in the effort to close this gap. Research has focused on the medical and psychological aspects of the ART children, reporting on a range of possible disabilities, hyperactivity, sense of vulnerability, and disclosure (Van den Akker 2006: 96). When focusing on the children themselves, scholars have followed children's rights' narratives, suggesting that the bioethical dilemmas are resolved in accordance with the child's welfare, best interests, and right to an open future. In practice, the examination has been too narrow, essentially substituting the parental-rights discourse with one that focuses on children, without looking at the broader familial picture or suggesting mechanisms to deal with the sociocultural root causes of some genetic selections, and furthermore, without actually listening to the child's own voice.

The dual-path model suggested is aimed to overcome at least some of these problems. It takes a case-by-case approach, acknowledging that diversity in circumstances and opinions may exist also among members of one family. By eliminating instances that substantially increase the child's morbidity (the medical/health path) and refocus on identity through the exploration of family relations, we capitalize the only space where children exercise rights. Such examination also illuminates, and allows, stepping away from the sociocultural prejudices and misconceptions about which medical intervention, from a child's perspective, are indeed justified, and about the importance of the genetic link to the child's sense of identity and family relations.

As I have shown, ART children do not necessarily share adults' attribution of importance to the genetic link or to the right to know. For children, the critical issue is whether or not they are—and always have been—wanted, and the corresponding positive, supportive, and nurturing relationship they develop with "their family" (Golombok et al. 1995: 297). And as studies have consistently found, ART children, including donor children, often enjoy these to a greater extent than non-ART children.

Positive attitudes and acceptance of ART, also in difficult bioethical dilemmas, often occur only when one encounters the situation (Van den Akker 2006: 92). Yet this does not need—and should not need—to be the case. Pronatalism is a universal culture, which scientific developments in reproduction aim to achieve. Perhaps a greater understanding and appreciation of children's views would change the discourse to the right direction. In a world where, on the one hand, the rates of divorce and remarriage is sky-rocketing, there is a visible rise in international and national adoption and in nontraditional family structures; and furthermore, also among traditional families a marked number of fathers (in the UK, one out of seven fathers) unknowingly raise children to whom they are genetically unrelated (McWhinnie 2001: 814).

On the other hand, a distinction between a genetic, social, and gestational parent can be made. Gametes are being sold, and genetic-related siblings and other individuals can be traced across the globe, so there is a need to reconsider if the old notion of the "family" still holds. Ultimately, the sociocultural barriers to the smooth reception of the diversity of families are to blame, and yet it is too often the children who suffer the result. This is a price that society should not be willing to accept.

NOTES

1. In IVF the egg is fertilized in a lab's Petri dish and then implanted in the womb.
2. In ICSI single sperms are mechanically injected into individual eggs to overcome a male's infertility.
3. In partial surrogacy the birth mother's egg is fertilized by the intended father's sperm. In full surrogacy the embryo implanted in the surrogate's womb (through IVF) has no genetic link to her.
4. In ooplasm transfer a small amount of the extranuclear material from a healthy egg donor is injected into the infertile woman's egg to increase the likelihood of fertilization.
5. Ooplasm transfer, womb implantation, and sperm creation are in the experimental stage.
6. Additional Protocol on the Prohibition of Cloning Human Beings; Article 11 of the Universal Declaration on the Human Genome and Human Rights.
7. Doctors have the discretion whether to provide medical treatment in nonemergency situations.

8. Actors can include: sperm donor, ova/egg donor, surrogate mother, intended parents, as well as relevant infertility clinicians and surrogacy agencies and more.

9. In 2005, 35 percent of ART births were multiple births (mostly twins), in comparison to less than 2 percent in the general population (Robertson 2009: 28; Goodwin 2005–2006: 6).

10. A single IVF cycle costs in the United States about $10,000. The price can double, depending on the clinic, and women often also need more than one cycle (Daar 2008: 36–37). Medication and other procedures, such as a preimplantation genetic diagnosis (PGD), add expenses.

11. Chromosomal abnormality occurs in 40 to 50 percent of pregnancies in women ages thirty to thirty-five, and in about 70 percent in women over forty (Carbone 2007–2008, fn. 104). Akker (2006: 96), though, dismisses such estimations.

12. Article 16, Universal Declaration of Human Rights; Article 23, International Covenant on Civil and Political Rights; Article 23, Convention on the Rights of Persons with Disabilities; Article 16, Convention on the Elimination of All Forms of Discrimination Against Women.

13. Women's fertility declines from early thirties and dramatically drops after the age of thirty-five. African American women have higher birthrates than white women until the age of twenty-five, but they lower at every age over twenty-five (Carbone 2007–2008: 1764).

14. Carbone 2007–2008: 1763–4, 1768; Storrow 2005–2006: 190. Infertility in developing countries is higher, reaching in some Sub-Saharan African states to 29 percent (Hoerbst 2009: 4).

15. Some religions have liberal attitudes toward ART—Baptists, Mormons, Presbyterian, Anglican Church, and Jehovah's Witness (Schenker 2003: 257).

16. See fn. 11.

17. In frozen embryo cases, couples who used ART split and now disagree about the created embryos' fate.

18. Before removing the woman's ovaries, her eggs were extracted, and following her husband's reassurance, they were fertilized with his sperm. The husband later withdrew his consent.

19. Thomas Beatie is a woman-to-man transgender who delivered in June 2008 a girl, conceived via IVF with anonymous sperm donor. He had chest reconstruction and testosterone therapy but kept his reproductive organs.

20. This aspect of children's rights builds on the feminist's "relational approach"/"ethic of care."

21. Autonomy is positioned on a scale: the traditional "autonomy from others" and autonomy *as* identity are the two extremes (Bilsky 1998: 145).

22. This includes all circumstances in which the likelihood of disability/genetic disorder is higher—multiple births, older mothers and gametes donors, and the multiple use of a gamete from one donor due to the potential future incest relations between siblings.

23. In cases such as Huntington's disease, Tay Sachs, and cystic fibrosis, the genetic carrier intrinsically involves significant health implications and deterioration up to death. Principally, however, persons with disabilities lead a completely healthy life but their impairment causes limitations.

24. This does not mean, though, that a child is necessarily better off to exist than not exist at all.

25. Articles 1, the Convention on Biomedicine and Human Rights and of its Additional Protocols; Preamble, Additional Protocol on the Prohibition of Cloning.

26. In Judaism, for example, a donor offspring may be a *mamzer* (bastard) who is excluded from participating and marrying within the community and also loses the father's religious status (Schenker 2003: 255–6; Wahrman 2005–2006: 131–33).

27. For example, for some, a Jewish man fulfills the commandment to procreate if he parents both a girl and a boy.

28. Some emphasize the importance of retrieving one's genetic origin for the collection of medical data (McWhinnie 2001: 815). As scientific developments increasingly allow for the diagnosis of *propensity* for inherited diseases, this rationale loses its force.

29. The financial incentive for gametes donation is stronger among men than women, and women have expressed greater interest in future offspring (Akker 2006: 93–94).

30. Donor offspring who discovered unexpectedly their conception story have consistently expressed a desire not to be *deceived* (Akker 2006: 96).

REFERENCES

Appel, J. M. 2006. "May Doctors Refuse Infertility Treatments to Gay Patients?" *The Hastings Center Report* 36 (4): 20–21.

Aulisio, M. P., T. May, and G. D. Block. 2001. "Procreation for Donation: The Moral and Political Permissibility of 'Having a Child to Save a Child.'" *Cambridge Quarterly of Healthcare Ethics 10*: 408–19.

Beatie, T. 2008. "Labor of Love." *Advocate* 1005:24.

Bilsky, L. 1998. "Child-Parent-State: The Absence of Community in the Courts' Approach to Education." In *Children's Rights and Traditional Values*, edited by G. Douglas and L. Sebba, 134–59. Burlington, VT: Ashgate Publishing Company.

Blyth, E., and L. Frith. 2009. "Donor-Conceived People's Access to Genetic and Biographical History: An Analysis of Provisions in Different Jurisdictions Permitting Disclosure of Donor Identity." *International Journal of Law, Policy & the Family* 23 (2): 174–91.

Caplan, A. L. et al. 2007. "Moving the Womb." *The Hastings Center Report* 37 (3): 18–20.

Carbone, J. 2007–2008. "If I Say 'Yes' to Regulation Today, Will You Still Respect Me in the Morning?" *George Washington Law Review* 76:1747–71.

Cohen, E. 2006. "Conservative Bioethics & the Search for Wisdom." *The Hastings Center Report* 36 (1): 44–56.

Daar, J. F. 2008. "Accessing Reproductive Technologies: Invisible Barriers, Indelible Harms." *Berkeley Journal of Gender, Law & Justice* 23:18–82.

Davis, D. S. 1997. "Genetic Dilemmas and the Child's Right to an Open Future." *Hastings Center Report* 27 (2): 7–15.

———. 2001. *Genetic Dilemmas: Reproductive Technologies, Parental Choices, and Children's Future*. New York: Routledge Publishing.

———. 2009. "The Parental Investment Factor and the Child's Right to an Open Future." *The Hastings Center Report* 39 (2): 24–27.

Deal, M. 2003. "Disabled People's Attitudes Toward Other Impairment Groups: A Hierarchy of Impairment." *Disability & Society* 18 (7): 897–910.

Degener, T. 2001. "Disabled Women and International Human Rights." In *Women and International Human Rights Law*, edited by K. D. Askin and D. M. Koenig, 267–93. Ardsley, NY: Transnational.

Dickson v. UK (Grand Chamber), Application no. 44362/04, European Court of Human Rights, Judgment of 4 December 2007.

Dwyer, J., and E. Vig. 1995. "Rethinking Transplantation Between Siblings." *The Hastings Center Report* 25 (5): 7–12.

Dwyer, L. 1999–2000. "Dead Daddies: Issues in Postmortem Reproduction." *Rutgers Law Rev.* 52:881–910.

Eisfeld, J. 2008. "'Sterile Yet?' Don't Be Alarmed, It's Standard Procedure!" *Magazine of ILGA-Europe, Equality* 8 (1): 21.

Evans v. the UK, Application no. 6339/05, European Court of Human Rights, Judgment of 7 March 2006.

Fasoulioties, S. J., and J. G. Schenker. 1999. "Social Aspects in Assisted Reproduction." *Human Reproduction Update* 5 (1): 26–39.

Feinberg, J. 1980. "The Child's Right to an Open Future." In *Whose Child? Children's Rights, Parental Authority, and State Power*, edited by W. Aiken and H. LaFollette, 124–53. Totowa, NJ: Littlefield, Adams.

Frith, L. 2001. "Gamete Donation and Anonymity: The Legal and Ethical Debate." *Human Reproduction* 16 (5): 818–25.

Golombok, S. et al. 1995. "Families Created by the New Reproductive Technologies: Quality of Parenting and Social and Emotional Development of Children." *Child Development* 66 (2): 285–98.

Goodwin, M. 2005–2006. "Assisted Reproductive Technology and the Double Bind: The Illusory Choice of Motherhood." *The Journal of Gender, Race & Justice* 9:1–54.

———. 2006–2007. "My Sister's Keeper: Law, Children, and Compelled Donation." *Western New England Law Rev.* 29 (1): 357–404.

Harris-Short, S. 2004. "An 'Identity Crisis' in the International Law of Human Rights? The Challenge of Reproductive Cloning." *International Journal Children's Rights* 11:333–68.

Hoerbst, V. 2009. "In the Making—Assisted Reproductive Technologies in Mali, West Africa." *Anthropology News*, February, 4–5.

Hull, Richard J. 2006. "Cheap Listening?—Reflections on the Concept of Wrongful Disability." *Bioethics* 20 (2): 55–63.

Hur, Y. M., and T. J. Bouchard. 1995. "Genetic Influences on Perceptions of Childhood Family Environment: A Reared Apart Twin Study." *Child Development* 66 (2): 330–45.

Jones, O. D. 1992–1993. "Sex Selection: Regulating Technology Enabling the Predetermination of a Child's Gender." *Harvard Journal Law and Technology* 6:1–62.

Kahn, J. P. 1991a. "Commentary on Zohar's 'Prospect for Genetic Therapy'—Can a Person Benefit from Being Altered?" *Bioethics* 5 (4): 312–17.

———. 1991b. "Genetic Harm: Bitten by the Body That Keeps You?" *Bioethics* 5 (4): 289–308.

Katz, K. N. 2006. "Parenthood from the Grave: Protocols for Retrieving and Utilizing Gametes from the Dead or Dying." *University of Chicago Legal Forum*: 289–315.

Kelle, H. 2001. "The Discourse of 'Development'—How 9-to-12-Year-Old Children Construct 'Childish' and 'Further Developed' Identities within Their Peer Culture." *Childhood* 8 (1):95–114.

Lauritzen, P. 1990. "What Price Parenthood?" *The Hastings Center Report* 20 (2): 38–46.

Leeb-Lundberg, S., S. Kjellberg, and G. Sydsjö. 2006. "Helping Parents to Tell Their Children about the Use of Donor Insemination (DI) and Determining Their Opinions about Open-Identity Sperm Donors." *Acta Obstetricia et Gynecologica Scandinavica* 85 (1): 78–81.

Lindemann, H., and J. Lindemann Nelson. 2008. "The Romance of the Family." *The Hastings Center Report* 38 (4): 19–21.

Lotz, M. 2009. "Procreative Reasons-Relevance: On the Moral Significance of Why We Have Children." *Bioethics* 23 (5): 291–99.

Mason, J., and B. Tipper. 2008. "Being Related—How Children Define and Create Kinship." *Childhood* 15 (4): 441–60.

McGee, G. 1997. "Parenting in an Era of Genetics." *The Hastings Center Report* 27 (2): 16–22.

McWhinnie, A. 2001. "Should Offspring from Donated Gamete Continue to Be Denied Knowledge of Their Origins and Antecedents?" *Human Reproduction* 16 (5): 808–17.

Nachmani v. Nachman, 49(1) P.D. 485 (1995) and 50(4) P.D. 661 (1996).

Norton, L. H. 2006. "Neutering the Transgendered: Human Rights and Japan's Law No. 111." *Georgetown Journal of Gender & the Law* 7:187–216.

Pannikar, R. 1982. "Is the Notion of Human Rights a Western Concept?" *Diogenes* 120:75–102.

Papaligoura, Z., and C. Trevarthen. 2001. "Mother-Infant Communication Can Be Enhanced after Conception by In-Vitro Fertilization." *Infant Mental Health Journal* 22 (6): 591–610.

Persson, I. 1995. "Genetic Therapy, Identity and the Person-Regarding Reasons." *Bioethics* 9 (1): 16–31.

Peters, P. G. 1998–1999. "Harming Future Persons: Obligations to the Children of Reproductive Technology." *Southern California Interdisciplinary Law Journal* 8:375–400.

Pfeiffer, D. 1999. "Eugenics and Disability Discrimination." In *The Psychological and Social Impact of Disability*, edited by R. P. Marinelli and A. E. Dell, 12–31. New York: Springer Publishing Company, Inc.

Ravitsky, V. 2004. "Posthumous Reproduction Guidelines in Israel." *The Hastings Center Report* 34 (2): 6–7.

Reeve, D. 2002. "Negotiating Psycho-Emotional Dimensions of Disability and Their Influence on Identity Constructions." *Disability & Society* 17 (5): 493–508.

Renteln, A. D. 2003. "Cross-Cultural Perceptions of Disability: Policy Implications of Divergent Views." In *The Human Rights of Persons with Intellectual Disabilities: Different But Equal*, edited by Stanley S. Herr, Lawrence O. Gostin, and Harold Hongju Koh, 59–82. New York: Oxford University Press.

Roberts, D. E. 1995. "The Genetic Tie." *University of Chicago Law Review* 62:209–73.

Robertson, J. A. 1996. "Genetic Selection of Offspring Characteristics." *Boston University Law Review* 76:421–82.

———. 2003. "Procreative Liberty in the Era of Genomics." *American Journal of Law & Medicine* 29:439–86.

———. 2004–2005. "Reproductive Technology in Germany and the United States: An Essay in Comparative Law and Bioethics." *Columbia Journal of Transnational Law* 43:189–227.

———. 2007–2008. "Assisting Reproduction, Choosing Genes, and the Scope of Reproductive Freedom." *George Washington Law Review* 76:1490–1513.

———. 2009. "The Octuplet Case—Why More Regulation Is Not Likely." *The Hastings Center Report* 39 (3): 26–28.

Robertson, J. A., J. P. Kahn, and J. E. Wagner. 2002. "Conception to Obtain Hematopoietic Stem Cells." *The Hastings Center Report* 32 (3): 34–40.

Sabatello, M. 2009. *Children's Bioethics: The International Biopolitical Discourse on Harmful Traditional Practices and the Right of the Child to Cultural Identity*. Leiden, The Netherlands: Martinus Nijhoff Pub.

Schenker, J. 2003. "Legitimizing Surrogacy in Israel: Religious Perspectives." In *Surrogate Motherhood: International Perspectives*, edited by Rachel Cook et al., 242–60. Oxford: Hart Publishing.

Schuz, R. 2003. "Surrogacy in Israel: An Analysis of the Law in Practice." In *Surrogate Motherhood: International Perspectives*, edited by Rachel Cook et al., 35–54. Oxford: Hart Publishing.

SH and others v. Austria, Application no. 57813/00, Grand Chamber of the ECHR, Judgment of November 3 2011.

Shakespeare, Tom. 2006. *Disability Rights and Wrongs*. New York: Routledge.

Shapiro, J. 2005–2006. "A Lesbian Centered Critique of 'Genetic Parenthood.'" *Journal of Gender, Race & Justice* 9:591–612.

Skloot, R. 2009, July 10. "Sally Has 2 Mommies and 1 Daddy—Infertility Update: Making Babies—and Birth Defects?" http://www.popsci.com/scitech/article/2003-04/sally-has-2-mommies-and-1-daddy.

Smerdon, U. R. 2008. "Crossing Bodies, Crossing Borders: International Surrogacy Between the United States and India." *Cumberland Law Rev.* 39 (1): 17–85.

Stalker, K., and C. Connors. 2004. "Children's Perceptions of Their Disabled Siblings: 'She's Different but It's Normal for Us.'" *Children & Society* 18 (3): 218–30.

Storrow, R. F. 2005–2006. "Family Tales: The Handmaid's Tale of Fertility Tourism: Passports and Third Parties in the Religious Regulation of Assisted Conception." *Texas Wesleyan Law Rev.* 12:189–211.

Van den Akker, O. 2006. "A Review of Family Donor Constructs: Current Research and Future Directions." *Human Reproduction Update* 12 (2): 91–101.

Vanfraussen et al. 2001. "An Attempt to Reconstruct Children's Donor Concept: A Comparison between Children's and Lesbian Parents' Attitudes towards Donor Anonymity." *Human Reproduction Update* 16 (9): 2019–25.

Wahrman, M. Z. 2005–2006. "Fruit of the Womb: Artificial Reproductive Technologies & Jewish Law." *Journal of Gender, Race & Justice* 9:109–36.

Waldman, E. 2003–2004. "The Parent Trap: Uncovering the Myth of 'Coerced Parenthood' in Frozen Embryos Disputes." *American University Law Review* 53:1021–62.

Walsh, F. 2009. "Scientists in Newcastle Claim to Have Created Human Sperm in the Laboratory in What They Say Is a World First." *BBC News*, July 7. http://news.bbc.co.uk/2/hi/health/8138963.stm.

Watson, N. 2002. "Well, I Know This Is Going to Sound Very Strange to You, but I Don't See Myself as a Disabled Person: Identity and Disability." *Disability & Society* 17 (5): 509–27.

X, Y, Z v. UK, Application no. 21830/93, European Court of Human Rights, Judgment of 22 April 1997.

Zahraa, M., and S. Shafie. 2006. "An Islamic Perspective on IVF and PGD, with particular Reference to Zain Hashmi, and Other Similar Cases." *Arab Law Quarterly* 20:152–80.

3

Cutting-Edge Debates

A Cross-Cultural Consideration of Surgery

Alison Dundes Renteln

ABSTRACT

Many bioethics controversies involve cutting. Sometimes individuals from different cultural backgrounds have objections to surgery. Although there is often a presumption in favor of surgical intervention in modern medical systems, it is not obvious that surgery is always advisable. In other situations individuals seek surgical procedures that may be unacceptable to medical professionals. In order to come to grips with the question of when surgery is appropriate, this chapter surveys scholarship on this topic in the fields of global bioethics, comparative religious ethics, folk medicine, and medical anthropology. After analyzing the relationship between diverse worldviews and surgery, I discuss various theoretical frameworks within which one can evaluate these conflicts. I then comment on the implications of a cross-cultural approach for training health care professionals. Finally, I argue that it is important to take culturally varying attitudes toward surgery into account to devise the most effective health policies.

INTRODUCTION

The field of bioethics has not benefitted sufficiently from the contributions of social scientists studying the cultural context of medical practices.[1] The ethical analysis of medical procedures often reflects the cultural presuppositions of leading scholars, many of whom are Anglo-American. Not only does this limited perspective obscure the double standards operating in biomedical ethics, but it increases the likelihood that Western bioethics will become less relevant as medicine becomes more global.

Insofar as bioethicists provide philosophical reasoning to support the practices of doctors, their analytic treatment of surgical procedures helps maintain physicians' cultural hegemony in medicine. This is a serious concern because ethnocentrism in biomedicine could lead physicians to impose their worldviews on others who may have different understandings of medicine and healing. Cultural bias in health care also runs the risk of preventing patients from seeking medical attention.

Bioethicists occupy a unique position in guiding medical professionals who see patients in vulnerable circumstances. Because individuals from different cultural backgrounds often seek treatment in medical institutions unfamiliar with their worldview, bioethicists ought to consider the relevance of cultural notions for medicine.[2]

In this chapter I focus on surgery because many conflicts arise from cultural differences surrounding cutting procedures. Western bioethicists typically analyze the advisability of surgical procedures on the grounds of either medical necessity or aesthetic enhancement. The fact that medical professionals tend to judge the reasonableness of procedures instead of deferring to patients' choices deserves careful consideration.

If the ethical analysis of surgical procedures privileges patient autonomy over the judgment of doctors, then ascertaining patient motivations becomes less critical. This cross-cultural consideration of surgery emphasizes the centrality of informed consent, so patient consent is viewed as the decisive factor in judging its reasonableness. This will likely necessitate a rethinking of the role of consent as a defense for surgeons who perform controversial operations.

As part of this inquiry into the role that consent plays, one must draw a sharp distinction between children and adults because children ordinarily lack the capacity to consent to surgery.[3] Because surgeries result in permanent changes and because children cannot make decisions in their own right, it is not obvious that there should be a presumption in favor of cutting. Furthermore, it is important to consider the circumstances under which the state, the family, or a guardian should be empowered to judge whether a particular surgery is in the best interests of the child.[4]

In this chapter, I offer some reflections on cultural conflicts in the context of surgery when patients and doctors do not share the same cultural background. I will present a set of surgical procedures that have been subject to differing cross-cultural interpretations. For surgeries in the first category, the minority community objects to the operation that the medical establishment (and sometimes the larger society) considers necessary. Within the second category of cutting, either the majority objects to the surgery that the minority regards as necessary or there is lingering unease in society about a commonly used procedure. After describing some of these types of cutting as well as rationales for and objections to them, I take up theoretical frameworks for analyzing them.

Bioethicists often analyze specific practices in light of whether they are consistent with the principle of nonmalificence or "do no harm." Not only must we consider what surgeries constitute "harms" but whether a patient's consent to an ostensibly harmful cutting shields the surgeon from moral criticism and liability. While some arguments assess consequences and harms of the surgery, others are rights based and include the rights to health and to essential surgery.

Ultimately we must reconcile the analysis of universal ethical principles with cultural relativism. In the section on theoretical frameworks, I argue that one can advocate universal standards and apply them to culturally specific contexts. I then assess the implications for the role of bioethicists and medical practitioners and suggest possible policies to resolve cultural conflicts related to cutting.

CULTURAL AND RELIGIOUS OBJECTIONS TO SURGERIES

Culture matters in bioethics because every individual is subject to enculturation.[5] By this largely unconscious process people acquire the categories of their society. Culture influences both cognition and conduct, so this naturally includes notions of illness and healing. Since the nineteenth century the fields of anthropology and cultural psychology have demonstrated the power of culture in shaping perceptions. If we accept the premise that cultural imperatives affect decision making, then we may assume that judgments about surgical procedures are likewise influenced by cultural factors.

Surgeries serve quite varied purposes such as curing people of health problems, solving crimes, improving physical appearance and mobility, ensuring marriageability, and matching a body with an identity. Because most individuals are not aware of their own cultural biases, it is easy to assume that some types of cutting are acceptable, while others are not.

AUTOPSIES

One of the most blatant examples of ethnocentric bias in the interpretation of cutting involves postmortem exams. There is a strong bias in modern medicine in favor of performing autopsies with little regard for the objections raised by members of ethnic minority groups.[6] Surprisingly, despite the literature on these objections in medicine and clinical ethics, most bioethics texts have ignored this topic.[7]

Cutting the dead seems mostly unobjectionable because the dead cannot speak for themselves and, at least in Anglo-American jurisprudence, they lack personhood.[8] The reasons for autopsies include investigations in which foul play is suspected, possible threats to public health, administering quality control in hospital standards, and avoiding insurance fraud. Despite these rationales, some ethnic minority groups have belief systems that prohibit autopsies. For example, the Hmong object to autopsies for several reasons, including the belief that the body, if mutilated, will remain in that condition for eternity in the afterlife.[9]

In a Rhode Island case, the medical examiner performed an autopsy after a young Hmong man died inexplicably while asleep in a hospital. There was public concern about his death because of a phenomenon known as Sudden Nocturnal Death Syndrome: young Hmong men had been dying in this way for no apparent reason.[10] The judge admonished medical examiners to know the worldview of those who reside in their communities:

> [I]t is reasonable to believe that when a medical examiner receives the body of a person who might be a Hmong, he should realize that an autopsy would violate the religious beliefs of the descendant's next of kin. This conclusion is strengthened if the Yangs' uncontested allegation that they expressed their opposition to an autopsy to the doctors at Rhode Island Hospital is true.[11]

One question is whether the state interest in performing an autopsy supersedes the family's right to religious freedom. Although states may pay lip service to cultural accommodation, sometimes by permitting a certificate of religious objection to prevent an autopsy from being performed,[12] a compelling state interest can override the religious objection. For example, in *Albareti v. Hirsh* a Muslim man working in a small grocery store died after being shot in the chest.[13] The medical examiner performed an autopsy over his parents' objections, and the court ruled in favor of the state on the basis of the need to solve the crime. As there was little doubt as to the cause of death, the postmortem exam did not seem necessary.[14]

These cases show unequivocally that a proautopsy bias exists among medical professionals and law enforcement in the United States and some "Western" countries. They presume that cutting is acceptable to determine the cause of death, even when there are strong religious objections. While those in North America and Europe may assume that the dead lack rights, in societies where the dead are regarded as persons, this cutting may be considered abhorrent. Interestingly, even in societies favoring autopsies, there is the principle that the dead deserve to be treated with respect.

Just as medical professionals see autopsies as morally unproblematic, they tend to think that those with disabilities need corrective surgery for their own good. In another Hmong case, a doctor decided that Kou Xiong, an eight-year-old boy born with clubfeet and a dislocated hip, should undergo surgery despite the vehement objections of his family and the entire Hmong community.[15] After the judge ordered the surgery, the family's attorney attempted a series of appeals but lost at every level. After all the litigation, the original judge decided to vacate his earlier ruling ordering the surgery.

The main reasons for the surgical procedure were to ease Kou's pain and improve his mobility. The Hmong objected to the operation because they believed that Kou had been born with the condition to atone for the sins of ancestors and that surgical intervention would have adverse consequences.[16] Even with the opposition of Kou, his family, and the Hmong community, the medical establishment and the legal system insisted on the operation. Ultimately no doctor would perform the surgery without parental consent. Moreover, there was no urgency, because he could have the surgery when he was older.

As the law in the United States draws a sharp distinction between life-threatening and non-life-threatening procedures, it is striking that the court ordered the surgery, given that having clubfeet is not life threatening.[17] That doctors can invoke the power of law to compel a child to undergo surgery in the absence of a life-threatening condition should give us pause.

This example reflects a cultural presumption that children with disabilities must have surgery to correct what society considers "abnormal" conditions.[18] One might argue that it is dangerous to authorize operations to improve "quality of life" because such a vague standard is difficult to apply. Any attempt to interpret the standard in medical decisions would benefit from an understanding of culturally varying attitudes toward persons with disabilities.[19]

This is not to say that bioethicists and surgeons should not try to persuade people from other cultures that there are benefits to surgery in appropriate circumstances. In fact, when there is a culturally sensitive intercultural exchange, some families may eventually decide that a procedure is worthwhile. In the absence of a life-threatening condition in which saving the lives of children is justifiably a paramount concern, medical professionals should be encouraged to tread carefully.

CULTURAL AND RELIGIOUS IMPERATIVES FOR SURGERY

Much more controversial than the surgeries discussed above are those that medical professionals find questionable. In the following I focus on genital cutting and facial surgery, although other surgeries such as scarification and body piercing engender controversy as well.

Female Genital Cutting

One of the most sensational procedures is female genital cutting, known variously as female circumcision, clitoridectomy, or female genital mutilation. For those unfamiliar with this surgery, it is almost incomprehensible because it involves removing parts of the genitalia of young girls.[20] Although I do not defend this custom, I would like to point out a few difficulties with the way the issue is treated in the scholarly literature and the popular press. First, the terminology itself is highly inflammatory. The word *mutilation* conveys the degree to which the cutting is viewed with contempt. As Leslie Obiora observes:

> Describing a vital aspect of African cultural identity as "mutilation" has proven offensive, if not psychically mutilating, to critical African constituencies like the Premier Group des Femmes D'Afrique who prefer to employ the term "female circumcision." This semantic tug-of-war is emblematic of the constellation of misunderstandings that surround the practice. Ironically, the catch-all phrase of "genital mutilation" favored by Westerner-influenced critics is potentially as much a misnomer as "female circumcision" because not all forms of the genital surgeries are impairing.[21]

Second, many types of surgery are subsumed under the single term. Some, like clitoridectomy, are far more extreme than others, but they are often referred to as though they were all identical.[22] Although there are those who condemn all forms of genital surgery, some engage in moral criticism entirely unaware of their oversimplification.

Third, the vast literature on the practice has been subject to trenchant criticisms. For instance, African women have campaigned for decades to eradicate the practice, and they are insulted when Western feminists give the impression that they were responsible for launching the campaign.[23] Moreover, the moral condemnation is sometimes regarded as cultural imperialism.[24] Finally, banning the custom outright has simply driven it underground.

For the most part, critics focus on the potentially serious health consequences of the procedure.[25] Yet when parents have their daughters circumcised in hospitals, this can be done without any complications. However, there is concern about the "medicalization" of female genital cutting because it may lend an air of legitimacy to the custom. As a UNICEF report put it: "The fact that certain medical professionals or health works are known to be involved in the practice may contribute to a general misconception that FGM/C is somehow acceptable."[26] Because of this posture, the WHO and the World Medical Association have condemned the practice and any involvement by medical professionals.

The risk of criminalizing the practice is that individuals who cannot go to hospitals may either perform it themselves[27] or take their daughters to countries where the operation is permitted. This policy has the unintended consequence of driving the custom underground where there is even less protection for girls.[28] Ultimately, the objection must be formulated in terms other than simply an adverse health impact and thus indicate that the surgery is objectionable for more than just medical reasons. Western commentators' primary objection is that it is designed to control the purity of women, and surgeons who participate in this reaffirm patriarchal and misogynist values.

This was made clear when the Harborview hospital in Seattle considered implementing a policy to allow girls to receive a symbolic cut in lieu of actual removal of tissue.[29] Because this compromise was objectionable to feminist legislators, the hospital rescinded the policy, even though it could have prevented girls from undergoing the traditional form of the surgery. Doriane Coleman explains poignantly:

> In their Pyrrhic victory . . . Harborview's opponents probably denied some Somali girls in Seattle the possibility of living a life free of the physical and emotional devastation caused by the traditional circumcision practiced by their community; in the name of ideological purity, they probably sacrificed some of the very girls they claim are the beneficiaries of their efforts. . . . Additionally, Harborview's opponents also squelched what was probably the most successful compromise of a cultural collision that has been publicly contemplated in this country.

Ultimately the strongest argument against female genital cutting is that it is performed on minors. Children do not have the legal capacity to consent to surgical procedures,[30] and the removal of a healthy body part should be presumed to be against the best interests of the child.

HYMENOPLASTY

Another debate about genital surgery concerns customary law requiring women to be virgins on their wedding day. When it comes time to marry, some of these women visit a surgeon's office and request a hymenoplasty.[31] They fear that without hymen reconstruction, they may be rejected by their husbands and families or be victims of honor killings.[32]

In the 1990s two Dutch doctors performed the hymen operation as an outpatient procedure in a hospital. Their defense was that they followed patients' wishes and their actions were permissible according to Dutch law. They distinguished hymen reconstruction from clitoridectomy:

> We reject any suggestion that this operation is analogous to traditional clitoridectomy. There are strong arguments for rejecting a request for clitoridectomy, but equally strong ones exist for accepting hymen reconstruction. Most importantly, hymen reconstruction, like male circumcision is an example of "ritualistic surgery." Our definition of ritualistic surgery, modified from that of Bolande, is "fulfillment of a person's need rather than a response to their medical condition." The ethics of hymen reconstruction could be compared to the ethics of cosmetic surgery, an accepted part of plastic and reconstructive surgery worldwide.[33]

However, some surgeons have ethical qualms about performing the surgery on the grounds that they are perpetuating a value system that requires women to be pure.[34]

There is also a question as to whether this surgery is medically necessary or only cosmetic. If health insurance only covers medically necessary procedures, this could be an awkward matter. Of course, it could be argued that the procedure is medically necessary if the woman might otherwise be killed.

Complications may develop if the husband discovers the deception. According to media reports, in one case a husband in France sought an annulment based on what he considered fraud. The judge ruled in his favor and was subsequently criticized for adhering to an "archaic" interpretation of Islamic law.[35] The Justice Ministry intervened to have the decision reversed.

The question as to whether surgeons should perform the hymen reconstruction procedure has generated a debate in biomedical ethics. As suggested above, some worry that doing so implicates the medical profession in perpetuating blatantly sexist marriage systems. Others fear that failure to operate may put the lives of the women seeking surgery in jeopardy.[36]

In a thoughtful consideration of the ethical issues, Rebecca Cook and Bernard M. Dickens take stock of feminist objections to the procedure while noting the risks of honor killings. They take up the legal issues associated with the surgery, highlighting the jurisprudential complexities. In Arab countries that have outlawed "hymen restoration," professional associations cannot officially take a position on it. Even where it is not illegal, legal systems generally do not accept consent to maim as a defense.

Moreover, Cook and Dickens deny that laws prohibiting female genital cutting apply to this custom, noting that the hymen restoration is performed on consenting adult women in safe circumstances, whereas female genital cutting is usually performed on girls in nonsterile conditions. They conclude that the procedure is lawful and usually requested by adult women able to give informed consent. In this sophisticated argument, exemplary for both its cultural sensitivity and nuance, they explain why bioethicists should take culture into account and why this sort of analysis can influence the practice of medicine.

COSMETIC SURGERY: ENHANCEMENT OR SELF-MUTILATION?

On what grounds other than medical necessity can surgery be justified? That hymenoplasty may protect women from death is a rather compelling justification, but is it enough that a person simply feels a strong desire for surgery?[37] In North America the field of cosmetic and plastic surgery, initially viewed with suspicion, has become an established branch of medicine and indicates a widespread acceptance of what some regard as self-inflicted cutting.[38] A vast literature on this subject conveys the impression that historically there has been a great anxiety about the legitimacy of enhancement procedures.[39] While some of the commentary reflects a negative tone, it is not generally considered to be a form of self-mutilation.

Even though plastic surgery is now considered reasonable, society may have to impose limits. Indeed, surgeons have an ethical obligation to evaluate the mental state of patients who request surgical procedures. For instance, in *Surgery Junkies*, Victoria Pitts-Taylor describes the case of a woman who, after undergoing dozens of procedures over a six-year period, sued her doctor on the grounds that he should have known she had body dysmorphic disorder.[40] Not only ought there to be concern when an individual seeks multiple surgeries within a short duration, but the type of surgery may also signal a possible problem. For example, some individuals want to emulate movie stars (regardless of whether the individuals whose traits are copied wish to share their facial identities).

Cosmetic surgery has also been used to change facial characteristics to adhere to the dominant standards of beauty or to conceal ethnic identity[41] and/or to conform to "white" aesthetic standards.[42] Elizabeth Haiken treats this subject in a discussion of "The Michael Jackson Factor: Race, Ethnicity, and Cosmetic Surgery":

> From the early twentieth century on, the reigning cultural norms of beauty have been understood to demand an absence of what surgeons call racial or ethnic stigmata, and cosmetic surgery has consistently focused on altering features that differentiate patients from a norm that is always implicitly, and often explicitly, understood to be not just Caucasian but Anglo Saxon or northern European.[43]

For example, Fred Korematsu had plastic surgery in an attempt to evade the infamous Executive Order 9066 that wrongfully incarcerated Japanese Americans in internment camps during World War II.[44] Historically, the use of cosmetic surgery both here and abroad for the purpose of "Caucasianization" did not immediately lead surgeons to question the ethical implications of these procedures.[45]

Just as hymenoplasty reinforces societal norms related to the purity of women, so, too, does cutting to achieve ethnic anonymity risk perpetuating nefarious social standards. The question is whether the motivation matters—whether plastic surgery is primarily designed to improve patients' individual appearances, or whether it is a culturally motivated form of self-mutilation.[46] There does appear to be an underlying double standard operating with regard to cultural constructions of specific types of surgery.

Another type of surgery that deserves mention is the surgical removal of organs for commercial purposes. While the ethical issue is whether to allow the sale of organs given the scarcity, the participation of medical professionals also raises serious ethical questions.[47] Although the sale of organs is illegal in many countries and prohibited by international instruments,[48] those who are desperate for resources for their families may nevertheless try to sell body parts. While it may seem prima facie unethical for surgeons to engage in these activities, the failure of medical professionals to remove the organs or tissue may put donors at greater risk.

Just as refusal to perform genital cutting and hymen restoration may seem ethically preferable, the consequences of that stance could result in greater harm to the patients. Preventing impoverished individuals from selling body parts may put them in a worse situation, financially speaking, than allowing them to do so.[49]

These surgeries show how complicated cutting can be in pluralistic societies. While we cannot settle the question of where to draw the line in all cases of cultural conflicts in bioethics, these examples permit us to consider how to approach the ethics of surgery when cultural differences are relevant to the analysis.

THEORETICAL APPROACHES: TOWARD THE CENTRALITY OF CONSENT

With regard to the question of when surgeries are ethically justifiable, there are various approaches one can take to these issues. Because surgery involves substantial risks, the degree to which it should be regulated to protect both patients and surgeons is a serious matter.

One view is that there should be minimal state interference insofar as liberal democracies usually empower individuals to exercise autonomous decision making in order to make choices about their own life plans. According to the principle of autonomy, the patient should be entitled to undergo any surgical procedure, regardless of whether it is medically necessary. As long as the patient has the capacity to consent to the surgery, noninterference by the state is the optimal policy and the surgeon should be able to perform surgery without risk of prosecution or lawsuit.

But autonomy is not an absolute principle, so there are objections to this line of reasoning. Patients, in exercising their autonomous decision making, cannot request unreasonable surgeries. For instance, if surgery would result in a person's death, that would be considered murder in legal systems prohibiting active euthanasia. In addition, it would be improper for a surgeon to remove a limb simply because a person desired this.[50]

Analysts have generally not supported consent as a defense in the context of the controversial surgeries discussed above. This is presumably because the dominant culture regards the surgeries as unreasonable. It is precisely because of cross-cultural differences in the interpretation of the cutting that the question of reasonableness comes to the fore and raises for surgeons the question of whether performance of such operations is ethically permissible.

When individuals having the capacity to consent request cutting required by cultural traditions, they may be accused of "false consciousness." That they have been brainwashed to desire the surgical procedure ostensibly undermines their autonomous decision making. Of course, the problem with this logic is that individuals from the dominant culture have likewise been socialized to think that particular surgeries are acceptable. Hence, we return to the problem of double standards.

Some fear that making consent the centerpiece of the analysis risks too much because individuals may request unreasonable surgical procedures. An alternative would be to analyze surgeries according to the principle of nonmaleficence. Intuitively appealing, it is not always self-evident that the cutting constitutes a harm. Moreover, whether a procedure is considered a harm may depend on the cultural upbringing of the person interpreting the surgical procedure. This means that if surgeons are bound by the principle of nonmaleficence, then it is critical to know whether the cutting constitutes a harm.

Some might disagree with relying on a nonmaleficence approach and argue that what matters instead of adherence to this principle are the consequences of the cutting. If the surgery interferes with a bodily function, reinforces negative societal attitudes, or endangers the patient's health in the long run, these might constitute reasons for not allowing an operation to take place. On this view, the analysis hinges on whether or not the cutting is considered an objective physical harm.

In a thoughtful consideration of what harms deserve to be criminalized, Dennis Baker contends that the harm principle ordinarily does not cover self-harm: "[S]elf-wrongs are not criminalizable because they do not wrong or harm others."[51] According to this line of reasoning, adults who seek surgeries that others consider harmful should be allowed to have them performed.

If adults are opting for what others regard as a form of self-harm or self-mutilation, then surgeons could be protected from liability and their actions seen as morally permissible simply by documenting the patient's informed consent. If a patient signs a waiver, is mentally capable of choosing to undergo the surgery, and is videotaped requesting the procedure, then surgeons arguably should be shielded from legal action. In essence, the question is whether consent should be a defense to self-mutilation.[52] If a competent adult patient requests a procedure and there is no coercion, duress, or mental disability involved, then the procedure should be considered ethically acceptable, based on Western principles of bioethics.

An approach focused on consent, admittedly, does not solve the problem of surgery for children. The reason, of course, is that children are regarded as lacking the capacity to consent. Although their families could invoke proxy consent, it remains to be seen in what cultural community children will finally choose to reside. In light of the irreparable nature of the cutting, surgeries involving the removal of healthy body parts, even if required by cultural and religious imperatives, should not be allowed.

These customs should be prohibited because children cannot consent to have any form of surgery. Children represent a special case in which paternalism is appropriate; the presumption in most cases should be against surgery, unless they have a life-threatening condition or serious health problem.[53]

Some have begun to ask whether a presumption against surgery precludes the possibility of male circumcision.[54] Scholars question this medical procedure based on some of the same criticisms made of female genital cutting, even though the two types of surgery are not comparable. Acting on this interpretation, some campaigned for a ballot measure to ban male circumcision in the boundaries of San Francisco in 2011.[55] The logic is that baby boys should be protected against an unnecessary cultural tradition that involves permanent removal of body tissue.[56]

With respect to adults, if we are likewise true to extant principles of autonomy and nonmaleficence, adults should be able to undergo the surgical procedures they request. To the extent that medical jurisprudence and professional ethics supports the logic of this position, legal systems should allow consent as a defense when surgeons fear repercussions for performing contested surgeries. Otherwise, it is unfair to require the doctors as a matter of professional ethics to provide the medical services that their patients demand. It is crucial that consent be formally recognized as a defense to allow surgeons to do their job and serve the interests of their patients.

There are other normative principles that may offer a way of analyzing culturally motivated surgeries that seem unreasonable to the medical establishment. Rights-based theories are sometimes used in bioethics debates as a way of dissecting the problem. At least two human rights may be pertinent—the right to health and the right to bodily integrity. Both are widely recognized in medical ethics as well as existing international human rights treaties that numerous states have ratified and are therefore legally binding.

The right to health is enshrined in Article 25 of the Universal Declaration of Human Rights and Article 12 of the International Covenant on Economic, Social, and Cultural Rights. Other treaty provisions guarantee a right to health for particular groups.[57] A body of literature emerged in the late twentieth century that emphasized the importance of this human right. Brigit Toebes, for instance, wrote a treatise that provided the definitive treatment of the subject.[58]

Other commentators, while recognizing that few legal systems formally recognize a right to health, contend that despite this lack of juridical recognition, states are morally obligated to provide access to health care. Dieter Giesen, for example, argues that protecting the autonomy of individual citizens is a central concern in common law and civil law systems. He says:

> [H]ealth is an essential prerequisite to the exercise of personal autonomy and human flourishing. To the extent that any society denies access to basic health care services, it disvalues individual autonomy and thereby exposes itself to serious moral criticism.[59]

The World Health Organization has affirmed its commitment to the protection of health and human rights. For our purposes, the question is whether such a right helps settle the question of whether states should guarantee, regulate, or ban the provision of surgical services. If we assume for the sake of argument that international law guarantees a right to health that states are obligated to provide, the question is whether this encompasses a right to surgery.[60]

Some scholars argue that this particular right should be interpreted to guarantee the right to essential surgery, even it is not currently construed in this way.[61] Their claim is based on research showing that many so-called developing countries lack the ability to provide surgical procedures to their citizens.[62]

If international law affords protection to a specific human right, that signifies that states have obligations to provide those rights. While it is not inconceivable that governments could do this, it is unlikely that all of them could fulfill this responsibility. Even if the human right to health guarantees surgery, this does not settle the question as to which surgical procedures must be provided.[63]

Presumably, this would not cover elective cosmetic or plastic surgical procedures. Generally speaking, states mandate coverage of medically necessary surgery because this is how health insurance companies function. However, an argument could be made that cosmetic surgery ought to be covered as well because it promotes physical and mental health.[64]

The other human right possibly relevant to the question of surgery is the right to bodily integrity.[65] This right is predicated on the concept of the inviolability of the patient as a human being. This raises the question of whether a person can choose to alter his or her body consistent with this principle. If a right to bodily integrity exists, to what extent can medical professionals cut their patients at the patients' own request?

With regard to children who cannot make choices on their own, the question is whether their parents or guardians can make the decision or whether this would be inconsistent with the right to bodily integrity. Some assume that children should not be subject to procedures. For instance, some of the San Francisco "intactivists" lobbied for the ballot measure banning male circumcision and campaigned "For Genital Integrity."[66]

The concept of integrity suggests that an individual's self-conception is based on a reasonable body image. If not, any bodily modification might be incompatible with the notion of integrity. Because the entire matter hinges ultimately on what constitutes "reasonable" changes in the body, this may ultimately be an insolvable puzzle.

REVISITING RELATIVISM

The reason why it is challenging to decide on the limits to surgical procedures is because there are culturally varying ideas about the scope of proper medical procedures and aesthetic standards. Scholars resist the notion that the cultural context matters for surgery because they fear that this will lead to a slippery slope. This reaction reflects a long-standing anxiety about cultural relativism.

Opponents of relativism mistakenly assume that it requires a posture of nihilism, or "anything goes." Their flawed interpretation erroneously casts the theory of relativism as a prescriptive theory and assumes that it endorses the value of tolerance. As I have explained elsewhere, one should not follow the early proponents of relativism down this path.[67] Reconceptualizing cultural relativism as a *descriptive* theory that recognizes the diverse moral codes across the globe avoids the logical difficulties found in the prescriptive version. Relativism as a descriptive theory does not require either acceptance or rejection of any particular customs as a moral posture. As Robert Redfield succinctly put it: "It cannot be proved from the proposition that values are relative, that we ought to respect all systems of values. We might just as well hate them all."[68]

Critics of relativism also shy away from this theoretical approach for another reason: the unwarranted assumption that relativism is fundamentally incompatible with universal ethical principles. While a relativist approach to morality is diametrically opposed to moral absolutism, it is entirely compatible with universalism. It is important to underscore the point that accepting relativism does not preclude the possibility of shared principles across diverse cultures. Rather than conceptualizing relativism as a set of entirely discrete systems, we should instead think of cultural relativism as a Venn diagram. The reality that there are many different worldviews is entirely consistent with the existence of shared principles or what might be called cross-cultural universals.[69]

With regard to bioethics, it is likely that all societies reject what they consider to be serious harms. Thus, avoiding serious harm may be a universal ethical principle or value. The problem is that they may disagree as to which specific practices should be designated as harms. There are those who consider it self-evident that some types of bodily change are harms, but this culturally biased outlook is precisely the problem. While it may be self-evident to people unaccustomed to plastic surgery that this is a form of self-mutilation, it seems a reasonable medical procedure to North Americans for whom this social practice has become institutionalized as a "normal" medical procedure.

As compared to other types of cutting, genital surgery is most fraught with controversy. In some ways it is peculiar because most opposed to the operation seldom confront it. By contrast, the results of cosmetic surgery such as facial surgery are quite visible. Yet those who inhabit the social worlds in which this is normal have become accustomed to the faces that have been altered, sometimes in drastic ways.

In the final analysis, it is not possible to provide a general ethical theory that is wholly consistent and avoids ethnocentrism. If anything is universal, it is the human instinct to favor one's own value system. Yet even if complete theoretical consistency is unattainable, we should nevertheless strive for greater transparency in our argumentation. If ensuring informed consent and protecting children are the paramount values, then we must make those values explicit. Condemning the surgeries of others as unreasonable is an untenable position if we consider some of the extreme surgical makeovers that occur within modern medical systems.

POLICY PROPOSALS

If bioethics is to remain relevant in the twenty-first century, it is crucial that the field take a broader cross-cultural approach to the examination of the topics of investigation. This can be accomplished in several ways. First, the analysis of any topic should include the consideration of scholars from other parts of the world. It should also incorporate research in the social sciences such as medical anthropology and folk medicine.

Second, bioethicists should actively seek out the folk views of the biomedical issue under consideration. With this global, more populist approach to bioethics, the reasoning about life-and-death matters will reflect a deeper understanding of community values. The arguments will be grounded in the actual belief systems by which ordinary people live their lives.

Third, hospitals and clinics that provide access to health care should be sure to have a member of the ethnic community(ies) on their ethics committees. When cultural clashes occur, members of the community should have the opportunity to share their views, so the decision about policy is not rendered in a vacuum.

Finally, we need a code of ethics for surgeons that address cultural conflicts.[70] It should contain provisions related to specific operations that patients request. Currently surgeons are expected to refrain from performing surgery that is inconsistent with "reasonable" practice. To protect their own professional integrity, they may decline a request, but they may be expected to refer patients who insist upon having surgery to their colleagues. Considering that surgical procedures can be a matter of life and death, it is time for global bioethics to provide more guidance.

CONCLUSION

It is not enough to identify ethnocentrism in the field of bioethics. There is also an obligation to think creatively to find ways to overcome these challenges. As we have seen, there are steps that bioethicists can take to expand their horizons by incorporating the scholarly contributions of their colleagues in medical anthropology, folk medicine, and comparative law. Furthermore, they can make a more concerted effort to recruit new voices to the discipline to diversify the perspectives.

With regard to clinicians, taking a global approach means reimagining institutions so that they reflect diverse cultural perspectives. Ethics committees at hospitals that have a large ethnic or religious community should always have representatives of those cultures. Medical professionals of all kinds—physicians, nurses, medical technicians, and other staff—should receive training to make them aware of different worldviews, values, and folk beliefs about healing.

It will remain important to draw a distinction between adults and children. Insofar as children cannot, for the most part, exercise autonomous decision making, society has the obligation to protect them from surgical procedures that would lead to irreparable changes. This presumption against cutting would disallow surgery for children except when they have a life-threatening condition or serious health condition. This would prevent or delay genital surgeries, female or male. It would also delay the piercing of ears, tattooing, and other customs until such time as children reach the age of adulthood.

While it may be in the best interests of the child not to have surgery, in democratic systems individuals are usually given the right to make their own life plans. This means that adults should be able to decide to have whatever surgeries they see fit. If this strikes a surgeon as unacceptable, he or she may decline but then is ethically obligated to refer the patient to another physician who may perform the surgery.

We tend to regard our own surgeries as normal and medically appropriate. It is only when we take a cross-cultural approach to analyze various types of cutting that we can appreciate our own ethnocentrism. Relativism is a highly effective theoretical framework that forces us to wrestle with our own preconceived notions of normalcy. Examining personal biases helps us reconsider our cultural presuppositions so we can design social policies that are more just.

In the twenty-first century, because of increasing migration and the influence of the international human rights movement, more demands are being made of medical professionals to perform surgeries that implicate different value systems. These demands force them to confront their own cultural precepts and determine what course of action is ethically correct. Bioethicists therefore must rise to the challenge and consider how to approach the cultural conflicts that inevitably arise in order to provide guidance to surgeons.[71] What these concrete cases reveal is that the analysis of surgery requires a more global approach that takes culture into account.

NOTES

1. Bioethics would be enriched by greater attention to medical anthropology and folk medicine. See, for example, the special issue "Cross-Cultural Medicine," *Western Journal of Medicine* 139 (6) (1983); "Cross-Cultural Medicine: A Decade Later," *Western Journal of Medicine* 157 (3) (1992). More interdisciplinary research would enhance the analysis of bioethicists. For a defense of bioethicists, see Leigh Turner, "Anthropological and Sociological Critiques of Bioethics," *Bioethical Inquiry* 6 (2009): 83–98.

2. A few books advocate taking a cross-cultural approach. One of the more interesting texts is the volume edited by Julia Tao Lai Po-Wah, *Cross-Cultural Perspectives on the (Im)possibility of Global Bioethics* (Dordrecht: Kluwer Academic Publishers, 2002). There is an elementary

textbook by Darryl R. J. Macer, ed., *A Cross-Cultural Introduction to Bioethics* (Bangkok: Eubios Ethics Institute, 2006). Kazumasa Hoshino, *Japanese and Western Bioethics: Studies in Moral Diversity* (Kluwer, 1997). Jonathan E. Brockopp and Thomas Eich, eds., *Muslim Medical Ethics: From Theory to Practice* (Columbia: University of South Carolina Press, 2008). For a more scholarly consideration of the relevance of culture and race to the study of bioethics, see Lawrence J. Prograis Jr. and Edmund E. Pellegrino, eds., *African American Bioethics: Culture Race, and Identity* (Washington, DC: Georgetown University Press, 2007). There are also significant works in the fields of transcultural medicine and psychiatry. See, for example, Bashir Qureshi, *Transcultural Medicine*, 2nd edition (Dordrecht: Kluwer Academic Publishers).

3. For a sophisticated treatment of this subject, see Maya Sabatello, *Children's Bioethics: The International Biopolitical Discourse on Harmful Traditional Practices and the Right of the Child to Cultural Identity* (Leiden: Martinus Nijhoff, 2009), 99–115. See also Priscilla Alderson, *Children's Consent to Surgery* (Buckingham, UK: Open University Press, 1993).

4. One of the challenges is interpreting the best interests of the child standard in a culturally diverse world. See Philip Alston, ed., *The Best Interests of the Child: Reconciling Culture and Human Rights* (Oxford: Clarendon, 1994).

5. Nobuo Shimahara, "Enculturation—A Reconsideration," *Current Anthropology* 11 (2) (1970): 143–54. Shimahara contends that enculturation should not presuppose the children learn culture in an entirely passive manner; instead of conceiving of enculturation as the unconscious acquisition of cultural categories, he suggests the process involves reflection and innovation on the part of children.

6. There is a substantial literature on this topic. See for example Roger E. Mittleman et al., "Practical Approach to Investigative Ethics and Religious Objections to the Autopsy," *Journal of Forensic Sciences* 37 (3) (1992): 824–9; Lauren R. Boglioli and Mark L. Taff, "Religious Objection to Autopsy: An Ethical Dilemma for Medical Examiners," *American Journal of Medicine and Pathology* 11 (1) (1990): 1–8; Henry Perkins, Josie D. Supik, and Helen P. Hazuda, "Autopsy Decisions: The Possibility of Conflicting Cultural Attitudes," *Journal of Clinical Ethics* 4 (2) (1993): 145–54; Henry S. Perkins, "Cultural Differences and Ethical Issues in the Problem of Autopsy Requests," *Texas Medicine* 87 (5) (1991): 72–77. Alison Dundes Renteln, *The Cultural Defense*, chapter 9, "The Dead" (New York: Oxford University Press, 2004); Renteln, "The Rights of the Dead: Autopsies and Corpse Mismanagement in Multicultural Societies," *South Atlantic Quarterly* 100 (4) (2001): 1005–7; Joseph Westermeyer, "Cultural Beliefs and Surgical Procedures," *Journal of the American Medical Association* 255 (23) (1986): 3301–2.

7. A general article on the cadaver contains a paragraph about varying attitudes toward the corpse related to autopsies. Christian A. Hovde, "Cadavers: General Ethics Concerns," in *Encyclopedia of Bioethics* 1, edited by Warren T. Reich, 139–43 (New York: Simon & Schuster MacMillan, 1978). See also Walter S. Wurzbuerger, "Jewish Perspective," 144–5.

8. In the field of bioethics there is recognition that there are divergent cultural conceptions of the body. See, for example, Thomas J. Csordas, "Body: Cultural and Religious Perspectives," in *Encyclopedia of Bioethics* (revised edition), edited by Warren T. Reich, *Encyclopedia of Bioethics* (1995), 305–12. For an anthropological interpretation of the person, see Richard A. Shweder and Edmund J. Bourke, "Does the Concept of the Person Vary Cross-Culturally?" in *Cultural Conceptions of Mental Health and Therapy*, edited by A. J. Marsela and G. M. White, 97–137 (Dordrecht: D. Reidel, 1982).

9. Not only do they fear that the autopsy will interfere with reincarnation, but some think that "American doctors want to eat the organs of the dead." They also continue to love the person as if he or she were still alive. Dia Cha, *Hmong American Concepts of Health, Healing,*

and Conventional Medicine (New York: Routledge, 2003), 36–38. For a discussion of the importance of cultural understanding when a Gypsy woman faced death, see Robert D. Orr, "Cross-Cultural Medical Ethics," *Medicine in the Americas: Medicine in a Multi-Ethnic Culture* 1 (1) (2000): 13–14.

10. Shelley Adler, "Sudden Unexpected Nocturnal Death Syndrome among Hmong Immigrants: Examining the Role of the 'Nightmare.'" *Journal of American Folklore* 104 (1991): 54–71. Adler explains: "The various forms of stress that characterize Hmong refugee life may actually have a direct effect on incidents of SUNDS" (66). She advocates the study of folk belief for its investigatory power: "Folkloristics has much to offer other fields of inquiry, including biomedicine, that will contribute to the advancement of knowledge and understanding of human behavior" (68).

11. In *Oregon v. Smith*, the U.S. Supreme Court rejected the compelling state interest test in cases in which a general statute has an incidental effect on religiously motivated actions. 494 U.S. 872 (1990). The judge vacated his earlier decision in *You Vang v. Sturner* (1990), 750 F. Supp 558. *You Vang v. Sturner* (1990). 728 F. Sup. 845 (DRI 1990), and expressed his "profound regret" at having to do so.

12. David L. Abney, "Blocking a Coroner's Autopsy in California Based on Religious Preference," *Daily Journal Report* No. 86–16, August 22, 1986, 3–8.

13. *Albareti v. Hirsch* (1993, July 7). *New York Law Journal* 21.

14. On the other hand, if family members realize that not performing the autopsy may undermine police efforts to apprehend the murderer, one wonders if they should have the right to choose to dispense with it.

15. Alison Dundes Renteln, *The Cultural Defense* (New York: Oxford University Press, 2004), 61–63.

16. After a first attempt at surgery in a refugee camp, two of Kou's siblings were born with cleft palates; this was attributed to the procedure. Li-Rong Lilly Cheng, "Asian-American Cultural Perspectives on Birth Defects: Focus on Cleft Palate," *Cleft Palate Journal* 27 (3) (1990): 294–300.

17. Alison Dundes Renteln, "Is the Cultural Defense Detrimental to the Health of Children?" *Law and Anthropology* 7 (1995): 27–106.

18. This same logic applies to the debate over deaf parents rejecting cochlear implants for their children. See Maya Sabatello, "Disability, Cultural Minorities, and International Law: Reconsidering the Case of the Deaf Community," *Whittier Law Review* 26 (2005): 1025–50. This presumption is inconsistent with evolving thinking in the disability rights movement where the focus is on equalizing opportunities for persons with disabilities rather than on rehabilitation. But see Dena Davis, "Cochlear Implants and the Claims of Culture: A Response to Lane and Grodin," *Kennedy Institute for Ethics Journal* 7 (3) (1997): 253–8.

19. Alison Dundes Renteln, "Cross-Cultural Perceptions of Disability: Policy Implications of Divergent Views," in *The Human Rights of Persons with Intellectual Disabilities: Different but Equal*, Stan Herr, Lawrence Gostin, and Harold Koh, eds., 59–81 (New York: Oxford University Press, 2003).

20. In England it was also advocated as a cure for various diseases including hysteria. Armando R. Favazza, *Bodies under Siege: Self-Mutilation and Body Modification in Culture and Psychiatry* (Baltimore: Johns Hopkins University Press, 1996).

21. L. Amede Obiora, "Bridges and Barricades: Rethinking Polemics and Intransigence in the Campaign against Female Circumcision," *Case Western Reserve Law Review* 47 (1997): 275–378, quotation on 290. See also Isabelle R. Gunning, "Female Genital Surgeries:

Eradication Measures at the Western Local Level—A Cautionary Tale," in *Genital Cutting and Transnational Sisterhood: Disputing U.S. Polemics*, edited by Stanlie M. James and Claire C. Robertson, 114–25 (Urbana: University of Illinois Press), especially 118.

22. Ellen Gruenbaum, *The Female Circumcision Controversy: An Anthropological Perspective* (Philadelphia: University of Pennsylvania Press, 2001).

23. See, for example, Marie-Angelique Savane, "Why We Are Against the International Campaign," *International Child Welfare Review* 40 (1979): 37, 39. Sandra D. Lane and Robert A. Rubinstein, "Judging the Other: Responding to Traditional Female Genital Surgeries," *Hastings Center Report*, (May–June, 1996), 31–40. Rogaia Mustafa Abusharaf, ed., *Female Circumcision* (Philadelphia: University of Pennsylvania Press, 2006).

24. A leader at Equality Now said: "There is a strong feeling that movement against this must be led by African activists." Barbara Crossette, "Mutilation Seen as Risk for the Girls of Immigrants," *New York Times*, March 23, 1998.

25. The surgery, when performed without antiseptic circumstances, can cause infection, death, problems urinating, difficult pregnancies, pain, and death.

26. *Innocenti Digest, Changing a Harmful Social Convention: Female Genital Mutilation/Cutting* (Rome: UNICEF, 2005), 17.

27. Obiora refers to a Dutch controversy in which African immigrants who had been turned away from medical facilities circumcised themselves. Somali immigrants requested a symbolic prick at the Harborview Medical Center in Seattle. See Doriane Coleman, "The Seattle Compromise: Multicultural Sensitivity, and Americanization," *Duke Law Journal* 47 (1998): 717–83.

28. Wanda Jones et al., "Female Genital Mutilation/Female Circumcision: Who Is at Risk in the United States?" *Public Health Reports* 112 (September–October 1997): 368–77. Reference to driving the custom underground on page 112.

29. Celia Dugger, "New Law Bans Genital Cutting in the United States: Violators Could Face Five Years in Prison," *New York Times*, October 12, 1996, 1, 6.

30. Indeed, consent is emphasized in the Testimony on Female Genital Mutilation of Dr. Nahid Toubia, a Sudanese physician, to the House of Representatives, Committee on Foreign Affairs' subcommittee on International Security, International Organizations, and Human Rights: "All professional organizations must pronounce it unethical for any of their members to undertake circumcising a girl under the age of consent" (September 28, 1993), 6. See also Jean F. Martin, "Article 7: Persons Without the Capacity to Consent," in *The UNESCO Universal Declaration on Bioethics and Human Rights: Background, Principles and Application*, edited by Henk A. M. J. Ten Have and Michele S. Jean, 139–59 (Paris: UNESCO, 2009).

31. It is said to be increasingly common, and the fee for it ranges from $300 in North Africa to $5,000 in private clinics in France. Bruce Crumley, "The Dilemma of 'Virginity' Restoration," *Time* (online), July 13, 2008. Another option is the use of an Artificial Virginity Hymen Kit. Jeffrey Fleishman and Amro Hassan, "Idea of Poseur Virgins Rattles Egypt," *Los Angeles Times*, October 7, 2009, A21.

32. According to one source, Mufti Ali Gomaa considered the "surgical reconstruction of the hymen of a raped girl lawful. This operation is illegal but frequently performed in Egyptian hospitals to remedy rape, and it is one that arouses considerable ethical problems. Previously many religious figures of Al-Azhar had condemned the operation, deeming it deception as the Koran requires the bride to be a virgin: If she is no longer a virgin, it is pointless lying to the husband." Dariusch Atighetchi, *Islamic Bioethics: Problems and Perspectives*, 117–18 (Dordrecht: Springer, 2007).

33. Ibid., 460.

34. A. Logmans, A. Verhoeff, R. Bol Raap, F. Creighton, and M. van Lent, "Ethical Dilemma: Should Doctors Reconstruct the Vaginal Introitus of Adolescent Girls to Mimic the Virginal State?" *British Medical Journal* 316 (February 7, 1998): 459–60. The writers disagree as to whether hymenopasty is comparative to female genital cutting or not.

35. Bruce Crumley, "The Dilemma of 'Virginity' Restoration," *Time*, (online), July 13, 2008.

36. Rebecca J. Cook and Bernard M. Dickens, "Hymen Reconstruction: Ethical and Legal Issues," *International Journal of Gynecology and Obstetrics* 107 (2009): 266–69.

37. It is important to distinguish between reconstructive surgery and purely cosmetic surgery. For individuals who have suffered accidents, the medical procedures serve the function of enabling them to rejoin society. For instance, James Partridge in his book *Changing Faces: The Challenge of Facial Disfigurement* (Grand Rapids, MI: Phoenix Society, 1997), writes of the enormous benefits he derived from a series of surgeries. Even though this surgery seems intuitively easier to justify because it is reconstructive, the need for it stems from the existence of societal stigma against people who look different. Ibid., 122–5. He says in discussing the pros and cons of surgery: "The impact of facial disfigurement can be greatly diminished by a course of surgery. You will have to draw on considerable reserves of stamina and even courage to stay the course, but the benefits of doing so are that your friends and family and public in general will not be appalled by your face or, hopefully embarrassed to be seen with you" (55). See also Michael Hughes, *The Social Consequences of Facial Disfigurement* (London: Ashgate, 1998).

38. Obiora comments on the double standard, 318–22. It is not my intent to review the vast literature about this subject but rather to suggest, as does Obiora, that we ought to consider carefully what cutting is designated as mutilation and what surgery is treated as "normal."

39. See, for example, Victoria Pitts-Taylor, *Surgery Junkies: Wellness and Pathology in Cosmetic Culture* (New Brunswick: Rutgers University Press, 2007). She notes: "In the United States in 2005, there were nearly two million aesthetic operations—more than quadruple the number in 1984" (3). See also the classic article by Kathryn Pauly Morgan, "Women and the Knife: Cosmetic Surgery and the Colonization of Women's Bodies," in *Cosmetic Surgery: A Feminist Primer*, edited by Cressida J. Heyes and Meredith Jones (Farnham: Ashgate, 2009 [originally published 1991]). See also Kathy Davis, *Reshaping the Female Body: The Dilemma of Cosmetic Surgery* (New York: Routledge, 1995). Rosemarie Tong and Hilde Lindemann, "Beauty under the Knife: A Feminist Reappraisal of Cosmetic Surgery," in *Cutting to the Core: Exploring the Ethics of Contested Surgeries*, edited by David Benatar, 183–93 (Lanham, MD: Rowman & Littlefield, 2006).

40. Pitts-Taylor, *Surgery Junkies*, 128. Although she eventually lost, the case raises the question as to whether a cosmetic surgeon has an obligation to look for the signs of body dysmorphic disorder (129). This scholar compares cosmetic surgery to adolescent self-cutters whose condition has been described as self-mutilation (144).

41. Sander Gilman, *Making the Body Beautiful: A Cultural History of Aesthetic Surgery* (Princeton: Princeton University Press, 1999).

42. Some challenge the presumption that surgery is designed to adhere to "white" aesthetic standards, arguing that the trend is toward "racial syncretism" (Amy Wilentz, "To Keep or Not to Keep Your Nose," *West Magazine*, July 9, 2006, 33–35, 43) or toward a culturally specific standard of beauty (Sam Dolnick, "Ethnic Differences Emerge in Plastic Surgery," *New York Times*, February 18, 2011). There are probably multiple motivations for the quest for cosmetic surgery.

43. Elizabeth Haiken, *Venus Envy* (Baltimore: Johns Hopkins University Press, 1998), 177. See also Aren Z. Aizura, "Where Health Meets Beauty: Feminity and Racialisation in Thai Cosmetic Surgery Clinics," *Asian Studies Review* 33 (3) (2009): 303–17.

44. Peter Irons, *Justice at War: The Story of the Japanese American Internment Cases* (New York: Oxford University Press, 1983), 94. Annie Nakao, "Overturning a Wartime Act Decades Later," *San Francisco Chronicle*, December 12, 2004, D3. One newspaper story about rhinoplasties mention of this issue in the context of German Jews: "Is it right to deny your Jewishness by changing your facial structure?" Wilentz, "To Keep or Not to Keep Your Nose," 33, 35, 43.

45. "Until recently, most surgeons have been as reluctant to confront the implications of cosmetic surgery in African American patients as they have to discuss implications in relation to Asian patients" (Haiken 1998: 214).

46. Some scholars reject the notion that the question for cosmetic surgery represents a form of self-rejection. At the center of the debate is Eugenia Kaw's article, "Medicalization of Racial Features: Asian American Women and Cosmetic Surgery," *Medical Anthropology Quarterly* 7 (1) (1993): 74–89. Inspired by Kaw, Cressida Heyes argues that feminist critiques should learn from critical whiteness theory. White women use cutting to appropriate features associated with other ethnic groups. Cressida J. Heyes, "All Cosmetic Surgery Is 'Ethnic': Asian Eyelids, Feminist Indignation, and the Politics of Whiteness," in *Cosmetic Surgery: A Feminist Primer*, edited by Cressida Heyes and Meredith Jones, 191–205 (Farnham: Ashgate, 2009).

47. Gilbert Geis and Gregory C. Brown, "The Transnational Traffic in Human Body Parts," *Journal of Contemporary Criminal Justice* 24 (2008): 212–24. Nancy Scheper-Hughes, "Illegal Organ Trade: Global Justice and the Traffic in Human Organs," in *Living Donor Organ Transplantation*, edited by Rainer Gruessner and Enrico Benedetti, 106–21 (New York: McGraw-Hill, 2008). R. R. Kishore, "Human Organs, Scarcities, and Sale: Morality Revisited," *Journal of Medical Ethics* 31 (2005): 362–5. S. E. Statz, "Finding the Winning Combination: How Blending Organ Procurement Systems Used Internationally Can Reduce the Organ Shortage," *Vanderbilt Journal of Transnational Law* 39 (2006): 1677–1709.

48. See the Declaration of Istanbul on Organ Trafficking and Transplant Tourism, *Lancet* 374 (9632) (July 5, 2008): 5–6.

49. It is beyond the scope of this chapter to delve into all of the arguments regarding coercion and global inequality. Suffice to say that some defend the libertarian argument regarding the sale of body parts.

50. Dennis Baker uses this example: "If a surgeon amputates a patient's legs to prevent gangrene spreading, this maintains a patient's dignity, but if she amputates them merely because the patient does not want her legs anymore, she would violate the dignity of the patient" (192). Dennis J. Baker, *The Right Not to Be Criminalized: Demarcating Criminal Law's Authority* (London: Ashgate, 2011).

51. Baker, *The Right Not to Be Criminalized*, 185. Surprisingly, he eventually rejects consent as a defense because it would violate the dignity of the patient at least for objectively repugnant harms that violate the dignity of the consenter.

52. This question of whether consent can serve as a defense has arisen in the context of female genital cutting. See, for example, R. D. Mackay, "Is Female Circumcision Unlawful?" *Criminal Law Review* (1983):717–22.

53. With respect to male circumcision, some medical professional associations like the American Academy of Pediatrics has tried to remain neutral. Others, for example, the Centers for Disease Control and Prevention, have been reconsidering their posture of neutrality.

See K. J. Dell'Antonia, "Debating Circumcision and Consent," *New York Times*, July 12, 2012.

54. See, for example, Debra L. DeLaet, "Framing Male Circumcision as a Human Rights Issue? Contributions to the Debate over the Universality of Human Rights," *Journal of Human Rights* 8 (2009) 405–26. Leslie Cannold, "The Ethics of Neonatal Male Circumcision: Helping Parents to Decide," in Benatar, *Cutting to the Core*, 47–61. Marie Fox and Michael Thomson, "Short Changed? The Law and Ethics of Male Circumcision," in *Children's Health and Children's Rights*, edited by Michael Freeman, 161–181 (Leiden: Martinus Nijhoff, 2006).

55. Anon, "Against the Cut: The 'Intactivist' Movement Takes on the Oldest Surgery Known to Man," *The Economist* 399 (8734) (2011): 34. Jennifer Medina, "Efforts to Ban Circumcision Gain Traction in California," *New York Times*, June 5, 2011, 18.

56. In Cologne, Germany, a court called the practice of male circumcision into question in that region. Although the court did not ban it and acquitted the doctor accused of endangering the health of a boy, it concluded that "the right [of] parents to raise their children in a religion does not override the right of a child to bodily integrity." Melissa Eddy, "In Germany, Ruling over Circumcision Sows Anxiety and Confusion," *New York Times*, July 13, 2012.

This decision led to public controversy and united religious minorities, Jewish and Muslim groups, in their opposition to the ruling. Melissa Eddy, "Germany: Circumcision Ruling Opposed," *New York Times*, July 13, 2012. Many Jewish leaders and organization condemned the court, alleging that this was yet another instance of anti-Semitic action by Germans against the Jewish people. In response, the prime minister's office, announced that Jewish and Muslim communities could continue to follow this tradition as long as it was "carried out in a responsible manner." Anon, "Angela Merkel Intervenes over Court Ban on Circumcision of Young Boys," *The Guardian* (Reuters), July 13, 2012.

57. These include children, indigenous people, migrant workers, prisoners, racial minorities, and women. See discussion in Brigit C. A. Toebes, "Toward an Improved Understanding of the International Human Right to Health," *Human Rights Quarterly* 21 (1994): 661–79, 664.

58. Brigit C. A. Toebes, *The Right to Health as a Human Right in International Law* (Antwerp: Intersentia, 1999).

59. Dieter Giesen, "A Right to Health Care? A Comparative Perspective," in *Justice and Health Care: Comparative Perspectives*, edited by A. Grubb and M. J. Mehlman, 287–304 (Hoboken, NJ: John Wiley & Sons, Ltd., 1995).

60. In much of the early literature on health and human rights, surgery is not an explicit part of the interpretation of the right to health.

61. To provide an authoritative interpretation of Article 12, in 2000 the human rights committee that enforces the instrument issued a policy statement, general comment 14, "The right to the highest attainable standard of health," which does not mention surgery. General Comment No. 14 (2000). E/C.12/2000/4, 11 August 2000. http://www.unhchr.ch/tbs/doc.nsf/; K. A. McQueen et al., "Essential Surgery: Integral to the Right to Health," *Health and Human Rights* 12 (2010): 137–52. McQueen is part of the Global Surgical Consortium, a nonprofit organization that is lobbying for emergency and essential surgery in poor countries. www.globalsurgicalconsortium.org.

There is also an organization, Surgeons Overseas, that since 2008 has provided surgical care for people in "developing" countries. See Jeffrey Leow et al., "Teaching Emergency and Essential Surgical Care in Sierra Leone: A Model for Low Income Countries," *Journal of Surgical Education* 68 (5) (2011): 393–6.

62. For commentary on the right to surgery as a key part of the right to health, see, for example, Doruk Ozgediz et al., "The Burden of Surgical Conditions and Access to Surgical Care in Low- and Middle-Income Countries," *Bulletin of the World Health Organization*, 2011, http://www.who.int/bulletin/volumes/86/8/07-050435/en/#. Doruk Ozgediz et al., "Surgery in Global Health Delivery," *Mount Sinai Journal of Medicine* 78 (3) (2011): 327–41; K. A. McQueen et al., "The Provision of Surgical Care by International Organizations in Developing Countries: A Preliminary Report," *World Journal of Surgery* 34 (3) (2011): 397–402; McQueen et al. "Essential Surgery," 145.

63. Scholars have devised a tiered system that prioritizes particular types of surgeries. See McQueen et al., "Essential Surgery," 141–43. Charles Mock et al., "Developing Priorities for Addressing Surgical Conditions Globally: Furthering the Link Between Surgery and Public Health Policy," *World Journal of Surgery* 34 (2010): 381–85.

64. Some countries do pay for cosmetic surgery in their national health insurance programs, and assessments of global health also make reference to it. If adults have the right to cut themselves, then should health insurance cover nontherapeutic procedures? If not, then this would mean that only the wealthy will have the ability to have the surgeries they desire. If the right to surgery is part of an international right to health, then accepting a class difference with regard to who is able to exercise the right is problematic.

65. Sibylle Kalupner, "The Human Right of Bodily Integrity and the Challenge of Intercultural Dialogue," Unpublished manuscript, 1–9.

66. See Doctors Opposing Circumcision Genital Integrity Policy Statement, http://www .doctorsopposingcircumcision.org/. In the 1990s an organization, NoCirc, lobbied to ban circumcision of boys and girls. The founders wrote one of the early articles on this topic: Marilyn Fayre Milos and Donna Macris, "Circumcision: A Medical or a Human Rights Issue?" *Journal of Nurse Midwifery* 37 (2), (Supp.): 87–96. Also, Dr. Toubia's international advocacy organization was called the Research, Action & Information Network for Bodily Integrity of Women. Jones et al., "Female Genital Mutilation/Female Circumcision," 370.

67. Alison Dundes Renteln, "Relativism and the Search for Human Rights," *American Anthropologist* 90 (1988): 56–72.

68. Robert Redfield, *The Primitive World and Its Transformations* (Ithaca: Cornell University Press, 1962), 146–47.

69. Alison Dundes Renteln, *International Human Rights: Universalism Versus Relativism* (Newbury Park: Sage, 1990). Others have suggested a similar idea; for example, John Rawls argued on behalf of what he termed "an overlapping consensus."

70. Evidently there has been little attention paid to this topic. In Laurence B. McCullough, James W. Jones, and Baruch A. Brody, eds., *Surgical Ethics* (New York: Oxford University Press, 1998), few pages deal with culture conflicts—pp. 124–29. They discuss patients who refuse surgery on religious grounds and when surgeons may refuse to perform operations. In James W. Jones, Laurence B McCullough, and Bruce W. Richman, eds., *The Ethics of Surgical Practice: Cases, Dilemmas, and Resolutions* (New York: Oxford University, 2008), of the seventy-one cases, only two are pertinent—one on the patient who is a Jehovah's Witness and one on truth-telling.

71. For exemplary bioethics scholarship that considers culture, see, for example, Patricia Marshall, "'Cultural Competence' and Informed Consent in International Health Research," *Cambridge Quarterly of Healthcare Ethics* 17 (2008): 206–15; Leigh Turner, "An Anthropological Exploration of Contemporary Bioethics: The Varieties of Common Sense," *Journal of Medical Ethics* 24 (1998): 127–33; Leigh Turner, "From the Local to the Global: Bioethics and the Concept of Culture," *Journal of Medicine and Philosophy* 30 (2005): 305–20.

4

Sex Determination and Sex Pre-Selection Tests in India[1]

Vibhuti Patel

ABSTRACT

Asian countries are undergoing a demographic transition resulting from a combination of low death rates and birthrates in their populations. This could be partly due to the vigorous promotion of small families by governments in South Asia and Southeast Asia. India adopted the two-child policy in 2004, while China, since 1978, has strictly implemented the "one child per family" policy. Historically, most Asian countries have had a strong preference for sons. This chapter examines the gender, sociocultural, and demographic implications of the deficit of women and the role of new reproductive technologies, with a focus on sex determination (SD) and sex preselection technologies (SP).

INTRODUCTION

Sex ratios in Europe, North America, the Caribbean, Central Asia, and even the poorest of regions—such as Sub-Saharan Africa —are favorable to women. In the South and Southeast Asia, the sex ratios are lower for women, as table III.4.1 reveals. The historical legacy of the preference for sons and neglect of daughters in Southeast Asia has taken a dangerous turn in which scientific technologies for SD such as amniocentesis, chorionic villus biopsy, foetoscopy, and sonography are being misused for the selective abortion of female fetuses.

"All countries of the region with the exception of Indonesia, Myanmar, Sri Lanka [*sic*] and Thailand have a higher male than female population, as evident in the sex ratio of the population. In some countries (Bangladesh and India) the relatively

Table III.4.1. Women per One Hundred Men in Selected Regions, Countries

Region	Women Per 100 Men	Country	Women Per 100 Men
Bangladesh	95.3	Latin America	100
Bhutan	98.2	Maldives	94.8
Caribbean	103	Myanmar	101.0
Central Asia	104	Nepal	97.8
China	94.4	South Asia	95
Democratic Republic of Korea	99.7	Southeast Asia	95
Europe and North America	105	Sri Lanka	101.2
India	93.5	Sub-Saharan Africa	102
Indonesia	100.5	Thailand	100.0
WORLD	98.5		

Source: United Nations. 1995. *The World's Women: Trends and Statistics;* World Health Organization. 2000. *Women of South East Asia: A Health Profile.* New Delhi.

higher proportion of males in the population is at least in part due to the higher female than male mortality during childhood and in the reproductive age group."[2] The lowest sex ratio adverse to females is found in India.

Among the Jains in Gujarat, Rajasthan, and Karnataka, the sex ratio has become dangerously low due to sex selection during the last two decades, although Jainism prohibits abortion. Preconception sex selection that does not involve abortion is quite popular among Jains. It is possible to preselect the sex of the fetus using in vitro fertilization (IVF), gamete intrafallopian transfer (GIFT), and zygot intrafallopian transfer (ZIFT), technologies that could be costly. Doctors are able to select an X chromosome from the egg of the woman and a Y chromosome from the sperm of a man to fertilize an egg to produce a male fetus. As a result of the use of these various technologies, Jain men are finding difficulty getting brides and are purchasing brides from non-Jain, poor families. Religious leaders are alarmed by this phenomenon and have been delivering religious sermons among the followers to prevent sex selection in the name of "racial purity."

Among the Sikhs, the female-to-male sex ratio is alarmingly low, and religious leaders have also issued notices and sermons to stop sex-selective abortions of female fetuses. Noble laureate Amartya Sen calls the adverse ratio of female-to-male the phenomenon of the "missing women,"[3] which is an indication of discrimination and stigmatization of mothers delivering daughters. The preference for sons is driven by the perception that boys are assets; the birth of boys symbolizes "sunrise" while that of girls, "sunset." Boys remain within the family and take care of parents in their old age, whereas girls marry and "go away." "Sex selection in society occurs in the context of entrenched values, interests, and cultural beliefs and practices. Their eradication requires investment in long-term strategies and economic and social development, and educational and cultural empowerment."[4]

POPULARITY OF SD AND SP

SD and SP tests are popular among upper-class, educated families who believe that small family norms mean a minimum of one or two sons in the family. The propertied classes do not desire a daughter/daughters because after the marriage of a daughter, the son-in-law may demand a share in the property.

However, even without these qualifying conditions, sex selection is practiced and advertised in very poor rural and tribal areas. Poor families dispose of daughters to avoid possible dowry harassment, which refers to the social stigmatization of parents who fail to marry off their daughters because they cannot afford an acceptable dowry. But they do not mind accepting dowry for their sons. The birth of a son is perceived to be an opportunity for upward mobility while that of a daughter is believed to result in downward economic mobility. The social price to pay for having an unmarried daughter in India is too high in terms of being taunted; parents with unmarried daughters and the daughters as well are made to feel worthless. Predominant cultural values treat marriage as a "be all" and "end all" of a woman's lifetime achievement and identity.

AGENTS HIRED TO BUY THE BRIDES AND FORCED POLYANDRY

Among certain communities in Madhya Pradesh, Haryana, Gujarat, Rajasthan, and Punjab, the sex ratio is extremely adverse for women. As a result, a wife could be shared by brothers or sometimes even by patrilineal parallel cousins.[5]

Recently, in Gujarat, there have been disturbing reports of the reintroduction of polyandry (a Panchali system where a woman is married to five men). In villages in Mehsana District, the problem of a declining number of girls has created a major social crisis as almost all villages have hundreds of boys who are left with no choice but to buy brides from outside.[6] Poor girls from tribal communities in Gujarat and Karnataka are purchased by the agents and married off to households where the woman has to provide sexual services to all male members of the extended family.

VIOLENCE AND HEALTH ISSUES OF WOMEN OVER THE LIFE CYCLE

As unborn children, women face covert violence in terms of sex selection and overt violence in terms of female feticide after the use of amniocentesis, chorionic villus biopsy, sonography, ultrasound, and imaging techniques.[7] Infertile couples approach IVF (in vitro fertilization) clinics for assisted reproduction attempting to produce sons. Doctors are advertising such messages aggressively: "Invest Rs.500 now, save

Rs.50,000 later"—that is, "If you get rid of your daughter now, you will not have to spend money on dowry."

Girls under five years of age in India face neglect in terms of medical care and education and the risk of sexual abuse and physical violence. As adolescents and adult women in the reproductive age group, they face the risk of early marriage, early pregnancy, sexual violence, domestic violence, dowry harassment, and torture in cases of infertility. If they fail to produce sons, they face desertion or a witch hunt. The end result is high maternal mortality.

NEW REPRODUCTIVE TECHNOLOGIES (NRTS) AND WOMEN

There are three main aspects to NRT-assisted reproduction, genetic or prenatal diagnosis, and the prevention of conception and birth. NRTs perform four types of functions: assisted reproduction; contraception; sex selection and genetic manipulation; in vitro fertilization (IVF) and subsequent embryo transfer, GIFT (gamete intrafallopian transfer), ZIFT (zygote intrafallopian transfer), and cloning-assisted reproduction.[8]

Contraceptive technologies prevent conception and birth. Amniocentesis, chorionic villus biopsy (CVB), and ultrasound and imaging are used for prenatal diagnosis.[9] Fetal cells are collected by the technique of amniocentesis and CVB. Gene technologies are welcomed for their potential of treating diseases, for diagnosis, and more. Genomics is "the science of improving the human population through controlled breeding" and "encompasses the elimination of disease, disorder, or undesirable traits, on the one hand, and genetic enhancement on the other. It is pursued by nations through state policies and programmes."[10] But we have to be critical and examine the scientific, social, juridical, ethical, and economic and health consequences of the NRTs. NRTs have made women's bodies a site for scientific experimentations.

In Mumbai, girls are selling their eggs for rupees 20,000 (approximately $163). Infertility clinics in Mumbai receive four to five calls per day from young women who want to donate their eggs.[11] NRTs in the neocolonial context of third-world economies and the unequal division of labor between the first- and the third-world economies have created a bizarre scenario and cutthroat competition among body chasers, clone chasers, intellect chasers, and supporters of femicide. It is important to understand the interaction among NRT developers, providers, users, nonusers, potential users, policymakers, and representatives of international organizations.[12]

INITIATIVES BY THE STATE AND NGOS

Due to active lobbying by women's groups and NGOs, the Prenatal Diagnostic Techniques (Regulation and Prevention of Misuse) Act was enacted in 1994 by the

Centre, the Government of India. But the violation of this legislation continues. While the Act only allows tests to identify deformity in the fetus, in 95 percent of cases, sex determination tests were used for sex-selective abortions of the female fetus.

In response to the public interest, a petition filed in 2001 by Dr. Sabu George, Centre for Inquiry into Health and Allied Themes Mumbai and MASUM—fought on their behalf by the Lawyers Collective (Delhi)[13]—the Supreme Court of India directed all state governments to effectively and promptly implement the Prenatal Diagnostics Techniques (Regulation and Prevention of Misuse) Act. Now it has been renamed "The Preconception and Prenatal Diagnostic Techniques (Prohibition of Sex Selection) Act."

The women's movement has emphasized women's rights, using slogans such as: Eliminate Inequality, Not Women; Destroy Dowry & Dehumanization, Not Daughters; Say "No" to Sex-Determination, Say "Yes" to Empowerment of Women; Say "No" to Sex Discrimination, Say "Yes" to Gender Justice; and Daughters Are Not for Slaughter.

DO WOMEN HAVE A CHOICE?

The ethical dilemma faced by gender-sensitive professionals is this: "Is the mother to blame for having her female fetus destroyed?" There are ethicists who have averred that aborting a female fetus or not allowing a female embryo to be conceived is a lesser evil than birthing a girl child and making her live a life of discrimination.

This question reflects the assumption that women have the freedom to choose. "It is a question of women's own choice." This is especially problematic when viewed in the light of feminists' advocacy throughout the world for the right of women to control their own fertility, to choose whether or not to have children, and to access facilities for free, legal, and safe abortions. But in the social context of countries such as India, this so called "choice" is not made in a social vacuum. These women are socially conditioned to accept that unless they produce one or more male children, they have no social worth.[14] They can be harassed, taunted, or even deserted by their husbands if they fail to do so. In effect, they really have no choice.

NOTES

1. *Asian Bioethics Review* 2 (1) (March 2010): 76–81. Used with permission.
2. WHO, "Women of South East Asia—A Health Profile," New Delhi, 2000, 4–5.
3. A. K. Sen, "Missing Women," *British Medical Journal* (1992):304.
4. H. L. Chee, "Genomics and Health: Ethical, Legal and Social Implications for Developing Countries," *Issues in Medical Ethics* X (1) (2002): 146–9.
5. L. Dubey, "Misadventure in Amniocentesis," *Economic and Political Weekly*, Bombay, 1983.
6. Sabu, George. "Millions of Missing Girls: From Fetal Sexing to High Technology Sex Selection in India," *The Times of India*, July 8, 2004.

7. V. Patel, "Girl Child: An Endangered Species?," in *The Girl Child in 20th Century Indian Literature*, edited by V. Kripal (New Delhi: Sterling Publications Pvt. Ltd., 1992), 9.

8. T. D. Nandedkar, and M. S. Rajadhyaksha, *Brave New Generation: Vistas in Biotechnology* (Delhi: CSIR, Department of Biotechnology, Government of India, 1995).

9. T. D. Nandedkar, and M. S. Rajadhyaksha, "Sex Selection," in *Routledge International Encyclopedia of Women: Global Women's Issues and Knowledge*, volume 4, edited by Cheris Kramarae and Dale Spender, 1818–9 (New York: Routledge, 2001).

10. Chee, "Genomics and Health," 146–49.

11. Special Correspondent, "Sex Selective Abortions and Declining Sex Ratio," *The Asian Age*, June 11, 2004.

12. FINRRAGE—Feminist International Network of Resistance to Reproductive and Genetic Engineering, Germany, 2000, and UBINIG: Women's Declarations on Reproductive Technologies and Genetic Engineering, Dhaka, 2004.

13. A. Basu, "Sex Selective Abortions," *Lawyers Collective*, 18 (11) (2003): 20–23.

14. R. Rapp, "The Ethics of Choice," *Ms. Magazine*, April 1984, 97–100.

5

Confucianism and Killing versus Letting Die

Cecilia Wee

ABSTRACT

Much of the Western contemporary debate on the permissibility of active euthanasia centers on whether there is any morally significant distinction between killing and letting die. Those who would prohibit active euthanasia but permit passive euthanasia point out that the former involves a direct *act* of killing, whereas the latter involves an *omission* (i.e., omitting to do that which may prolong life). This argument turns on a commonly accepted view in the West that there is a morally significant difference between an act and an omission (even in contexts where the eventual outcomes are the same). In this chapter I will argue that this distinction between act and omission—active and passive euthanasia—may not carry the same moral weight in Confucianism. I begin with an outline of Confucian role-morality. Drawing in part from classical Confucian texts, I then argue that, on such a role-based morality, the distinction between acting and omitting to act may be largely irrelevant to moral decision making. This is then brought to bear on end-of-life decisions: I suggest that, to the Confucian, the distinction between killing and letting die may not play the same role in end-of-life decisions that it has done in the West.

INTRODUCTION

Medical ethics, particularly in Western countries, has traditionally held that there is a clear distinction between passive and active euthanasia—between withholding or ceasing treatment so as to allow a patient to die and taking direct action aimed at killing the patient. While the former is held to be permissible, at least in certain circumstances, the latter has been seen as wholly impermissible. Put another way, while it is acceptable in some cases to let a patient die, it is never acceptable to kill a patient.

The difference in the perceived ethical permissibility of active and passive euthanasia is partly rooted in a well-entrenched distinction—most notably set out by James Rachels. This is the moral (and in many cases also legal) distinction between an action and an omission to act. The scenario is as follows: Consider someone (person "A") who wants another person dead and deliberately kills that person. By taking the other's life, "A" would be deemed morally culpable and might well be guilty of murder. In contrast, consider another person ("B") who stands by rather than saving the individual's life, when that could be done easily and at no great risk. "B" would generally be thought less morally culpable than "A" for the other's death and would not likely be seen as having murdered the person.

This suggests that a moral difference exists between acting to obtain an outcome and (knowingly) failing to act. This distinction underpins the permissibility of withdrawal of treatment in end-of-life situations that a patient faces and the nonpermissibility of an act designed to directly kill the patient.

In view of the debate, it would be helpful to put in some caveats concerning the scope and concerns of this chapter. These will help clarify the contrast between Western and Confucian views on the subject. The distinction between act and omission—active and passive euthanasia—may not carry the same moral weight in Confucianism. In the second half of this chapter, I will set out my argument.

First, note that the distinction between active and passive euthanasia used here is rather broad. The actual range of options pertaining to end-of-life situations should perhaps more appropriately be classified as follows:

1. passive euthanasia
2. indirect euthanasia (pain-relieving treatment under the nonintended risk of abbreviation of life)
3. assisted suicide (e.g., procuring and/or providing a deadly medicine)
4. active euthanasia

This chapter will merely contrast active euthanasia with passive euthanasia and include (3) and (4) under active euthanasia and (1) and (2) under passive euthanasia. Therefore, my primary focus will be to contrast (1) and (4).

Second, while the distinction between act and omission is widely accepted as grounding the difference between active and passive euthanasia, the two concepts may not stand in a one-to-one relation with each other. One objection is that the term *passive euthanasia* is a contradiction in terms. This is because euthanasia, by definition, causes death, and omission, by definition, cannot cause anything. Passive euthanasia would then be that which causes death but cannot cause anything.[1] The viability of this objection hinges on the question of whether omissions can have a causative effect—which some commentators think possible.

The discussion above assumes that passive euthanasia always involves an omission to act. Another objection as to why active and passive euthanasia do not stand in a one-to-one correlation with action and omission comes by way of the point that passive euthanasia does not always involve an omission to act. For example, we usually include under the category of passive euthanasia the case of "pulling the plug" on a patient's ventilator, which involves an *action* by some agent. "Pulling the plug" and thus allowing the patient to die tends to be viewed differently from a direct killing such as stabbing someone to death. In the latter case, the outcome would be death regardless of whether the individual in question is healthy. In the former case, the outcome is the death *specifically* of a terminally ill person.

Frances Kamm has likened the case of "pulling the plug" on a patient whose life is being prolonged solely by the ventilator to a situation in which one has been saving someone from drowning and then decides to stop. Both cases count as *omissions* to save, despite one's action (see Kamm 2008).[2]

Another case in which passive euthanasia involves an action would be when euthanasia involves extraordinary treatment (such as putting the patient on a ventilator) that is then discontinued at the same time that ordinary treatment (such as providing nutrition) is continued. In this situation, passive euthanasia arguably involves not just pure omission but *action* (in the provision of nutrition).

However, the relevant contrast in the present debate concerning end-of-life decisions is that of the action of *killing* versus the omission of letting the patient die. The action of providing nutrition is aimed at the (ordinary) *sustenance* of life, and hence it is not germane to the specific action-omission contrast at issue here.

The distinction between active and passive euthanasia may not map directly onto the distinction between action and omission. Nevertheless, there are reasonable grounds, and some intuitive plausibility, to holding that passive euthanasia is an omission, in relevant contrast to active euthanasia, which is an action. I hold the view that passive euthanasia is indeed an omission to act while active euthanasia is an action.

Let me now come to the third caveat. As can be seen above, it is not always easy to distinguish clearly between actions and omissions—that is, pulling the plug on the ventilator that keeps a patient alive can be both an action and an omission. But even if we assume that there is a distinction between an action and an omission, there remains the question as to whether there is any *moral* difference between the two.

The debate here is well established. For example, it has been argued that the moral distinction between action and an omission derives from the fact that an action can cause an outcome but an omission cannot. Agents are causally responsible (and hence morally responsible) for the outcomes of their actions, but they are not causally or morally responsible for omissions. On the other hand, as indicated above, some commentators argue that omissions can be causal as well, and we can thus be morally responsible for acts of omission. Whether we believe that there is a moral difference between an action and omission to act may ultimately depend on the ethical theory that one holds. The Utilitarian, for instance, would say there is no relevant moral difference between an action and an omission to act, as Utilitarianism enjoins that one should always pursue (whether by action or omission to act) that which maximizes the overall balance of pleasure over pain.[3]

In this chapter I shall not engage with the recent debate and controversy on the distinction (moral, metaphysical, or both) between actions and omissions. That the American Medical Association has maintained that passive euthanasia is permissible but active euthanasia is not goes to show how well entrenched is the assumption of the moral difference between action and omission.[4] The pervasive Western assumption of moral difference between action and omission is much less likely to obtain in a person who comes from a role-based morality such as Confucianism. Because of this divergence, the distinction between active and passive euthanasia, along with the action-omission distinction, plays an important role in determining end-of-life medical decisions in the West. However, it would not likely have the same role in such decisions in societies with a strong Confucian background.

Bioethical decision making in countries influenced by Confucianism differs markedly from that which obtains in Western countries. On this basis, some writers have advocated the development of a distinctive Confucian bioethics that draws on the fundamental metaphysical and moral beliefs of the tradition (see, for example, Fan 1999, Lee 2007). If indeed there is no morally significant difference between active and passive euthanasia in Confucianism, this can be addressed when developing a Confucian bioethics.

I will give a brief account of Confucian morality as a role-morality and then discuss role-moralities in the context that they are most frequently associated with in the West—viz., the professions. In contexts where there are well-specified professional role-obligations, there may be no moral distinction drawn between an act and an omission to act. Confucianism is then shown to be similar to the professions in having highly specific sets of role-obligations. I then argue that the distinction between act and omission is similarly absent in such Confucian contexts. This is used to explain why end-of-life decisions in Confucian societies may differ from those in the West.

CONFUCIANISM AS A ROLE-MORALITY

The view that Confucianism is essentially a role-morality is well accepted and pervasive (e.g., Rosemont 1986 and Nuyen 2007). In addition, various commentators have argued that there are important similarities between Confucianism and Aristotelian virtue ethics (e.g., Sim 2007), feminist care ethics (e.g., Li 2000), and Kantian deontology (e.g., Wawrytko 1982). It is not clear whether the view that Confucianism is a role-morality is ultimately incompatible with any of these other positions. Roger Ames (2008) and Henry Rosemont (2007) have argued that it is not thus compatible. This issue is not easily settled. What is certainly true is that the view of Confucianism as a role-morality has considerable textual and historical support and that it is very likely an accurate representation of Confucianism *as it is actually practiced* (Ho 1998).

According to Confucius, there is one true path ("the Way") that all humans should try to follow. Its crucial component is the cultivation and development of the appropriate inward attitudes and feelings toward others, which are then expressed in appropriate outward behaviors. However, unlike the rival Mohist school that advocates the development of an attitude of universal and impartial concern toward all mankind, Confucians hold that the appropriate attitudes and behaviors toward others should be subject to gradations. In general, these should differ according to the relation to the person in question. Confucianism is well known for emphasizing the importance, indeed the primacy, of the family. More generally, what is accorded to any given person would depend on the *role* one inhabits with respect to that person: what is appropriately accorded to one's father, elder brother, friend, political leader, and others would thus be quite different.

There are of course certain general virtues or attributes that Confucius and his followers thought the ethical person should possess and make an effort to cultivate. These virtues would include sincerity (*cheng*), trustworthiness (*xin*), conscientiousness (*zhong*)—and especially benevolence (*jen*). Benevolence is held to be the key or overarching virtue, without which one cannot be an effective political leader or attain moral sagehood. These attributes or virtues may be expressed in different behaviors, and they may receive somewhat different emphases, depending on the role that one occupies in respect of the person in question. There are also virtues that tend to be role specific; for instance, the virtue of filiality (*xiao*) obviously applies specifically to sons and daughters.

It has been argued that Confucian role-morality is rooted in the Confucian conception of the self, which sees the self as relational and as embedded within a set of social, and more especially, familial relations.[5] This conception of the self differs from the standard Western conception of the self or person as an independent individual having autonomy and choosing freely to enter into the various associations he or she enters.[6]

Confucians see themselves primarily as a part of a larger whole(s). They are *members* of a particular family, a particular institution, and a particular society. They are, thus, embedded in a wider network of specific relationships. It then behooves them to cultivate the appropriate internal attitudes and outward behaviors in respect to each of these roles.

Let us now turn to professional ethics, where an action, at least to some extent, is regulated by the specific role that she has undertaken as a professional. I will argue that, in the context of such professional roles, the moral or ethical gap between act and omission to act is usually less than in ordinary, nonprofessional contexts.

PROFESSIONAL ROLES AND THE MORAL DIFFERENCE BETWEEN ACTION AND OMISSION

Writers on professional ethics have emphasized the link between the specific role that a professional plays and what is ethically or morally expected of her in virtue of occupying that role. Being in a certain profession generates certain role-obligations, which are often embodied in a code of ethics. While such obligations may include the observance of professional etiquette, they would also, and importantly, include the moral and ethical obligations that a professional has in virtue of being a member of that profession (Beauchamp and Childress 1996: 6).

A substantial portion of the literature on professional role-morality concerns the potential conflicts that might arise between the specific moral obligations that a professional has in her professional role and the (more) universal moral norms that should be observed. We will not be concerned here with how the moral obligations of particular professions stand in relation to the wider set of moral norms, whether genuine conflicts may arise between the two, and if so, what the potential means of resolution are.[7] These issues lie beyond the scope of the chapter. Instead, that these issues arise at all makes evident that the moral obligations of the professional are different from—extend beyond—the broader moral norms that people are expected to observe in the community. In this section, I highlight two ways in which the presence of such professional role-obligations can impact on the moral assessment of omissions to act by the professional.

The first is that an omission or failure to observe a professional role-obligation is often taken to be a more significant moral failure than other comparable omissions to act in contexts that do not involve such role-obligations. Consider a doctor who, in the course of treating a patient for a minor problem, discovers a tumor needing urgent excision. The doctor fails to inform the patient of the tumor and the need for urgent surgery. Compare this with someone who notices that there are some loose tiles on a neighbor's roof that should be fixed urgently, as they could be dislodged and cause serious injury. The person fails to inform the neighbor of the loose tiles.

We would tend to assign the doctor a higher degree of moral culpability for her failure to inform than we would the neighbor. This is because the doctor, in her professional role, has well-specified role-obligations toward her patients. The same does not apply to neighbors, where the issue of what one owes to, or ought to observe in respect of, a neighbor is much less specific. One's attitude toward a neighbor can acceptably range from the stance of "Am I my brother's keeper?" to one of some degree of concern and responsibility. This contrasts with the doctor, who, in embarking on her profession, is required to have a reasonably clear idea of what is or is not morally acceptable in the doctor-patient relationship.

The second way in which omissions to act by professionals differ from omissions in a nonprofessional context can be made clear through the following example. Suppose Doctor C conspires with a patient's relative to ensure the patient's demise so that the latter can inherit vast wealth. To bring this about, she deliberately prescribes a drug that she knows full well will result in the patient's death. Now Doctor D is similarly in conspiracy with a patient's relative to ensure the patient's demise. To bring this about, she deliberately withholds a drug, knowing full well that, given the patient's condition, this will result in her certain death.

In the situation outlined above, *both* doctors would be seen to be morally culpable for their respective patients' deaths. Moreover, it is not intuitively evident that there is any clear difference in the *level* of moral culpability of the two doctors, although one doctor brings about the death by deliberately acting and the other by deliberately omitting to act. While physicians are bound by the obligation to not kill but are allowed to let die in end-of-life contexts, they are also bound by the obligation to prolong the life and well-being of the patient. All other things being equal, the deliberate transgression of this obligation, whether by omission or by commission, would be counted as a moral failure.

The cases of doctors C and D thus stand in some contrast to the cases mentioned in the introduction, where the level of moral culpability between persons A and B is intuitively judged to be quite different. What underpins the difference in our intuitions in the two cases is again that the doctors (C and D) are acting in their professional roles and, in that capacity, have a particular set of obligations which A and B, judged to be acting in their personal capacity, do not.

"Ordinary" morality, underpinned by "ordinary" intuitions, generally assigns less culpability to one who fails to act to bring about an outcome than one who acts to bring it about. A direct action aimed at a negative outcome is a much more serious overall threat to the peace and security of humans in a society than an omission to act to bring about that outcome (see Nesbitt 1999).[8] However, matters are different when an individual is acting in a professional capacity and is governed by well-specified role-obligations. In such contexts, transgressions of such obligations, whether by omission or commission, are, *certeris paribus*, regarded quite equally as transgressions.

In sum, professional roles generally come with specific obligations embodied within and emphasized by a code of ethics. In such a context, an omission to act would clearly count as an ethical failure, where an omission in ordinary, nonprofessional contexts might not.

PROFESSIONAL ROLE-MORALITY AND CONFUCIAN ROLE-MORALITY

I now turn back to the role-based ethics of Confucianism, which enjoins the cultivation of the appropriate inward attitudes that will then be expressed as appropriate outward behaviors. These appropriate attitudes and behaviors would differ according to the specific relationship that obtains between oneself and the person in question.

Suppose that Mei-ling is both a daughter and a sister. As a daughter, she would be expected to cultivate certain attitudes and behaviors in respect of this role; they would not be quite the same as the attitudes and behaviors that should be cultivated in her role as a sister. Moreover, the respective behaviors by which Mei-ling expresses her filiality and sisterhood would include not only general sorts of behaviors that manifest concern for parent and sibling. Confucianism also indicates that her appropriate inward attitudes would also be expressed by the fulfillment of some well-specified requirements, including the observance of various rituals and rites.

There are thus similarities between professional role-morality and Confucian role-morality. First, both emphasize the role that an individual inhabits in relation to another and on the role-obligations that obtain as a result. Second, these role-obligations are well specified in Confucianism, as in professional role-morality.

These features suggest that Confucian morality would differ significantly from "ordinary" morality in the West. Consider the question of what a son should morally owe to his father. In "ordinary" morality, there seems to be relatively wide latitude for one's answers to this question, just as there is for one's answers to what one owes a neighbor. One son may maintain that he owes it to his father to turn up annually for Thanksgiving; another might think he is obliged to regularly visit his parent once a month; and so on.

In contrast, the role-obligations of a son are quite clearly specified in the Confucian tradition. As Ho notes, the "stringent demands" that must be fulfilled for one to be filial include "providing for the material and moral well-being of one's aged parents, performing the ceremonial duties of ancestral worship . . . ensuring the continuity of the family line, and in general conducting oneself so as to bring honor and avoid disgrace to the family name" (Ho 1998: 11). Inhabiting the role of son thus brings with it very specific role-obligations, and the tradition is quite emphatic on the need to observe these specific obligations. In these respects, Confucian morality is more akin to professional morality than "ordinary morality."

There is also a degree of latitude as to how a Confucian child should manifest filiality, just as there is a degree of latitude as to how a professional such as a doctor should meet her obligation to her patients. For example, a Confucian child may manifest filiality by deciding to take her parents on an overseas holiday; similarly, a doctor may decide on prescribing one specific course of treatment for a patient rather than another.

Specific obligations that a Confucian child is expected to fulfill to her parents could change over time in accord with changes in tradition, just as a doctor's specific obligations can change over time in accord with changes in the accepted code of medical ethics. Nevertheless, both the Confucian child and the doctor are subject, at any given point in time, to very specific obligations in many areas in which "ordinary" (Western) morality does not enjoin any specific obligation.

Given these similarities, we might expect to find that there is less of a moral distinction in Confucianism between actions and omissions to act, particularly in contexts where these are transgressions of a particular role-obligation. And indeed, there is textual evidence in classical Confucian texts that this is the case. While there are certainly examples of moral transgression that involve a specific action in Confucian texts, there are a number of texts in which an *omission to act* is treated as moral failure. In the *Book of Mencius*, Mencius notes: "There are three ways of being a bad son. The most serious is to have no heir" (4A: 26).

Here it is the *omission* of providing an heir that is considered a transgression of one's role-obligation as a son. Again, Mencius also notes: "No one considers the *neglect* of parents and the *denial* of relationships between prince and subject, and between superior and inferior as laudable" (*Mencius* 7A: 34, emphasis mine).

Once again, moral transgression is expressed in terms of what one has omitted or failed to do. The failure to look after one's parents and to observe the role-obligations that obtain in the relations between prince and subject, and superior and inferior, are deplored because one has *omitted* to behave in the morally appropriate way. Confucius notes: "Faced with what is right, to leave it undone shows a lack of courage" (*Analects* 2:24). This encapsulates the general Confucian position that an *omission* to do what is right (which of course includes what is demanded by one's various role-obligations) is morally wrong.

There are significant similarities between professional role-morality and Confucian role-morality. Both emphasize role-obligations that pertain to the particular role one inhabits, and in both cases, these role-obligations are fairly well specified. Finally, both would hold that transgression of these role-obligations constitute a moral breach, whether the transgression is caused by a direct action or an omission to act.

In the next section, because the Confucian sees no moral distinction between a transgression of one's role-obligation by omission and one by direct action, she will not see any moral difference between letting die and killing in end-of-life situations. Letting die in this context is quite as bad as killing for the Confucian.

END-OF-LIFE ISSUES AND THE
CONFUCIAN MORAL PERSON

Empirical studies have suggested that, in countries with a strong Confucian background, families are often reluctant to withdraw life support for family members in end-of-life situations (Hui 1999). To understand why this may be so, we need to take into account not just the role-obligations of family members but the overall Confucian attitude toward the body.

The Confucian, and more generally East Asian, uses a different metaphysical framework than that which obtains in the West in the understanding of the "body." The predominant conception of the person in the West is as an autonomous individual having a dichotomy between mind and body. After all, the autonomous decisions by the individual are often seen as *mental* decisions, as taking place in the individual's mind—and this is seen as conceptually distinct from what takes place in the body.

This distinction is not found in Confucianism. There is no corresponding concept in Confucianism of what we would call the individual "mind" as the locus not only of one's autonomous choices, but as the repository of a lifetime of thoughts, feelings, experiences, and memories (Rosemont 2007).

Part of what underwrites the movement to define "death" as brain death is the assumption that, with the cessation of brain function, there is a cessation (or, if one believes in an afterlife, a departure from the body) of the *ego* or "I." That is, there is an end or departure of a particular consciousness with its own specific thoughts, choices, life experiences, memories from the body, and therefore, to all intents and purposes, an end to a *lived* life in that particular body.

Confucians do not have an equivalent concept of mind *qua ego* or a discrete experiencing "I" that is conceptually distinct from the body. Thus, brain death, commonly seen as concomitant with the end or departure of a consciousness in the West, may not be accorded the significance that it holds in the West. Absent the contrast of mind and body, the individual live body of someone in a vegetative state is not seen as an empty husk—it remains significant despite this cessation of brain function. Confucianism also holds a reverent attitude toward the body: "Being reverent about the body (*shen*) is of the greatest importance. The body is a branch of one's parents, so how could one be irreverent in this regard?"[9]

The Confucian body is seen as a branch whose foundational trunk are the parents. The reverence for one's body is seen implicitly as a form of family reverence. Failure to take care of one's body is a dishonoring of one's parents. Failure to take care of one's parents' bodies might well be seen as a dishonoring of one's ancestors or family line. Given this Confucian attitude toward the body, we can now come back to the role-obligations of the Confucian family member.

Confucianism emphasizes the primacy of family: Patient autonomy does not receive the same emphasis that it does in the West (Fan and Tao 2004). Family members rather than the patients make many significant medical decisions, including end-of-life decisions (Fielding and Hung 1996, Li and Chou 1997). Patient confidentiality also takes a back seat. Bad medical news is usually first conveyed by the doctor to family members who then decide whether the patient should be told of her condition. In the medical context, family members are expected to honor their role-obligations to the patient. Thus, in making a decision for a parent, the appropriate attitude to keep in mind is that of filiality or *xiao*.

One significant role-obligation of a Confucian child (especially a son) is to ensure his parents' well-being and to take care of them in their old age. This is often held to include keeping one's parents alive for as long as possible. For example, *The Twenty-Four Paragons of Filial Piety*, written by the Yuan dynasty scholar Guo Jujing, abounds with stories of paragons who went to extreme lengths to prolong their parents' or in-laws' lives.[10] Keeping one's parents—and more specifically parents' bodies—alive using life support is seen as an expression of filiality (Hui 1999, Tse and Tao 2004).

For the Confucian, as for the professional, an omission to meet one's role obligation is viewed as a significant moral transgression. Given that the Confucian's primary obligation is to one's parent or other family member, *not* keeping the latter alive is a serious moral transgression. This is the case even if the family member is brain dead or in a persistent vegetative state. The two reasons for this view is that (1) there no clear conception here that the family member's life is over because her lived, experienced life is over and (2) there is generally a reverence for the body in Confucianism. Withdrawal of a ventilator or life support ("letting die") would be seen as a failure or omission to keep that member alive and could be almost as bad as directly killing a family member in similar circumstances.

Where the West has had a tendency to assume that there is a morally significant difference between killing and letting die, Confucianism tends to see no difference in the two in contexts such as these. Moreover, in the West there is the line of argument that, if it is morally permissible to let die in appropriate contexts, it should also be morally permissible to kill in those contexts.

In Confucianism, the assimilation apparently goes in the other direction. The Confucian assimilates letting die to killing, maintaining that, inasmuch as it is morally impermissible to kill one's parents, then, given one's role-obligations, it is also impermissible to let them die.

In November 2008, a Seoul Western District Court ordered doctors to remove life support from a woman who was "in a persistent vegetative state." This made international news because, prior to this, South Korean courts, and indeed, the general populace, had generally been against the withdrawal of life support for such patients. This in turn has been widely attributed to the Confucian background of South Koreans. In addition, it was thought comparable to a 1997 case in which a father had requested the removal of a ventilator, an extraordinary means of life support, from his son who was similarly in a vegetative state.

The doctors who acceded to his request and took the patient off life support were subsequently convicted of "abetment to murder." The withdrawal of life support, and the consequent *letting die*, of the patient, was deemed to be a direct act of *murder*—thus the conviction. While none of those involved was jailed, the very conviction of "abetment to murder" indicates there was no clear-cut distinction between omission (to keep alive) and direct action (to kill) in this case. Confucianism, as shown above, entails a role-morality with well-specified obligations regarding end-of-life situations. In such contexts, an omission to preserve life could be seen as impermissible as, and not entirely distinguishable from, a direct killing.[11]

NOTES

1. See, for example, Garrard and Wilkinson (2005) for a discussion of this particular claim. McLachlan (2008) provides a response.

2. See also McMahan (2002). McMahan provides some fine-grained distinctions with respect to the question of whether the withdrawal of ventilator support counts as a killing or a letting die.

3. See, for example, Singer (1979), 147–53. It is also likely that adherents of other moral theories, such as Kantians and virtue ethicists, would accept that (at least under specific conditions) there may be no relevant moral difference between an action and omission. I thank an editor for this point.

4. Helpful further readings on the issues I have discussed above can be found in Beauchamp and Childress (1996), Foot (2002), and Singer (1979).

5. Confucian scholars argue that the Confucian self is *metaphysically constituted* by the roles that she inhabits with respect to the various others in her life. See, for example, Rosemont (2007).

6. This conception of the self is also being reevaluated in the West. See Mackenzie and Stoljar (2000).

7. See Andre (1991), Bowie (1982), Gibson (2003), and Veatch (1972).

8. Nesbitt's point here occurs in a response to Rachels (1999). Rachels's seminal paper [of 1975] uses a specific example (usually called the example of the "nasty cousins") to argue that, under appropriately specific conditions, there is no moral difference between killing and letting die. Nesbitt responds by revisiting the example and arguing that the example does not show that there is no moral difference between killing and letting die. A response to Nesbitt is to be found in Kuhse (1999). Kuhse argues that Nesbitt's conclusions from the example are not germane to the case of active versus passive euthanasia, and she provides other examples that she considers more closely analogous.

9. See Legge (1894: 288).

10. These include the Emperor of Han, who unfailingly tasted the daily prescriptions for his sick mother, and Lady Tang, who saved her ailing mother-in-law from death by daily expressing her own milk for the latter.

11. I would like to thank C. L. Ten, Henry Rosemont Jr., and the editors of this volume for their very helpful comments on earlier drafts of this chapter.

REFERENCES

Ames, R., and H. Rosemont. 2008. "Family Reverence (*xiao*) as the Source of Consummatory Conduct (*jen*)." *Dao* 7:9–19.

Ames, R., and H. Rosemont, trans. 2009. *Xiaojing: The Chinese Classic of Family Reverence.* Hawaii: University of Hawaii. (See esp. 34–59.)

Andre, J. 1991. "Role Morality as a Complex Instance of Ordinary Morality." *American Philosophical Quarterly* 28 (1) (1991): 73–80.

Beauchamp. T. L., and J. F. Childress. 1996. *Ethical Issues in Death and Dying,* 2nd edition. Upper Saddle River: Prentice Hall.

———. 2001. *Principles of Biomedical Ethics.* New York: Oxford University Press.

Bowie, N. E. 1982. "'Role' as a Moral Concept in Health Care." *Journal of Medicine and Philosophy* 7:57–63.

Confucius. 1979. *The Analects,* edited by D. C. Lau. Harmondsworth: Penguin.

Fan, R., ed. 1999. *Confucian Bioethics.* Dordrecht: Kluwer.

Fan, R., and J. Tao. 2004. "Consent to Medical Treatment: The Complex Interplay of Patients, Families and Physicians." *Journal of Medicine and Philosophy* 29:139–48.

Fielding, R., and J. Hung. 1996. "Preferences for Information and Involvement in Decisions during Cancer Care among a Hong Kong Chinese Population." *Psycho-Oncology* 5:231–329.

Foot, P. 2002. *Moral Dilemmas.* Oxford: Clarendon Press.

Garrard, E., and S. Wilkinson. 2005. "Passive Euthanasia." *Journal of Medical Ethics* 31:64–68.

Gibson, K. 2003. "Contrasting Role Morality and Professional Morality: Implications for Practice." *Journal of Applied Philosophy* 20 (1): 17–29.

Ho, D. Y. F. 1998. "Interpersonal Relationships and Relations Dominance: An Analysis Based on Methodological Relationalism." *Asian Journal of Social Psychology* 1:1–16.

Hui, E. 1999. "A Confucian Ethic of Medical Futility." In *Confucian Bioethics,* edited by R. Fan. Dordrecht: Kluwer.

Kamm, F. 2008. "Physician Assisted Suicide, Euthanasia and Intending Death." In *Physician Assisted Suicide: Expanding the Debate,* edited by M. P. Battin, R. Rhodes, and A. Silver. New York: Routledge.

Kuhse, H. 1999. "Why Killing Is Not Always Worse—and Sometimes Better—Than Letting Die." In *Bioethics: An Anthology*, edited by H. Kuhse and P. Singer, 227–30. Oxford: Blackwell.

Lee, S. C. 2007. *The Family, Medical Decision-Making and Biotechnology: Critical Reflections on Asian Moral Perspectives*. Dordrecht: Netherlands.

Legge, J. 1894. *The Chinese Classics*. University of Hong Kong reprint of Shanghai edition.

Li, C. 2000. *The Sage and the Second Sex: Confucianism, Ethics and Gender*. Chicago: Open Court.

Li, S., and J. L. Chou. 1997. "Communication with the Cancer Patient in China." *Annals New York Academy of Sciences* 809:243–8.

Mackenzie, C., and N. Stoljar, eds. 2000. *Relational Autonomy: Feminist Perspectives on Autonomy, Agency and the Social Self*. New York: Oxford University Press.

McLachlan, H. V. 2008. "The Ethics of Killing and Letting Die: Active and Passive Euthanasia." *Journal of Medical Ethics* 34:636–8.

McMahan, J. 2002. *The Ethics of Killing*. New York: Oxford University Press.

Mencius. 1970. *Mencius*, trans. by D. C. Lau. Harmondsworth: Penguin.

Nesbitt, W. 1999. "Is Killing No Worse Than Letting Die?" In *Bioethics: An Anthology*, edited by H. Kuhse and P. Singer, 231–325. Oxford: Blackwell.

Nuyen, A. T. 2007. "Confucian Ethics as Role-Based Ethics." *International Philosophical Quarterly* 47 (3): 315–28.

Rachels, J. 1999. "Active and Passive Euthanasia." In *Bioethics: An Anthology*, edited by H. Kuhse and P. Singer, 227–30. Oxford: Blackwell.

Rosemont, H. 1986. "Kierkegaard and Confucius: On Finding the Way." *Philosophy East and West* 36 (3): 201–12.

Rosemont, H. 2007. "On the Non-Finality of Physical Death in Classical Confucianism." *Acta Orientalia Vilnensis* 8 (2).

Sim, M. 2007. *Remastering Morals with Aristotle and Confucius*. Cambridge: Cambridge University Press.

Singer, P. 1979. *Practical Ethics*. Cambridge: Cambridge University Press.

Tse, C., and J. Tao. 2004. "Strategic Ambiguities in the Process of Consent: Role of the Family in Decisions to Forgo Life-Sustaining Treatment for Incompetent Elderly Patients." *Journal of Medicine and Philosophy* 29:207–23.

Veatch, R. M. 1972. "Models for Ethical Medicine in a Revolutionary Age." *Hastings Center Report* 2:5–7.

Wawrytko, S. 1982. "Confucius and Kant: The Ethics of Respect." *Philosophy East and West* 32 (3): 237–57.

6

Understanding the Concept of Vulnerability from a Western Africa Perspective

Peter F. Omonzejele

ABSTRACT

This chapter examines several definitions of vulnerability and found such definitions incapable of sufficiently protecting the interests of vulnerable research subjects in the West African region. Hence, we derived a refined definition of the concept of vulnerability that involves identifying the specific nature of vulnerability of potential research subjects in that region. Some categories of research subjects were indicated in the West African setting, and reasons were advanced why those categories hold a special form of vulnerability in that setting. The indicated categories of potential research subjects in the West African setting were classified into identifiable types (contextual or intrinsic) of vulnerability to demonstrate how our refined definition would apply in practice in that region.

INTRODUCTION

Bioethics is the discipline that addresses ethical issues in medicine and in the life sciences. The ethics of the conduct of medical research (research ethics) among humans is an important aspect of that discipline. This is because even in the twenty-first century medical progress relies on ongoing research on human beings. As a result, an interaction between researchers and research subjects is extremely important even where drugs and treatment already exists. And clearly, it is even more important in the discovery of treatments for hitherto unmanageable diseases. Without research subjects' participation in medical research, researchers cannot know the efficacy or side effects of a new drug, both of which are essential before one can bring a drug to the market.

However, the conduct of medical research among vulnerable populations raises serious moral concerns. This is because potential research subjects who are perceived to be vulnerable could be taken unfair advantage of, as they are usually unable to negotiate genuine informed consent in the research setting. This is often the case when studies are conducted in areas in which illiteracy and serious poverty thrives; such circumstances are often responsible for the vulnerability of potential subjects in West African countries in the research setting.

The word *vulnerable* is derived from the Latin word *vulnerare*, which means to "wound" (*Oxford Encyclopaedic Dictionary*, 1995), and as with most etymological derivations, this is inadequate for the purposes of definition. The concept of vulnerability is a complex concept to define. According to the *New Oxford Dictionary of English*, to be vulnerable means to be "exposed to the possibility of being attacked or harmed, either physically or emotionally." For instance, a European visiting any West African country is vulnerable to malaria attacks in a way the native West Africans are not.

On the other hand, a West African visiting any European country during the winter is vulnerable to the cold-related infections in a way that native Europeans are not. Broadly speaking, as a people we are all vulnerable one way or another, since we are all exposed to one sort of risk or another, from which we cannot protect ourselves.

We shall examine the definition of the concept of vulnerability in the Council for International Organisations of Medical Sciences (CIOMS) document and argue that the application of the concept of vulnerability in the CIOMS document as it currently stands does not sufficiently protect potential research subjects in West African countries due to the prevailing circumstances in that region, and hence, the need for a refined definition of the concept. This is important if we aim to protect this category of potential research subjects in that region from exploitation and harm in the medical research setting.

WHAT IS VULNERABILITY?

We could preliminarily define vulnerability as follows. To be vulnerable means to be under threat of harm or under threat of exploitation leading to harm. If we are dealing with vulnerability in medical research, we are therefore referring to the possible exposure to harm or exploitation within medical research. As already indicated above, vulnerability to harm and exploitation in the research setting is more pronounced in developing (African) countries often occasioned by social, cultural, and economic circumstances.

To define more precisely what vulnerability means in developing (West African) countries, we need to move beyond our preliminary definition. To do so, let us look at the definition used by the Council for International Organisations of Medical Sciences (CIOMS 2002). According to CIOMS, vulnerable research subjects are "those who are relatively or (absolutely) incapable of protecting their own interests because they may have insufficient power, intelligence, education, resources, strength, or other needed attributes to protect their own interests" (the reference for this is located in the bibliography).

This quote implies that to be vulnerable is to be relatively or (absolutely) incapable of protecting one's own interests, or in other words, of protecting oneself from the threat of harm. An already refined definition would therefore be: to be vulnerable means to be incapable of protecting one's interests under threat of harm or under threat of exploitation leading to harm.

The CIOMS guidelines appreciate that there are different categories of research subjects: those that are vulnerable and those that are not. Those that are vulnerable cannot protect themselves from harm, hence the need for guidelines to protect such subjects. Vulnerable research subjects can be further categorized into subsectors based on the nature of protection they require. The above-quoted CIOMS guidelines list insufficient power, intelligence, education, resources, and strength as characteristics that make research subjects vulnerable.

For instance, somebody with insufficient education and intelligence may be unable to protect their interests because of his/her inability to refuse or give consent. Insufficient (especially due to severe poverty) resources may limit a subject's capacity to protect their interests because of a lack of alternatives. An opportunity for exploitation arises from one party lacking any *alternative* to the solution offered by the would-be exploiter, thereby coercing the exploited (the vulnerable) into acceptance.

Benn (1988: 138) supports this suggestion. An important characteristic of the exploiter, he maintains, is that he makes an otherwise unattractive offer that the exploited person cannot reject, because the latter is vulnerable, has no alternative, and is in need of the object or service offered. For instance, if someone offers a woman whose child is dying from pneumonia antibiotics at an exorbitant price knowing that the woman cannot get the needed antibiotics elsewhere, there is no doubt that he is trying to exploit the woman. Where there is an urgent and compelling need, and a third party offers the only way of meeting the need, the third party holds the power to coerce.

It is important to identify the possible nature of vulnerability of research subjects. This requires two steps: first to identify what exactly vulnerability means, and second to identify which subjects are vulnerable. Going by our working definition of vulnerability as the incapacity to protect one's own interests under threat of harm or under threat of exploitation leading to harm, it would then be necessary to understand which categories of research subjects fall under this definition and why. Before we look into categories of vulnerable research subjects, let us further define the concept of vulnerability for the purposes of this chapter. In addition to the preliminary definition already given, it is necessary to introduce one more distinction; namely, the distinction between contextual and intrinsic forms of vulnerability.

Contextual forms of vulnerability refer to situations in which the inability to protect one's own interests emanates from social, cultural, political, or economic circumstances. The cause of making somebody vulnerable is extraneous. For instance (and as we shall see below in our examples), married African women and people who are seriously economically disadvantaged fall into the extraneous category of vulnerability. The lack of choices for access to essential medicines in, for instance, rural Rwanda is a social, political, and economic circumstance affecting Rwandan citizens rather than vulnerability related to specific people.

If some of the affected citizens were to receive political asylum in the United Kingdom, their access to essential medicines would be guaranteed. Intrinsic forms of vulnerability, on the other hand, exist when the nature of vulnerability is imbedded in the research subjects themselves, such as in the case of incompetent mentally ill[1] or children.

Consequently, the concept of vulnerability can be defined as a contextual or intrinsic state of being incapable of protecting one's own interests under threat of harm or under threat of exploitation leading to harm. A proper appreciation of the concept of vulnerability must necessarily take those two forms into reckoning.

THE APPLICATION OF OUR REFINED DEFINITION IN THE WEST AFRICAN CONTEXT: THE INCOMPETENT MENTALLY ILL

The incompetent mentally ill are vulnerable research subjects in ways that competent research participants are not. The most pronounced form of their vulnerability is that of incompetence, the inability to do certain things because of their lack of mental capacity. According to Lott (2005: 42–45), the limitations of using incompetent mentally ill in research revolves around their lacking in mental faculty required to consent to involvement in clinical research trials.

This makes them vulnerable and exposed to exploitation, and therefore it requires special protection for them. The incompetent mentally ill do not have the capacity to balance risks and benefits in matters that concern them, and they are therefore incapable of protecting one's own interests under threat of harm or under threat of exploitation leading to harm. Hence, the usual protective mechanism of securing informed consent that is to be freely given by research subjects is not helpful in research involving the incompetent mentally ill.

Informed consent that is a philosophical idea based on the principle of autonomy (Moreno, Caplan, and Wolpe 1998: 690) poses special problems in research involving the incompetent mentally ill because of the subject's impaired mental faculties. To give informed consent, research subjects are expected to make autonomous decisions. In the West African setting, this may imply securing family or community consent depending on the ethnic group and the nature of research to be conducted.

Whatever the mode of securing the required consent, an incompetent mentally ill cannot actively participate in the informed consent process, yet it is crucial to secure some form of consent (be it first person, proxy, etc.) from all research subjects, including the incompetent mentally ill.

Proxy consent is normally obtained when the research subjects cannot decide for themselves regarding participation in research. The inability to decide could be a result of a research subject being unconscious and a new unapproved drug is thought to be of potential benefit to him/her, or where a research subject is unable to understand or appreciate disclosures in terms of risks and benefits to him/her, such as is the case with an incompetent mentally ill person.

Whatever the reason for the incompetence of the research subject, proxy decision makers need to be those who regard the interests of such incompetent research subjects as paramount. Hence, most proxy decision makers are family members or those who know such incompetent research subjects well enough to know what the person would have wanted had she or he been able to make the decision herself/himself.

According to Andanda (2005: 16), the moral foundation of informed consent is the moral principle of respect for autonomy. She explains that the requirement for autonomy has two aspects, which are:

> Firstly, the requirement that those who are capable of deliberating on their personal choices should be treated with respect for their capacity for self-determination; and secondly, persons with diminished or impaired autonomy, or those who are in dependent or in vulnerable positions, should be protected against harm and abuse.

What is special about involving mentally incompetent research subjects in West Africa? In other words, where are special vulnerabilities, if there are any? We shall restrict ourselves to Nigeria, where I have previously undertaken research on the subject (Omonzejele 2004).

In Nigeria, the causes of mental health problems can be regarded as those prevalent in the West, but they could also be said to be caused by evil casting and machinations. Based on this view, traditional healing that could involve the use of oracles and divination are used side by side with Western therapies. In many cases, patients, or better put, relatives of such patients prefer to use traditional medicines for mental health care, which they regard as more effective than the Western option. This preference is responsible for the engagement of the services of traditional psychiatrists by many state governments in Nigeria and other West African countries.

Suggested cures tend toward spiritualism in combination with Western treatments. Mental ill health is stigmatized and so constitutes embarrassment to family members and the community of the sufferer (Omonzejele 2004). This brings about conflicts of interests between the incompetent mentally ill and his family members/community who are supposed to give proxy consent on his behalf to participate in research or not. For instance, they could consent on his behalf more willingly to enlist in research than they would do with those who are not mentally incompetent whom they perceive to be of more value to the family and the community.

This means that the incompetent mentally ill who is already vulnerable has the potential for further damage in a marginalized region such as West Africa, where he is perceived to be "an embarrassment" to family members. Within the African context, she or he would have to be regarded as specifically vulnerable and therefore needing further protection according to our definition of intrinsic vulnerability.

To summarize, the incompetent mentally ill are vulnerable research subjects for medical research because they are intrinsically unable to protect their own interests through the channel of giving first-person voluntary informed consent. In West African countries, they are additionally at risk of being volunteered for potentially harmful research by proxy consent given the heavy stigmatization of mental illness in the region.

CHILDREN AS RESEARCH SUBJECTS

In like manner with the incompetent mentally ill in the research setting, it is impossible to secure first-person consent from children (minors) when they are required to enlist in a study. The reason is that by their very nature they cannot evaluate risks. Nevertheless, it is important to enlist children into research when there is the need to develop drugs that are exclusively meant to ameliorate children's medical condition. In such circumstances, their parents make the needed decision for them. For instance, that was the case in the Kano meningitis trials.

In 1996, Pfizer, a big multinational pharmaceutical company, conducted a meningitis study in Kano, Nigeria. According to Stephens (*Washington Post*, December 17, 2000), Pfizer tested trovafloxacin (trade name Trovan), an antibiotic, "amid a terrible epidemic in a squalid, short-staffed medical camp lacking basic diagnostic equipment." Macklin explains that the said trial resulted in the death of eleven children, while two hundred became deaf, blind, or lame as a result of the trial (Macklin 2004: 99).

The study resulted in litigation between Pfizer and the Federal Republic of Nigeria. The Nigerian government on behalf of the subjects argued that the vulnerability of the research subjects in the study was taken advantaged of by Pfizer. Pfizer, on the other hand, claimed that they secured proxy (substituted) consent from the guardians of the children involved in the study, but they (Pfizer) could not substantiate their claim.

Besides, it is very likely that the children's parents/guardians may not have been sufficiently aware of the risks involved in the trial (that is, if they were even aware that their wards were involved in a study in the first place) since Kano is located in Northern Nigeria where illiteracy levels are very high. This brings the quality of proxy consents given on behalf of minors to participate in research to question in the West African setting.

How does this state of affairs pose special vulnerability for children in the research setting in West African countries? Let us use the Pfizer study to address this question. Minors by their nature suffer from intrinsic vulnerability and so cannot (and are usually not expected to) sensibly access risks and benefits in most important matters. Most people would agree that the decision to enlist in a study is an important issue (sometimes) with far-reaching consequences.

This implies that investigators have to rely on their guardians/parents to give proxy/substituted consent on behalf of their wards after evaluating the risks and benefits associated with a study before giving consent (or otherwise) for their wards' participation in research. In this way, guardian/parents are able to protect their wards from being recruited into harmful and exploitative research. But this line of reasoning only works well in affluent countries where there is easy access to basic health care, with high literacy levels and low poverty levels.

But in West African countries the reverse is the case, due to lack of access to basic health care, high illiteracy, and high poverty levels. For instance, in the Pfizer Kano meningitis study, the parents of the children had no alternative to what Pfizer had to offer to their children who suffer from the medical condition. This means that whatever risks are involved in a study, parents whose children are afflicted with a condition for which they cannot access care elsewhere would consent to enlist their children into a study irrespective of associated risks as the only way of accessing care.

Additional risk with recruiting children into research in the West African region is that of the high poverty levels in that region that could result in guardians/parents placing their own interests before that of their children in the research context. For instance, guardians-parents could give substituted consent for their wards to enlist in risky research if investigators promised to reward such parents-guardians with monetary incentives.

To sum up, children are vulnerable research subjects in the research context because as with the incompetent mentally ill, they (children) are intrinsically unable to protect their own interest in terms of giving voluntary first-person consent. In the West African context, they are further at risk because those who are in a position to give substituted consent on their behalf may consider their own interests over those of the children they were supposed to protect (in terms of making sure they do not come to harm).

THE POOR AS RESEARCH SUBJECTS

Medical research is generally conducted across different economic groups, at least in most cases. However, undertaking clinical research among poor people raises ethical problems not usually associated with those who are relatively well off. This is because the poor often volunteer to participate in research as the only way of accessing drugs that they cannot afford otherwise.

Poverty is pandemic, thus not restricted to any continent. But the density of poverty differs from one continent (region) to another. For instance, poverty is much more pronounced in developing (West African) countries, hence conducting medical research in such regions poses special moral concerns because of the vulnerability of such research populations. According to Dickens and Cook (2003: 79–86):

> Concerns have arisen with special regard to developing countries, however, that commercially inspired sponsors of studies from developed countries may take advantage of them as host sites to test products intended for sale in affluent markets. These countries may allow studies that recruit suitable participants who are more willing to participate, perhaps for inexpensive inducement, less understanding of study risks, and for instance, less likely and able to pursue grievances and litigation in the event of injury, than developed-country residents.

Economic depravity responsible for the vulnerability of research subjects in developing countries is sometimes not appreciated in its entire ramification. In African countries most research subjects participate in research for goods they cannot access otherwise, including money. For instance, if money is offered to a research subject in a West African country where drought and hunger thrive, such a subject might not evaluate risks associated with a study properly.

Rather, the subject would be more interested in the money she or he was offered to meet some of his/her urgent needs than in the evaluation of risks. This is because their economic circumstances potentially expose impoverished subjects to exploitation as money offered to them can serve as undue inducement for them to participate in risky research.

Current statistics of the level of poverty in developing countries are worrisome. According to a United Nations Development Programme (UNDP: 2005) report, about 850 million people are undernourished, most of whom reside in developing countries. The report goes on to state that a significant number of deaths in developing countries were linked to poverty. Specifically, UNDP *Statistics* indicate that Sub-Saharan Africa accounts for 20 percent of births but 44 percent of child deaths:

> Almost all childhood deaths are preventable. Every two minutes four people die from malaria alone, three of them children. Most of these deaths could be prevented by simple, low-cost interventions. Vaccine preventable illnesses—measles, diphtheria and tetanus—account for another 2–3 million childhood deaths. For every child who dies, million more will fall sick or miss school, trapped in a vicious circle that links poor health in childhood to poverty in adulthood. Like the 500,000 women who die each year from pregnancy related causes, more than 98% of children who die live in poor countries. They die because of where they are born.

Using World Health Organisation statistics, Pogge (2002: 98) captures the situation quite clearly when he states that one-third of all human deaths is poverty related. Diseases such as pneumonia, starvation, tuberculosis, and more "could be prevented or cured cheaply through food, safe drinking water, vaccinations, dehydration packs and medicines." This state of affairs has serious moral implications for conducting medical research in developing countries, especially as it relates to securing voluntary informed consent. This is because research subjects in poor nations could be easily induced into participating in risky research when offered incentives.

Incentives could be offered to research subjects in poor countries through several ways. For instance, incentives could be the prospect of financial compensation. But incentives could also be offered in nonfinancial form. According to Lott (2005: 45–46):

> Non-financial rewards that could potentially improve the standard of living of impoverished individuals may also be overly coercive. These rewards might include food, shelter, clothing, medical treatment, etc. Again, the depressed level of economic subsistence characterizing the developing world may turn these simple rewards/basic entitlements into forceful incentives for the poor. Researchers conducting trials among the poor of the developing world must not assume that the incentives structure characterizing the poor of their home (developed) countries applies as equally to the poor in the developing world.

It is worthy of note that, though there are poor people in developed countries, the pressure on people in *developing* countries in terms of voluntary informed consent is radically different. For instance, access to essential drugs is not an incentive for the poor in the United Kingdom, as a national health system exists. But access to essential drugs is a strong incentive for the poor in West African countries such as Nigeria, Ghana, Mali, Liberia, Sierra Leone, or Togo.

Though there are people in some developed countries who have no access to essential drugs, poverty in developing countries is much more prevalent, especially where such developing countries are on the African (West African) continent. This implies that the problem of lack of access to medication is more prevalent in poor nations.

To reiterate, the poor in Britain (and in many developed countries) can access most essential drugs through their public health systems and are therefore not under pressure to participate in medical research in order to access those drugs. The same cannot be said for research subjects in West African (developing) countries, who may enlist in a study as the only way of accessing essential medicines. This means potential research subjects in the West African region are vulnerable in a way potential subjects in developed countries are not.

Hence, the need for a refined definition of the concept of vulnerability in order to fully capture and appreciate the nature of the specific form of vulnerability of potential research subjects in the West African region. For instance, there is the possibility that pregnant women in West Africa may wish to enlist in research as the only way of receiving free antenatal and postnatal care, irrespective of potential risks to themselves. Because they are responsible for two lives, their own and their babies, this imposes an additional burden.

As already stated, oftentimes people in poor (West Africa) nations enlist in medical research as the only way to access essential medicines, irrespective of risks associated with such research. This has significant implications for securing genuine and voluntary informed consent as it exposes research subjects in West African (developing) countries to potential exploitation. When there is no alternative, one can easily be induced into research studies with high risks. This form of vulnerability could be subsumed into our definition of contextual vulnerability.

PRISONERS IN WEST AFRICA AS RESEARCH SUBJECTS

Prisoners are people who have been stripped of their freedom and confined to particular surroundings, where their day-to-day activities are monitored by those responsible for their care. In terms of involvement in research studies, they are vulnerable subjects due to their restricted autonomy.

According to Lott (2005: 37), prisoners, due to their confinement for whatever punitive or rehabilitative reasons, stand in an unequal power relationship with prison authorities, which could be described as coercive. DeCastro (2003: 171–5) states that coercive conditions make prisoners vulnerable as clinical research subjects, as their circumstances militate against voluntary decision making.

One reason for this is that most prisoners can only get parole based on the recommendations of those who look after them. This is an important factor when prisoners are confined in an unhealthy and deplorable prison situation, as it is often the case in most African prisons due to a shortage of resources for maintaining prisons and prisoners.

Lott (2005: 37–39) advanced several reasons why consent given by prisoners to participate in clinical trials may not be considered as voluntary, the most relevant of which is prospect of reward. Lott (2005: 38) also states that one of the reasons for the vulnerability of prisoners as research subjects is their belief that if they co-operated in clinical research they might get rewards for their consent. According to Lott:

> Prisoners may be unduly influenced by potential gains offered by research participation, such as reduced prison time or "extra" perks (more/better food, increased access to entertainment or exercise facilities, increased free time, etc.). These rewards can easily cloud prisoners' judgments and prevent them from adequately assessing the potential risks involved in the proposed research, leaving them unable to give informed consent.

He argues further that, although populations who are not confined could be affected by prospects of rewards as well, prisoners are at a higher risk and more vulnerable to abuse. This is because what nonprisoners normally take for granted could be considered as a reward to prisoners for being "good" prisoners.

The prospect of reward may be an even stronger inducement for prisoners to participate in research when such prisoners are imprisoned in Nigeria (Africa). This is because funding for prison services is limited and prisoners often live in deplorable conditions. Hence, if a prisoner thought he could have regular access to bathing soap instead of one bar a month, or if he thought he could have three meals a day instead of the usual one or two, he is very likely to be induced to participate in risky research even when he is conscious of the potential harm of the research to him.

This further exposes already vulnerable research subjects to potential damage in a way prisoners in wealthy nations tend not to be. Monetary and nonmonetary advantages derived from pleasing authorities or researchers influence their decision making on whether a clinical trial is a risk to their health and well-being or not. We could subsume this sort of vulnerability in the research setting within our definition of contextual vulnerability.

WEST AFRICAN MARRIED WOMEN AS RESEARCH SUBJECTS

In most African countries marriages are only recognized on the payment of the so-called bride-price, known as *labola* in South Africa, *roora* in Zimbabwe, *mahari* in East Africa, and generally referred to as *head-money* in West African countries. The bride-price is the payment either in cash or kind that family members of the groom make to the family members of the bride in order to marry the latter's daughter. The bride-price is the last and most important marriage rite, which takes place only after all other rites (such as consultations, "wine carrying," etc.) have been performed to the satisfaction of both families.

The execution of the bride-price "ranges from a mainly ritualistic transfer of tokens of esteem to an outright purchase in which the man reserves a right to ask for a refund from the woman's parents if he backs a claim that her behaviour is unsatisfactory" (Bishai, Falb, Pariyo, and Hindin 2009: 147). West African women who live with their men in a "marriage-type" union without the payment of the bride-price are regarded as concubines to such men. Their families do not consider themselves as in-laws. And neither are such women treated respectfully—they are usually not invited to nor partake in traditional functions, at least not in the capacity of a married woman.

Most West African women would not opt for the nonpayment of their bride-price due to its traditional and social implications, not even by women who want to use this as a way of asserting their individuality and autonomy. In any case, women are not in a position to determine if they want the bride-price to be paid or not, because it is paid to the bride's kindred.

The payment of the bride-price is taken so seriously that, where a couple lived together (and perhaps had children), and where the woman died before the payment of her bride-price, this price has to be paid even in death, otherwise she will not receive befitting burial rites as accorded to married women. The payment of the bride-price gives husbands and husbands' family members controlling influence over married West African women. This is because the payment of the bride-price gives husbands and husband's family members the impression of having "purchased" their wives. Hence, the bride-price places West African women in an inferior power relationship in marital unions, and native laws and customs tenable in West African countries support the linked male superiority.

This unequal relationship means that West African women are marginalized in terms of giving first-person voluntary informed consent, as they are required to get approval from their husbands before they could enlist in medical research. This state of affairs could also work the other way round, where the husband may make his wife partake in risky clinical research in order to get money.

West African married women can be considered vulnerable research subjects in the medical research setting because they are unable to protect their own interests through the channel of giving first-person voluntary informed consent. The reason for this is extraneous (that is contextual); through customs and laws expressed in bride-price payments, husbands and their families "buy" the bride and her rights to, for instance, take part in clinical trials.

Consequently, what is clear is that West African women who fall under the bride-price tradition usually require the consent of their husbands or other male members of his family before enrolling in medical research (Omonzejele 2008: 124). This means that at least two people need to consent before a West African woman can participate in a study. This sort of vulnerability falls within our definition of contextual vulnerability.

CONCLUSION

What we have achieved in this chapter is to refine the definition of the concept of vulnerability in the research context in order to identify specific forms of vulnerability in the medical research setting. This, in turn, we believe, would potentially assist investigators to devise and come up with an appropriate mode of protection required by subjects who fall within an identifiable (contextual or intrinsic) form of vulnerability in order to prevent exploitation and harm in the medical research setting.

To demonstrate how our refined definition works in practice, we applied it to circumstances in the West African region where we categorized subjects who are unable to protect their own interests, such as the poor, prisoners, and married African women in that region as contextually vulnerable. The incompetent mentally ill in that region was categorized as being intrinsically vulnerable.

NOTE

1. Those incompetent mentally ill for whom treatment would be available, but is not under current circumstances (due to severe poverty, for instance), fall into both categories.

REFERENCES

Andanda, P. 2005. "Informed Consent." *Developing World Bioethics* 5 (1).

Benn, S. 1988. *A Theory of Freedom*. Cambridge: Cambridge University Press.

Bishai, D. K., G. Falb, G. Pariyo, and M. Hindin. 2009. "Bride Price and Sexual Risk Taking in Uganda." *African Journal of Reproductive Health* 13 (1).

Council for International Organization of Medical Sciences. 2002. International Ethical Guidelines for Biomedical Research Involving Human Subjects. http://www.cioms.ch/publications/layout_guide2002.pdf.

DeCastro, L. D. 2003. "Human Organs from Prisoners: Kidneys for Life." *Journal of Medical Ethics* 29.

Dickens, B. M., and R. J. Cook. 2003. "Challenges of Ethical Research in Resource-Poor Settings." *International Journal of Gynaecology and Obstetrics* 80.

Lott, J. 2005. "Vulnerable/Special Participant Populations." *Developing World Bioethics* 5 (1).

Macklin, R. 2004. *Double Standards in Medical Research in Developing Countries*. Cambridge University Press.

Moreno, J. D., A. L. Caplan, and P. R. Wolpe. 1998. "Informed Consent." In *Encyclopedia of Applied Ethics*. San Diego: Academic Press.

Omonzejele. P. 2004. "Mental Healthcare in African Traditional Medicine and Society: A Philosophical Appraisal." *Eubios Journal of Asian and International Bioethics* 14 (5).

———. 2008. "African Women as Clinical Research Subjects: Unaddressed Issue in Global Bioethics." *Studies on Ethno-Medicine* 2 (2).

Pogge, T. 2002. *World Poverty and Human Rights*. Cambridge: Polity Press.

United Nations Development Programme. 2005. *Statistics*. http://hdr.undp.org/reports/global/2005/pdf/HDR05_chapter1.pdf.24.

7

Ethics of Aboriginal Research[1]

Marlene Brant Castellano

ABSTRACT

This chapter proposes a set of principles to assist in developing ethical codes for the conduct of research within the Aboriginal community or with external partners. It places the discussion of research ethics in the context of a cultural worldview and the struggle for self-determination as peoples and nations. It affirms that Aboriginal Peoples have a right to participate as principals or partners in research that generates knowledge affecting their culture, identity, and well-being. To provide context and rationale for the principles presented, the chapter outlines features of the current public dialogue on research ethics, how ethics are framed in Aboriginal cultures, and how Aboriginal perceptions of reality and right behavior clash with norms prevailing in Western research. Current initiatives of Aboriginal communities and nations, research-granting councils, and institutions to establish ethical guidelines for Aboriginal research are highlighted as evidence that the development of workable ethical regimes is already well begun.

INTRODUCTION

In September 1992, the Royal Commission on Aboriginal Peoples (RCAP) brought together about eighty Aboriginal Peoples who were involved in research as academics, lawyers, graduate students, project staff and consultants, community leaders, and Elders. We met at a workshop at Nakoda Lodge in Alberta to shape the emerging research agenda of RCAP. As codirector of research, I was the chairperson of the initial session in which numerous participants voiced harsh criticism of past research and serious skepticism that RCAP research would serve them any better. "We've been researched to death!" they protested. The workshop was not off to a promising start, until an Elder who had opened the meeting spoke quietly from a corner of the room. "If we have been researched to death," he said, "maybe it's time we started researching ourselves back to life."

That piece of wisdom has been repeated often in the past ten years. It was prophetic of the change that would gather remarkable momentum in just a decade. Aboriginal knowledge has always been informed by research, purposeful gathering of information, and thoughtful distillation of meaning. Research acquired a bad name among Aboriginal Peoples because the purposes and meanings associated with its practice by academics and government agents were usually alien to the people themselves, and the outcomes were, as often as not, misguided and harmful.

Aboriginal Peoples in organizations and communities, as well as universities and colleges and some government offices, are now engaged in transforming Aboriginal research into an instrument for creating and disseminating knowledge that once again authentically represents us and our understanding of the world.

Researching ourselves may mean self-initiated action, or it may mean entering into effective partnerships. In either case, the ground rules that should guide new practices are not immediately evident. Where Aboriginal expectations diverge from past practice, resistance from the academic research establishment is to be expected.

This chapter proposes a set of principles to assist in developing ethical codes for the conduct of research internal to the Aboriginal community or with external partners.[2] The context and rationale for these principles is developed in early sections outlining the current dialogue on research ethics, how ethics are framed in Aboriginal cultures, and how Aboriginal perceptions of reality and right behavior clash with prevailing norms of Western research. Efforts of Aboriginal communities and nations, as well as research-granting councils and institutions, to establish ethical guidelines for Aboriginal research are highlighted as evidence that the development of workable ethical regimes is already well begun.

In this chapter, research means activity intended to investigate, document, bring to light, analyze, or interpret matters in any domain, to create knowledge for the benefit of society or of particular groups. Aboriginal refers to First Nations, Inuit, and Métis Peoples as referenced in the Canadian Constitution. Indigenous is used interchangeably with Aboriginal, usually in international contexts. Where sources refer to specific groups, such as First Nations, the terminology of the source is retained.

Aboriginal research means research that touches the life and well-being of Aboriginal Peoples. It may involve Aboriginal Peoples and their communities directly. It may assemble data that describes or claims to describe Aboriginal Peoples and their heritage. Or, it may affect the human and natural environment in which Aboriginal Peoples live. Ethics refers to rules of conduct that express and reinforce important social and cultural values of a society. The rules may be formal and written, spoken, or simply understood by groups who subscribe to them.

The language, images, and perspectives in this chapter are those of a Mohawk woman and academic of a certain generation. I suggest that the principles I articulate are relevant more broadly to Aboriginal research, though readers from other cultures, particularly Métis and Inuit colleagues, will undoubtedly need to do some translation to connect my words with their own worldviews and experiences.

AN ACTIVE DISCOURSE ON RESEARCH ETHICS

International concern about research ethics arose from revelations in the Nuremberg trials of atrocities committed in experimentation on humans by the Nazis during the Second World War. To prevent future violations of human rights in the name of science, Western nations developed the Nuremberg Code representing broad international agreement on ethical standards in medical research.

The Nuremberg Code was replaced by the Helsinki Declaration, which was adopted in 1964 and subsequently updated.[3] Ethical codes place emphasis on informed consent and are intended to strike a balance between the risk incurred by participants and the potential benefit of the research to society.

The federal government is a major funding source, directly and indirectly, of research involving human subjects. It relies on other agencies to ensure that an ethical balance between benefit and risk is maintained in much of the research that it funds. This leaves open questions about the adequacy of safeguards of the public interest.

Aboriginal Peoples interested in research share the concerns cited above and welcome the current review of principles and processes for governing research involving human subjects. However, even if ethical oversight of research sponsored by public institutions is made more consistent, up-to-date, and enforceable, there is a danger that concerns particular to Aboriginal Peoples will be neglected or made subject to inappropriate regulation.

It is essential that Aboriginal Peoples and their organizations put forward not only concerns but also solutions to the ethical problems that too often have made research affecting them inaccurate and irrelevant. Reframing ethical codes and practice is necessary to ensure the social benefit that motivates research also extends to the Aboriginal Peoples whose universe is being studied.

AN ABORIGINAL PERSPECTIVE ON ETHICS

Descriptions of Aboriginal societies seldom speak of the ethics that support order, cohesion, and personal responsibility in those societies. Anthropological studies document customs that sometimes have the character of law. Dr. Clare Brant, a Mohawk physician who became the first Aboriginal psychiatrist in Canada, wrote an influential paper titled "Native Ethics and Rules of Behavior." In it, he used the language of ethics to illuminate some powerful, unspoken assumptions that guide behavior that he observed in his Iroquoian, Cree, and Ojibway patients.

Brant's elaboration of the ethic of noninterference, which inhibits argument and advice giving as normal means of communication, is particularly relevant for researchers and professionals offering services to Aboriginal Peoples. While noninterfering behavior may be perceived as passive and irresponsible, Brant points out that it is consistent with teaching based on nonintrusive modeling rather than direct instruction that attempts to shape the behavior of the learner.[4] Elder Peter Waskahat speaks of the foundations of knowledge and the connections between land, family, spirituality, values, and everyday living:

> We had our own teachings, our own education system teaching children that way of life was taught by the grandparents and extended families; they were taught how to view and respect the land and everything in Creation. Through that the young people were taught how to live, what the Creator's laws were, what were the natural laws, what were these First Nations' laws, and so on, the teachings revolved around a way of life that was based on their values.[5]

When Aboriginal Peoples speak about maintaining and revitalizing their cultures, they are not proposing to go back to igloos and teepees and a hunter-gatherer lifestyle. They are talking about restoring order to daily living in conformity with ancient and enduring values that affirm life. The relationships between individual behavior, customs and community protocols, ethics, values, and worldview are represented [by] the symbol of a tree.

The leaves represent individual behaviors. Protocols and community customs are small branches, while ethics, the rules governing relationships, are the large branches. Values, deeply held beliefs about good and evil, form the trunk of the tree. The worldview or perception of reality underpinning life as it is lived, like the roots of the tree, is not ordinarily visible. The whole of the tree is rooted in the earth that supports us. In this symbolic representation, I suggest that the earth is like the unseen world of spirit as vast, mysterious, and friendly, if we learn how to respect the laws that govern it.

Some nations have codified their ethical systems. The Iroquois's Great Law of Peace teaches the importance and the requirements of cultivating a "good mind" in order to live well and harmoniously in the world. The potlatching ceremonies of West Coast nations were public means of validating genealogies, family responsibilities, inheritance rights, and land tenure. Many other nations transmitted their ethical codes orally and nonverbally through family and community relationships. Public ceremonies reinforce the community's worldview and provide instruction for living. Skills for decoding complex messages from the social and natural environment are embedded in traditional languages.

The persons most knowledgeable about physical and spiritual reality, the teaching and practice of ceremonies, and the nuances of meaning in Aboriginal languages, are Elders. Elders typically have been educated in the oral tradition, apart from the colonizing influence of the school system. They carry credentials that are recognizable within Aboriginal society, but invisible to those who assess expertise on the basis of formal education. They enjoy respect as sources of wisdom because their way of life expresses the deepest values of their respective cultures. In many cases, they have exceptional skills in transmitting these values to those who seek their counsel.

Within Aboriginal communities, the struggle has gone beyond survival as small enclaves set apart from non-Aboriginal Canada. The struggle now extends to applying cultural ways in the management of lands and economic activity; the structures of governance; the provision of health, education, justice, and other human services; and relations with the larger Canadian society and the world community. The struggle is to live and thrive as peoples and nations maintaining and expressing distinctive worldviews and contributing uniquely to the Canadian federation. In the language of the United Nations Working Group on Indigenous Populations, this is the pursuit of self-determination.

Indigenous peoples have the right of self-determination. By virtue of that right they freely determine their political status and freely pursue their economic, social, and cultural development.[6] Fundamental to the exercise of self-determination is the right of peoples to construct knowledge in accordance with self-determined definitions of what is real and what is valuable. Just as colonial policies have denied Aboriginal Peoples access to their traditional lands, so also colonial definitions of truth and value have denied Aboriginal Peoples the tools to assert and implement their knowledge. Research under the control of outsiders to the Aboriginal community has been instrumental in rationalizing colonialist perceptions of Aboriginal incapacity and the need for paternalistic control.

Aboriginal scholars who have been educated in Western universities and who are conversant with Aboriginal ways of knowledge seeking are challenging Western assumptions and methodologies of research. In the study of Elders' language referred to earlier, the authors explain:

> The Elders' comments allude to formal and long-established ways, procedures, and processes that First Nations persons are required to follow when seeking particular kinds of knowledge that are rooted in spiritual traditions and laws. The rules that are applied to this way of learning are strict, and the seekers of knowledge are required to follow meticulous procedures and processes as they prepare for and enter the "quest for knowledge journey."

In the world of Aboriginal knowledge, a discussion of ethics cannot be limited to devising a set of rules to guide researcher behavior in a defined task. Ethics, the rules of right behavior, are intimately related to who you are, the deep values you subscribe to, and your understanding of your place in the spiritual order of reality. Ethics are integral to the way of life of a people.

The fullest expression of a people's ethics is represented in the lives of the most knowledgeable and honorable members of the community. Imposition of rules derived from other ways of life in other communities will inevitably cause problems, although common understandings and shared interests can be negotiated. This is the ground on which Aboriginal Peoples stand as they engage in dialogue about research ethics that will limit the risks and enhance the benefits of research affecting their lives.

"JAGGED WORLDVIEWS COLLIDING"

Leroy Little Bear coined the phrase *jagged worldviews colliding* to describe the encounter of Aboriginal philosophies and positivist scientific thought.[7] Aboriginal worldviews assume that human action, to achieve social good, must be located in an ethical, spiritual context as well as its physical and social situation. Scientific research is dominated by positivist thinking; it assumes that only observable phenomena matter.

Little Bear points out that much externally sponsored research has documented customs but missed the deeper significance of those customs: "[Anthropologists] have done a fairly decent job of describing the customs themselves, but they have failed miserably in finding and interpreting the meanings behind the customs. The function of Aboriginal values and customs is to maintain the relationships that hold creation together."[8]

Research was defined earlier in this chapter as knowledge creation for social benefit. If researchers and those researched have vastly different notions of what constitutes social benefit and how it is achieved, the research is unlikely to satisfy the needs and expectations of participants on both sides of the divide. This section outlines some of the issues that arise in devising ethical regimes that are appropriate for Aboriginal research.

SHOULD ETHICS BE RESTRICTED TO RESEARCH ON HUMAN SUBJECTS?

In Aboriginal knowledge systems, the boundary between material and spiritual realms is easily crossed. Similarly, the boundaries between humans, animals, plants, and natural elements are also permeable. This is represented in traditional stories of communication between humans and other beings and the transformation of persons into animals and sea creatures, or vice versa.

Because many Aboriginal societies maintain primary dependence on a healthy natural environment in order to meet their needs, industrial development that sacrifices environmental values directly infringes on their well-being and human rights. Ethical regimes for Aboriginal research must therefore extend beyond current definitions of research involving human subjects to include research that affects Aboriginal well-being. This includes environmental research that will impact their physical environment or archival research that may perpetuate negative or inaccurate representations of Aboriginal Peoples.

MAINTAINING A BALANCE BETWEEN REDUCTIONIST ANALYSIS AND HOLISTIC VISION

The prevailing model of scientific inquiry reduces the scope of analysis to smaller bits of reality that can then be analyzed with greater specialization. This is referred to as a reductionist approach. Research that takes measures to exclude variables or influences from the environment that might contaminate cause-effect sequences is applauded as more reliable than data about complex and unexplainable lived experience.

Social sciences exploring human experience have adopted the scientific method as the hallmark of their credibility even though human behavior is subject to many variables that interrupt linear cause-effect sequences. The science of ecology has emerged as an approach to understanding the interdependence of elements and processes in the natural world, to some extent countering the dominance of reductionist research. However, the role of intuitive insight or vision in scientific breakthroughs is regularly downplayed in Western disciplines and institutions.

In contrast, the heart of Aboriginal science acknowledges the spirit of the plant, animal, or the land and the importance of relationships in supporting life. Gregory Cajete, a Tewa educator, writes:

> Native peoples through long experience and participation with their landscapes have come to know the language of their places. In learning this language of the subtle signs, qualities, cycles and patterns of their immediate environments and communicating with their landscapes Native people also come to know intimately the "nature" of the places which they inhabit. Learning the language of place and the "dialects" of its plants, animals, and natural phenomena in the context of a "homeland" is an underlying foundation of Native science.[9]

Aboriginal science does not ignore analysis of the particular. In fact, the perception of patterns is synthesized from multiple keen observations. Holistic awareness and highly focused analysis are complementary, not contradictory. There are examples of effective partnership between communities and scientists. The Sandy Lake Health and Diabetes Project in northwestern Ontario has brought together clinical treatment, community-based prevention strategies, and participation in genetic studies.[10]

The Akwesasne Mohawk community enlisted scientists from Cornell University to assist in verifying the nature and degree of pollution that was destroying the health of their crops and animals. Too often, however, perceptions and concerns at the community level are dismissed as anecdotal while priority setting for research proceeds on a different track. The Aboriginal ethic is that all aspects of the world we know have life and spirit and that humans have an obligation to learn the rules of relating to the world with respect. We enter into mutual dialogue with the many people and other beings with whom we share the world.

Knowledge is not a commodity that can be purchased and exploited at will. Information can be gathered by individuals to shape personal perceptions. Aboriginal societies traditionally were respectful of the unique vision of individuals. However, individual perceptions had to be validated by community dialogue and reflection before they became collective knowledge, the basis of collective action. This was the function of the many councils responsible for family, clan, village, or nation affairs. Research that seeks objectivity by maintaining distance between the investigator and informants violates Aboriginal ethics of reciprocal relationship and collective validation.

If the researcher assumes control of knowledge production, harvesting information in brief encounters, the dialogical relationship with human and nonhuman sources is disrupted and the transformation of observations or information into contextualized knowledge is aborted. Attempts to gain an understanding of Aboriginal life and concerns from an objective, short-term, outsider vantage point have produced much research that Aboriginal Peoples reject as distortions of their reality.

Where Aboriginal Peoples control access to research sites—for example, research on First Nations territories—organizations and local governments are increasingly insisting on community control. This may mean assuming full responsibility for conducting the research, or it may mean collaborative research in which the respective responsibilities of community and outside researchers are set out in a contract. Some initiatives to achieve balanced, mutually respectful partnerships between Aboriginal communities and researchers are described in a later section of this chapter.

VOLUNTARY CONSENT

In many cases research in Aboriginal communities and on Aboriginal matters is initiated by agencies that Aboriginal Peoples receive essential services from. Governments that control the resources on which the community depends often fund the research. Rightly or wrongly, many Aboriginal Peoples fear that refusing to consent to research may result in loss of funding for essential needs. They are at a disadvantage in negotiating conditions that would alter the imbalance in power between researchers and the community and give adequate recognition to community priorities and approaches to knowledge creation.

Privacy of health data collected routinely in the delivery of services has become a major concern in health research, especially with the possibility of sharing masses of data electronically across borders. Once information is transferred, it becomes difficult to monitor the secondary or tertiary purposes for which it is used.

FROM GUIDELINES TO GOVERNANCE

The discussion on ethics of Aboriginal research over the past decade has clearly demonstrated that more appropriate and enforceable protection of Aboriginal Peoples' interests in research activities is required. Aboriginal Peoples are wary, however, of regulations that seek to include them as an addendum to protocols based on Western assumptions about the construction and distribution of knowledge. This section proposes some principles flowing from the previous discussion that could guide the development of appropriate ethical regimes.

CREATING KNOWLEDGE AN ABORIGINAL RIGHT

Aboriginal Peoples in Canada enjoy constitutional protection of rights to maintain their identity and participate as collectives in Canadian society. Creating and sharing knowledge that authentically represents who you are and how you understand the world is integral to the survival of a people's identity. The Royal Commission on Aboriginal Peoples, in its analysis of the foundations and exercise of self-government, proposed, "All matters that are of vital concern to the life and welfare of a particular Aboriginal people, its culture and identity" fall within the core of Aboriginal jurisdiction.[11]

The Government of Canada has acknowledged the inherent right of self-government, although the substance of the right has not been defined. This leads to the first principle in devising an ethics regime for Aboriginal research.

Principle 1: Aboriginal Peoples have an inherent right to participate as principals or partners in research that generates knowledge affecting their culture, identity, and well-being. This right is protected by the Canadian Constitution and extends beyond the interests that other groups affected by research might have.

Fiduciary Obligations

The restricted capacity of Aboriginal nations and communities to protect their interests and rights in the face of more powerful governments and institutions has led to case law defining fiduciary obligations of the Canadian government. A duty to consult, which could affect how research is conducted, has been recognized in decisions of the British Columbia Court of Appeal. NAHO (National Aboriginal Health Organization) is currently preparing a paper exploring related issues in Federal Government Fiduciary Obligations to Aboriginal Peoples and Health.[12]

Principle 2: The Government of Canada has a fiduciary obligation to guard against infringement of Aboriginal rights in research activities, particularly in institutions and activities for which it is responsible. Aboriginal Peoples must endorse the appropriateness of particular safeguards through their representative organizations.

Diversity of Aboriginal Cultures

In the Speech from the Throne on September 30, 2002, Governor General Adrienne Clarkson announced the government of Canada's intent to "work with provinces to implement a national system for the governance of research involving humans, including national research ethics and standards." Ethical codes developed by Aboriginal Peoples recognize the diversity of Aboriginal communities and the primacy of community authority in deciding what matters are appropriate for research, the protocols to be respected, and how resulting knowledge should be distributed.[13]

The situation of the Métis deserves specific attention. Although they are recognized in the Constitution as one of the Aboriginal Peoples of Canada, they are excluded from federal and most provincial legislation protecting their Aboriginal rights and access to culturally specific services. They generally lack resources to develop organizational and governance infrastructure and to conduct or partner in research undertakings. A search for examples of community-based research protocols did not turn up examples of Métis-specific documents.

Principle 3: Action by the government of Canada to establish ethical standards of research should strike a balance between regulations that restrict infringement of Aboriginal rights and those that respect the primacy of ethical codes originating in affected communities, including Métis communities.

The Scope of Ethics Regimes

Ethics that govern research only on human subjects is too restricted to provide the protections sought by Aboriginal Peoples. The report to the Commission on Human Rights from the seminar on draft principles and guidelines for the protection of the heritage of Indigenous People provides a useful model for defining the scope of ethical regulation. The report proposes that heritage broadly defined should be the object of protective measures.

Principle 4: Ethical regulation of research affecting Aboriginal Peoples should include protection for "all knowledge, languages, territories, material objects, literary or artistic creations pertaining to a particular Aboriginal Peoples, including objects and forms of expression which may be created or rediscovered in the future based upon their traditions" as cited in emerging international norms.

Harmonization of Ethical Protection and Intellectual Property Law

A study of intellectual property and Aboriginal Peoples sponsored by Indian and Northern Affairs Canada underlines the inadequacy and inappropriateness of existing intellectual property regimes in protecting traditional Aboriginal knowledge. National and international rules governing copyright, trademarks, patents, and licensing procedures consistently conflict with Aboriginal culture norms or are practically inaccessible. Canadian rules are designed to conform to international standards.

Principle 5: "The federal government, in collaboration with Aboriginal peoples, [should] reviews its legislation on the protection of intellectual property to ensure that Aboriginal interests and perspectives, in particular collective interests, are adequately protected."[14]

Administrative Infrastructure

Implementation of an ethics regime in Aboriginal research requires more than the clear statement of principles. Legislation at best sets out boundaries for protection of heritage rights. As noted earlier, the administration of existing guidelines is in the hands of research ethics boards (REBs) located in universities and research institutes from which Aboriginal communities are generally distant socially and culturally. The Indian Act, which sets parameters for program funding for registered Indians, makes no provision to support research administration or ethics enforcement in its administrative regimes.

In its submission to Health Canada on Governance of Research Involving Human Subjects, NAHO recommended the creation of a system of Aboriginal research ethics boards (AREBs) to address local, regional, and national Aboriginal concerns. The brief further recommended that a national committee be formed consisting of Aboriginal experts who would develop ethical standards that could provide a reference point for AREBs and minimum standards for institutional REBs.[15]

Principle 6: Development and implementation of ethical standards for Aboriginal research should be in the hands of Aboriginal Peoples, as experts in devising minimum standards for general application and as majority members on Aboriginal-specific research ethics boards serving local, regional, and national communities.

Costs of Implementing an Ethical Regime

Briefs submitted in 2002 noted that establishing the relationships and ground rules for research in Aboriginal communities required time and effort prior to finalizing a research proposal.[16] Granting councils generally do not fund up-front costs of developing a research plan, thereby placing serious limitations on respectful—that is, ethical—research practice in or with Aboriginal communities.

Aboriginal involvement in research to support evidence-based decision making in service planning is generally not recognized in the administration budgets of Aboriginal communities and organizations.

Principle 7: The costs of community consultation, development of research plans, negotiation and implementation of ethical protocols, and skills transfer should be recognized in budget formulas for research grants and project planning whether conducted by researchers internal or external to Aboriginal communities.

Education for Ethical Practice

Ethics of consent, safety, and social benefit in research has evolved over decades. Ethical practice is advanced through a combination of institutional regulation, peer monitoring, and communication in the venues where researchers meet and confer with one another. Establishing research practices that respect Aboriginal worldviews, priorities, and authority will also be an evolving process.

Aboriginal communities that have taken up the challenge of conducting and monitoring research have promoted a broad base of local involvement in field research, management committees, and board governance. By their actions, they have demonstrated that research is too important to be left to a small group of academics, even if the experts are Aboriginal. Aboriginal community researchers, in concert with their peers in graduate schools and universities, are now talking about reinstating Aboriginal research methodologies to explore processes that have been neglected or poorly represented in past research. The terminology used for this process is community control, borrowing the language that has driven parallel moves to assert Aboriginal authority over government institutions, education, health, and social services.

Aboriginal initiative is essential to reform research practice and bring it into conformity with Aboriginal notions of ethical behavior. Aboriginal assertiveness is already evident in the surge of activity devising community research codes and the demands for effective partnership in major research undertakings.

Principle 8: Responsibility for education of communities and researchers in ethics of Aboriginal research rests with Aboriginal communities and organizations, government funders, granting agencies, professional associations, research institutions, and individual researchers working collaboratively.

CONCLUSION

This chapter places the discussion of ethics governing Aboriginal research in the context of a cultural worldview and the struggle for self-determination as peoples and nations. Self-determination has been seen as a political goal expressed most notably in self-government that recognizes a degree of autonomy in relation to Canadian state institutions. The language of self-government has obscured the reality that Aboriginal Peoples are engaged in a struggle to reestablish ethical order in their communities and nations.

This order reaffirms fundamental values that are rooted in their traditional construction of reality, sometimes called a worldview. Efforts to regain control of education, health, justice, and more are only in part about the power to govern. They are fundamentally about restoring order to daily living in conformity with ancient and enduring principles that support life.

Aboriginal Peoples are digging deep into their traditional teachings, reviving their ceremonies, and working to conserve their languages. As they take control of community services and institutions, they are proving that traditional teachings offer a sturdy ethical framework for restoring vitality to community life. Aboriginal academics, professionals, service providers, and political leaders are rediscovering and updating traditional values in the practice of education, the arts, health services, justice, and government. They are also challenging the assumptions of research rooted in a scientific worldview that clashes with their concepts of reality and right relationships.

It would be wrong to suggest that all Aboriginal Peoples hold traditional world-views with the same degree of tenacity. However, applied research, going on spontaneously and autonomously in Aboriginal communities and organizations, is demonstrating that when learning, healing, or rehabilitating is aligned with traditional ethics and values, it takes on astounding energy. The leaves of a tree, connected to their vital source, display health and vigor.

The active discussion of research ethics now going on in government and in granting councils opens up an opportunity for Aboriginal Peoples to engage in dialogue on how research can be adapted to achieve social benefit as they define it. The principles proposed in this paper start with an affirmation of the right of Aboriginal Peoples to generate and disseminate knowledge for and about themselves. This is not to say that all dialogue should halt until complex questions about rights and responsibilities are definitively resolved. Starting with such an affirmation simply underlines that governance of research touches on fundamental issues of Aboriginal culture, identity, and well-being.

Establishing and enforcing ethical practice in Aboriginal research will require a continuing commitment to implementing protective legislation, administrative infrastructure, and the education of the many participants in research. It is my hope that the articulation of issues and principles in this chapter will advance the dialogue that is already underway.

UPDATE (BY WANDA TEAYS)

At the author's request, an update on recent changes has been added:

In December 2010 three major research agencies of the Canadian federal government adopted an updated policy statement, *The Tri-Council Policy Statement: Ethical Conduct for Research Involving Humans* (TCPS).[17] The revised guidelines include a chapter titled, "Research Involving the First Nations, Inuit and Métis Peoples of Canada."

Aspects of this policy statement are relevant to the discussion on research protocol involving Aboriginal peoples and are worthy of mention. From what is set out below, we can see that steps have been made to address the concerns raised in this chapter and better appreciate the concerns Castellano has raised.

The key points of the TCPS Guidelines for Research involving the First Nations, Inuit, and Métis People of Canada include the following:

- *The Principle of Concern for Welfare is broader*, requiring consideration of participants and prospective participants in their physical, social, economic, and cultural environments, where applicable, as well as concern for the community to which participants belong.

- *This Policy acknowledges the important role of Aboriginal communities* in promoting collective rights, interests, and responsibilities that also serve the welfare of individuals.
- *Aboriginal peoples are particularly concerned that research should enhance their capacity to maintain their cultures, languages, and identities* as First Nations, Inuit, or Métis peoples, and to support their full participation in, and contributions to, Canadian society.
- *The interpretation of Concern for Welfare in First Nations, Inuit, and Métis contexts may therefore place strong emphasis on collective welfare* as a complement to individual well-being.
- *Justice may be compromised* when a serious imbalance of power prevails between the researcher and participants [and thus must be guarded against].
- *In the case of Aboriginal peoples, abuses stemming from research have included*: misappropriation of sacred songs, stories, and artifacts; devaluing of Aboriginal peoples' knowledge as primitive or superstitious; violation of community norms regarding the use of human tissue and remains; failure to share data and resulting benefits; and dissemination of information that has misrepresented or stigmatized entire communities.

The TCPS Guidelines acknowledge that mutual trust and communication takes time, not to mention mutually beneficial research goals, collaboration in research, and ensures "that the conduct of research adheres to the core principles of Respect for Persons, Concern for Welfare—which in this context includes welfare of the collective, as understood by all parties involved, and Justice."

Among the new requirements is the "Recognition of the Role of Elders and Other Knowledge Holders." Such knowledge holders should participate in the design and execution of research, as well as the interpretation of research results. In this way, research will be understood within the context of cultural norms and traditional knowledge. Moreover, "Community advice should also be sought to determine the appropriate recognition for the unique advisory role fulfilled by these persons" (Article 9.15).

The TCPS guidelines also recognize the importance of privacy and confidentiality. Article 9.16 sets out the specifics and emphasizes that "researchers shall not disclose personal information to community partners without the participant's consent." To examine the entire document in order to get a more detailed presentation of the changed policy(ies), see the Council Policy Statement: Ethical Conduct for Research Involving Humans, December 2010. This is available online at http://www.pre.ethics.gc.ca/eng/resources-ressources/news-nouvelles/nr-cp/2010-12-07.

ACKNOWLEDGMENT

I wish to thank the National Aboriginal Health Organization (NAHO) for providing the stimulus and the forum for exploring these important matters.

NOTES

1. © 2004 National Aboriginal Health Organization. Reprinted with permission. Access the NAHO website at: http://www.naho.ca/jah/english/jah01_01/journal_p98-114.pdf.

2. This paper was commissioned in 2002 by the National Aboriginal Health Organization to assist in developing an organizational position on research ethics. Documentary research and conceptual development were substantially advanced by conversations with NAHO staff, particularly Richard Jock, Yvonne Boyer, and Gail McDonald. Analysis and interpretation, errors, and omissions are entirely the responsibility of the author.

3. Y. Boyer, "Aboriginal Health—a Constitutional Rights Analysis," *Ottawa: National Aboriginal Health Organization* (2003), http://www.naho.ca/documents/naho/english/publications/DP_rights.pdf.

4. C. C. Brant, "Native Ethics and Rules of Behavior," *Canadian Journal of Psychiatry* 35 (August 1990): 534–39.

5. H. Cardinal, and Walter Hildebrandt, *Treaty Elders of Saskatchewan* (Calgary: University of Calgary Press, 2000), 6.

6. United Nations, Economic and Social Council, Draft Declaration on the Rights of Indigenous Peoples (1994) E/CN.4/Sub.2/1994/2/Add.l.

7. L. B. Leroy "Jagged Worldviews Colliding," in *Reclaiming Indigenous Voice and Vision*, edited by Marie Battiste (Vancouver: University of British Columbia Press, 2000), 77.

8. Ibid., 81.

9. G. Cajete, *Native Science, Natural Laws of Interdependence* (Sante Fe, NM: Clear Light Publishers, 2000), 284.

10. National Council on Ethics in Human Research (NCEHR), "Research Involving Aboriginal Individuals and Communities: Genetics as a Focus, Proceedings of a Workshop of the Consent Committee, November 19 to 21, 1999" (Ottawa: NCEHR, 2001, 51).

11. Royal Commission on Aboriginal Peoples (RCAP), *Report of the Royal Commission on Aboriginal Peoples*, Vol. 2, "Restructuring the Relationship" (Ottawa: Canada Communications Group, 1996), 215.

12. Y. Boyer, "Aboriginal Health: A Constitutional Rights Analysis," Ottawa: National Aboriginal Health Organization, 2003, http://www.naho.ca/documents/naho/english/publications/DP_rights.pdf.

13. Mi'kmaw Ethics Watch, *Principles & Guidelines for Researchers Conducting Research with and/or among Mi'kmaq People* (2000); Kahnawake Schools Diabetes Prevention Project, *Code of Research Ethics* (Kahnawake, Quebec: Kateri Memorial Hospital Centre (1997); and Brian Schnarch, "Ownership, Control, Access and Possession (OCAP) or Self-Determination Applied to Research *Journal of Aboriginal Health* 1 (1) (Ottawa: National Aboriginal Health Organization, 2003).

14. Royal Commission on Aboriginal Peoples (RCAP), *Report of the Royal Commission on Aboriginal Peoples*, Vol. 3, "Gathering Strength," 601.

15. National Aboriginal Health Organization (NAHO), "Governance of Research Involving Human Subjects, Research Brief" (Ottawa: National Aboriginal Health Organization).

16. Social Sciences & Humanities Research Council (SSHRC), "A Discussion Paper for the Roundtable Consultation" (Ottawa: SSHRC, 2002).

17. Canadian Institutes of Health Research, Natural Sciences & Engineering Research Council of Canada and Social Sciences and Humanities Research Council of Canada, "Tri-Council Policy Statement: Ethical Conduct for Research Involving Humans," November 29, 2010, http://www.pre.ethics.gc.ca/eng/resources-ressources/news-nouvelles/nr-cp/2010-12-07.

Discussion Topics: Part III

Wanda Teays

1. How much truth should doctors and nurses share with patients? To what degree should cultural values shape truth-telling?
2. The notion of the duty to inform has tended to focus on diagnosis. The California case of *Arato vs. Avedon* (1993) raised the issue of whether the doctor has to inform the patient of a dire prognosis. Mark A. Rothstein (2011) pushes the issue further, arguing that times have changed and access to information is not so burdensome as it once was. He, thus, asserts that doctors have a duty to notify patients of new medical information. Share your thoughts about whether it's time to change our expectations around doctors' duties to inform, in light of Rothstein's observations:

   Physicians generally have had no ethical or legal duty to notify patients about new medical information discovered after a visit, notwithstanding the health care benefits to patients that might flow from receiving the information. The rule was based on the relatively high burdens that notification would impose on physicians compared with the likelihood of benefits to patients. This established view, however, no longer may be appropriate in light of new physician-patient relationships and the reduced burden of patient notification using new types of health information technology (HIT).

   As a result, there is a duty to inform patients and former patients about relevant, medical development subsequent to their episode of care. It concludes by recommending the recognition in ethics and law of a limited, ongoing duty to notify patients of significant information relevant to their health.
3. To what extent should cultural diversity and religious beliefs play a role in the development of guidelines for handling patients with terminal illnesses?

4. To what extent should cultural diversity and religious beliefs play a role in the development of guidelines in hospital bioethics committees? Should bioethics committees be required to have representatives from the major cultures and religions of the community that those committees (or hospitals/institutions) serve?

5. Maya Sabatello looks at the notion of "family" in her chapter in this unit. Consider, for example, the case of the NASA scientist who used IVF with a nineteen-year-old embryo in her quest for a child. Read the following and then answer the questions below. Nancy Josephson Liff (2013) reports:

> NASA scientist Kelly Burke used a donated embryo that is believed to be the second oldest cryopreserved human embryo in history. Baby Liam has biological siblings born many years earlier. They were created from the same embryo cycle, using IVF. Those sibs are fraternal twins. Liam's sibs will be able to vote by the time the new arrival turns one later this year.
>
> Liam's story actually began more than nineteen years ago when a young woman donated her eggs at the Reproductive Science Center (RSC) in San Francisco. At that time, doctors transferred two donated embryos into the uterus of an Oregon woman who was seeking fertility treatment. Fraternal twins resulted from that cycle. Doctors froze the remaining embryos for use later on. The unused embryos were kept frozen until 2012 (Josephson 2013).

> *Answer the following:*
> a. What sorts of limits—if any—do you think should be put in place?
> b. Given the unknown risks of using embryos, eggs, and sperm that have been frozen for years or even decades, at what point should societal interests be factored into policies regarding such assisted reproduction?

6. When the "octomom," Nadya Suleman, a single parent with six children, gave birth to eight infants in 2011, the California Medical Board revoked her fertility doctor's medical license. "The California medical board said [Dr. Michael] Kamrava, who had implanted 12 embryos into Suleman with eight of them resulting in live births, made an 'extreme' departure from the standard of care." In their view, Kamrava did not exercise sound judgment (Dobuzinskis, June 1, 2011). *Answer the following:*

Discuss the ethical issues from any three of these perspectives—that of the fertility doctor (Kamrava), the medical profession in general, the parent (Suleman), the children (the eight infants and/or their siblings), or society in general.

7. Do you think it is right to restrict or even prohibit egg donation or sales? Read the following excerpt from *Science Daily* (2011), and then share your thoughts:

> Women who have become pregnant after egg donation should be categorized as high-risk patients. Why that is the case, and which consequences egg donation may have for women is the subject of a review article by Ulrich Pecks and co-authors from the University Hospital Aachen in *Deutsches Ärzteblatt International*.

The authors support their assessment with data from recent publications and with a case series they encountered in their own hospital. Viewing patient files they found that within the past 4 years, 8 women who had received donated eggs had to be treated for pregnancy-induced hypertension. Three of these pregnancies had to be terminated prematurely because of the threat to the mother's life. The other 5 cases showed a milder course of pregnancy-induced hypertension.

Egg donation has been in use for more than 25 years to treat unwanted childlessness. Since the German law on the protection of embryos explicitly forbids the procedure, couples often use medical institutions in neighboring European countries. After successful embryo transfer, the pregnant women are subsequently cared for in Germany in accordance with statutory maternity provision. Because of the risk of a hypertensive disorder of pregnancy, the authors recommend that the patients are closely monitored by doctors with a specialization in maternofetal medicine (*Science Daily*).

8. In her chapter on cross-cultural aspects of surgery, Alison Dundes Renteln suggests a code of ethics for surgeons that would address cultural conflicts. *Answer the following:*
    a. In light of some of the controversies that Renteln discusses in her chapter, do you think such an ethics code is advisable?
    b. What should be the protocol when a patient and surgeon disagree?
9. If a patient cannot speak for himself/herself and has no advance directives, but the hospital knows the patient's religious affiliation, should doctors be allowed to turn to a representative (priest, minister, imam, rabbi, etc.) about patients' medical care—that is, in regarding end-of-life decisions?
10. Share your concerns regarding the autonomy of minors seeking an abortion. *Answer the following:*
    a. What is the global picture on minors' rights to abortion? See what you can find out by looking at the laws in one or more countries from different continents. If there are restrictions, what form do they take?
    b. A 2013 report on the state of Arizona stated that 25 percent of abortion requests by minors that go before the Juvenile Court are denied—for example, because of her "maturity." Share your thoughts on the cultural or other influences on maturity and how that might impact this issue.
11. Looking at many issues in bioethics and health care, we often find people at polar opposites, with the middle path seemingly out of reach. In an article, "Debating the Moral Status of the Embryo," *Harvard Magazine* shared the views of professor of government Michael Sandel:

Sandel suggests that a more expansive view of the moral status of nature can help us see beyond the stark dualism between persons and things. "Personhood isn't the only warrant for respect," he says. "We consider it a failure of respect when a thoughtless hiker carves his initials in an ancient sequoia, not because we think the sequoia is a person, but because we consider it a natural wonder worthy of appreciation and awe, modes of regard inconsistent with defacing it for the sake of petty vanity.

"To respect an old-growth forest," he continues, "doesn't mean that no tree may ever be harvested for human purposes. Respecting the forest may be consistent with using it, but the purposes should be weighty and appropriate to the wondrous nature of the thing" (July–August 2004).

Answer the following:

  a. Is his comparison of ancient sequoias a useful way to look at the debate around embryos' moral status?

  b. Are there other analogies that might help us reach some common ground on this topic? Share your ideas.

12. In his chapter on human subjects, Peter Omonzejele argues that "vulnerability to harm and exploitation in the research setting is more pronounced in developing (African) countries often occasioned by social, cultural, and economic circumstances."

Answer the following:

  a. Assuming that is the case—and he offers examples to illustrate his point—what should Western researchers and pharmaceutical companies do to provide more protection for vulnerable research subjects?

  b. As Omonzejele notes, one condition that makes human subjects more vulnerable is poverty. What sorts of steps could be taken to better protect poor people in developing countries so they are less susceptible to exploitation in the research setting?

  c. Omonzejele states that prisoners are another vulnerable research group. They tend not to elicit as much sympathy as the poor. In addition, by their incarceration, the use of prisoners in experimentation is not as easily monitored. What sorts of steps could be taken to address their vulnerability as research subjects?

13. Native Americans, members of the First Nation, and other indigenous groups have raised issues around the Human Genome Project, other DNA research of native peoples, and the patenting of genetic material obtained from these research projects.

Answer the following:

  a. How might governments around the world follow the policy guidelines set down by the government of Canada (as discussed in Marlene Brant Castellano's essay in this unit)?

  b. Castellano shows that there are significant issues in researching Aboriginal people—not to mention major differences in both worldview and values. Would one way to address those be to rethink the role and composition of IRBs (Institutional Research Boards)? Share your thoughts.

14. Scott Stonington and Pinit Ratankul's chapter in part 1 and Cecilia Wee's chapter here in part 3 both examine cultural issues in decision making around euthanasia.

Answer the following:

a. What do you think might be a way to factor in cultural considerations when looking at such important medical issues as those centered on the end of life?

b. Would some form of cultural sensitivity suffice to bridge the differences between caregivers and the patient and his or her family? If not, what else could be put in place—that is, in terms of cultural protocols?

WORKS CITED

Arato v. Avedon (1993) 5 Cal.4th 1172, 23 Cal.Rptr.2d 131; 858 P.2d 598.

Dobuzinskis, Alex, "'Octomom' Doctor Loses California Medical License," *Reuters*, June 1, 2011, retrieved from www.reuters.com/article/2011/06/01/us-octomom-idUSTRE7507TL 20110601.

Josephson Liff, Nancy, "NASA Scientist Has Baby from an Embryo Frozen 19 Years Ago," What to Expect, August 26, 2013, retrieved from www.whattoexpect.com/wom/pregnancy/ 0826/nasa-scientist-has-baby-from-an-embryo-frozen-19-years-ago.aspx.

Rothstein, Mark A., "Physician's Duties to Inform Patients of New Medical Discoveries: The Effect of Health Information Technology," *Journal of Law, Medicine, and Ethics*, Vol. 39, No. 4, 2011, retrieved from http://papers.ssrn.com/sol3/papers.cfm?abstract_id=1971245.

Sandel, Michael, "Debating the Moral Status of the Embryo," *Harvard Magazine*, July-August 2004, retrieved from http://harvardmagazine.com/2004/07/debating-the-moral-statu.html

Science Daily, "Egg Donation: The Way to Happy Motherhood, with Risks and Side Effects," *Science Daily*, January 25, 2011, retrieved from www.sciencedaily.com/releases/2011/01/11012 4074013.htm.

IV

PUBLIC HEALTH

Introduction to Part IV: Public Health

Wanda Teays

The impact of public health concerns on the field of bioethics is both deep and wide ranging. Bioethics is fundamentally about health—our bodies, procreation and birth, disease and suffering, pain and death. It is about access to health care, the allocation of resources, and just versus unjust medical practices. It is about vulnerable populations used in research and experimentation, as sources of human organs, or as "gestational carriers" bearing children for contracting couples. We are not immune from its reach. Just one traveler from China brought SARS to the West, and just a few infected blankets brought smallpox to Native Americans.

Health is a basic good, and so it is vital that we give thought to different perspectives on the concept of "health" and look at the way it is understood across nations and cultures. The chapters in this book show how often health issues are human rights issues. Given the range of health inequities, questions of justice in health care merit our attention. Throughout this book, we see that is the case, as the chapters discuss important issues on health and human rights.

In the Preamble to the Constitution of the World Health Organization (WHO), health is defined as "a state of complete physical, mental and social well-being, and not merely the absence of disease or infirmity." WHO further asserts that governments are responsible for providing "adequate health and social measures." We might ask if access to health care is a fundamental right. A great deal follows from the answer to that question.

WHO's definition of health has brought with it considerable debate, given its social and ethical implications. In addition, it provides neither a discussion of the nature of mental or social well-being nor guidelines as to how they might be achieved. The very generality of the definition, as Daniel Callahan (1973) observes, has resulted in a concept that may be too broad. By including social problems as "health" problems, lines of responsibility have been blurred, leaving medical professionals in the difficult position of dealing with the "sick." Callahan's recommendation is to pull in the reins and, thus, he offers the following definition: "Health is a state of physical well-being." That state need not be "complete," he argues, but it must be adequate. He adds that neither mental well-being nor social well-being should be required for someone to be considered in good health.

Callahan's call for a narrower concept of health has its adherents. There are arguments for both sides, and depending upon our goals, a more restrictive versus more expansive definition of "health" may be preferable. One key factor is whether the issue is individual health or public health—the broader framework may require, at least in some circumstances, the more expansive approach to health.

Callahan points out that a person can be depressed (poor mental health, however temporary) and yet be in good physical health. Of course, if that person singularly or collectively turns to violence or terrorism to release pent-up anger or depression, we now have a public health problem. This should not escape the attention of bioethics.

When looking at public health on the global scale, it is easier to see why WHO suggested a broader approach to health. In many cases, physical well-being, mental well-being, and social well-being are intertwined. For example, according to the National Institute of Mental Health, mental health disorders are the leading cause of disability in Canada and the United States. In addition, social well-being may impact an individual's physical health and create a public health crisis—as Sanghamitra Padhy shows in her insightful discussion of Bhopal's gas explosion.

Limited health care delivery is also a public health concern, as Udo Schüklenk and Darragh Hare show in their important chapter. Moreover, dangerous work conditions, pollution, exposure to toxic chemicals or tainted water may all play a part in both social well-being and physical health. Disease control and prevention is one of the central concerns of public health policies. As a result, WHO's three types of well-being (physical, mental, and social) work in consort to mitigate—or exacerbate—global health problems.

Our assumptions, culture, traditions, and values, as well as biases and prejudices, transform what we consider good health. They also affect who has moral standing or whose health concerns are considered most pressing. This can result in disparities regarding access to resources and personnel, treatment options, decision making, and policy considerations.

In the opening chapter, Schüklenk and Hare examine moral responsibility for global health resources and the public health inequities concerning such issues as pandemic diseases and health care worker migration. Lawrence O. Gostin and Ames Dhai continue the discussion of health inequities in the next chapter. Their focus is on global health, calling for a shift of priorities and international collaboration. They make a compelling argument that we pay more attention to survival needs—systemic health problems—than the high-profile, heart-wrenching cases. Getting to the root of profound health inequalities is vital to achieving that goal.

Issues of health equity are also on the front burner in the United States, with the controversies around the implementation of the Affordable Care Act (ACA, also known as "Obamacare"). In his chapter, Peter Tan sets out a historical overview and analysis of the Act from the point of view of virtue ethics. He provides valuable insights into the ACA and its repercussions. That his chapter leads us back to concerns about justice and human rights is not surprising, given their centrality to a global bioethics.

The three cases on public health continue the thread of human rights and afford new insights, first, with Rosemarie Tong's thoughtful treatment of the ethical issues around long-term care of the elderly. Because of changing demographics, we need to acknowledge the health concerns and human rights issues that arise. Tong considers the societal pressures of a growing aging population. She presents various government policies designed to protect the rights of the elderly and looks specifically at China. China's one-child-per-family policy has led to questions about future eldercare. Because women have shouldered more of the burden of aging relatives, Tong asserts that men will need to play more of a role in eldercare to ensure global justice.

Continuing the case studies on vital public health issues, Michael Boylan examines public safety and risk assessment. Calculations of risks often require weighing trade-offs of various public goods. One essential element in such a calculation is the concept of public safety. Boylan examines this pressing concern within a context of various fallacies in risk assessment and then suggests a positive direction to public policy. His examples—such as that of a task force for preventative strategies and policies concerning avian flu—show the importance of risk assessment, proper planning, and prompt action in public health.

The final chapter is Sanghamitra Padhy's discussion of the public health concerns born of environmental disasters. The devastation in 2012 by the second-most-deadly hurricane in U.S. history (i.e., Hurricane Sandy in the northeastern United States) demonstrates the public health aspects of such crises. Natural and human-caused catastrophes often cross national boundaries and require a global response. Her analysis of Bhopal (gas explosion), Chernobyl (nuclear explosion), and Fukushima (earthquake, tsunami, and leaked radiation) calls for bioethicists to recognize that public health concerns are inevitable in the face of environmental catastrophes.

This collection of essays in part 4 gives us insight into the moral conflicts around public health. They also help us understand how morality, religion, and culture can intersect and call for closer examination and reflection. The valuable insights here in this section and in the book as a whole help broaden our understanding of bioethics and deepen our appreciation for the global impact of the issues examined here.

REFERENCE

Callahan, Daniel. 1973. "The WHO Definition of 'Health.'" *The Hastings Center Studies* 1 (3): 77–78.

1

Issues in Global Health Ethics

Udo Schüklenk and Darragh Hare

ABSTRACT

This chapter provides a brief overview of major ethical challenges in international health. This overview aims to demonstrate that current health inequities are not simply an unfortunate incident but that they are unjust and that they ought to be addressed. Among the issues reviewed is the question of whose moral responsibility global health resourcing is. What are the moral obligations, if any, of nation-states, international institutions, transnational NGOs, and large multinational corporations in this context? Infectious disease control poses its own ethical challenges. HIV/AIDS and influenza will be used as examples of paradigmatic pandemic diseases that require a concerted global response. It is, for instance, conceivable that the provision of a forthcoming pandemic influenza vaccine would preserve more lives if it was deployed in certain developing countries first. What are the moral obligations of developed world governments under such circumstances? Can we reasonably expect people who are HIV infected to take side-effect-prone AIDS medicines where this might not be of clinical benefit to them but where this would render them for all intents and purposes noninfectious? Does the public interest trump private interests in cases of pandemic diseases?

This chapter will proceed to a moral evaluation of health worker's migration issues. It is well known that, for instance, more Malawi-trained health care workers work in countries other than Malawi. What are the moral obligations of health workers to the societies that enabled their training? What are the obligations of net recipient countries (usually located in the developed world)? Is free-riding on developing countries' training of health care professionals ethically acceptable? Issues in global health ethics will conclude with a cursory discussion of at least some pertinent issues in international, multicenter clinical research studies. Questions to be addressed include standards of care in a trial, as well as post-trial, care both with regard to therapeutic and nontherapeutic clinical research.

PREVENTABLE SUFFERING AND GLOBAL HEALTH

Gross inequities in health treatment and health outcomes exist throughout the world. These inequities are determined by a complicated combination of local circumstances and international policies, and it is beyond the scope of this chapter to examine in detail the specific statistics relating to them. However, there is a clear geographical pattern: health outcomes, health care systems, and access to health care in the developing world fall far below the standards that are enjoyed by the developed world. This provides important questions for all manner of academic disciplines, from economics to immunology to anthropology to public policy and beyond. Many of the issues that arise have clear ethical dimensions, and we will consider some of the most topical.

Inequities between countries are inevitable. Some countries are stronger than others in terms of geographical area, natural resources, location, and population size. Such differences are unavoidable, and in broad terms they are morally neutral. However, inequities in health outcomes and access to health care do not fall into the same category. Rather, many if not all of them are the direct and indirect products of historical and contemporary exploitation in the form of colonialism and oppressive economic policies.[1]

Why should we be concerned about health in the first place? Why does health matter? Even though having good health is not synonymous with living a happy or worthwhile life, there is a strong link between good health and the ability to pursue one's preferences: The satisfaction of preferences is made easier by good health and more difficult by illness. Improving health and access to health care, therefore, must be one priority for any initiative designed to prevent suffering and improve the quality of people's lives. Those living in the developing world are disadvantaged in comparison to those living in the developed world.

This is typically characterized by poorer health generally and by diminished life expectancy.[2] However, it must be borne in mind that poor population health is not simply a symptom of substandard health care systems, but it is also almost invariably indicative of extreme poverty. Social inequality in societies with two-tier health care systems or private health care delivery infrastructure translates into significant differences in terms of health outcomes, and these differences are usually to the detriment of the poorer members of society.

Similarly, while investment in health services is obviously crucial to improving health outcomes, interventions in other policy areas can lead to dramatic health improvements. For example, education, social inclusion, and safe and sanitary built environments all have beneficial impacts on individual and public health. In some circumstances, these can improve health outcomes to a greater degree than clinical interventions. Similarly, basic primary care facilities in many developing countries can be more effective in terms of health outcomes than state-of-the-art facilities such as high-tech transplant centers. However, it is important to recognize that, even when adjustments are made to account for population size and cost of living, developed countries spend approximately thirty times more per person on health care than developing countries.[3]

These international disparities are largely a consequence of the global economic system. A minority of the world's population lives in material abundance while a significant proportion suffer severe harm as a result of extreme poverty. It is morally significant that this harm—of which poor health outcomes are only one manifestation—is preventable: the resources necessary to address global poverty and thereby to reduce substantially the suffering it causes exist.

The relationship between global economics, poverty, and suffering was brought into sharp focus by the events following the earthquake that struck Haiti in January 2010. This earthquake caused devastating damage to towns, villages, and cities, and more than 150,000 Haitians were killed.[4] Much of the destruction, death, and suffering, however, was preventable. Due to the extreme poverty in Haiti, its building safety standards are much lower than in the developed world, and buildings are therefore less resilient; if an earthquake of the same magnitude had struck Japan, for example, less damage would have been done to the built environment and fewer people would have died or been injured. The poverty in Haiti is preventable. At its root is interference by its formal colonizers and the United States.[5] When seen in this light, much of the suffering caused by the earthquake was not merely unfortunate, it was unjust. It was not so much a result of the—unavoidable—earthquake, but of the poverty that meant that building safety standards in Haiti were so low.

There is now widespread acceptance that the developed world has a moral obligation to address the suffering caused by extreme poverty by providing aid to the developing world. As we shall see later in this chapter, different models of moral reasoning support this conclusion. There is disagreement about the nature and extent of this obligation, which specific harms should be addressed, and how aid interventions ought to be prioritized. Competing answers to these questions can translate into enormously divergent policy solutions. But before we take a closer look at these policy issues, it will be useful to examine and discuss the competing theoretical frameworks that underpin them.

POLITICAL VERSUS HUMANITARIAN RATIONALES

A large proportion of aid to the developing world is delivered by means of intergovernmental transactions. These transactions involve the transfer of money, resources, or expertise by a government or intergovernmental organization in the developed world to a government or governments in the developing world. The actors involved in delivering this type of aid are governments, but there is continuing disagreement among political philosophers about whether the obligation to provide aid has its roots at the governmental level or whether this obligation actually belongs to individual citizens in the developed world.

These competing ideas take a variety of forms, and they have been loosely categorized into two discrete strands.[6] The first line of reasoning is the political rationale, which holds that the obligation to provide aid lies essentially with governments or nation-states. Pogge has suggested that governments or nation-states are responsible for providing aid as a form of reparation or compensation for historical wrongs.[7] This can be taken to mean, for example, that certain European countries have an ethical obligation to provide assistance to certain West African countries due to the manifold social, economic, and environmental harms inflicted on one country by another during colonialism. Furthermore, the political rationale goes beyond just compensation for past wrongs. It also addresses ongoing wrongs such as foreseeable extreme poverty caused in the developing world by present global economic arrangements.

Some objections to the political rationale have been made. Firstly, the idea of international aid as reparation for specific, definable harms, if applied strictly, might exonerate or severely reduce the obligations of some nations in the developed world. That is, while some developed countries have a clear history of colonialism or exploitation, others do not. This latter group, with no clear history of exploitation, could claim that they are therefore not morally required to provide aid to the developing world.

Secondly, major changes to geopolitics mean that some of the nation-states involved in historical injustices no longer exist. This raises the problem of how aid transactions should be carried out on behalf of now nonexistent developed countries or as compensation to now nonexistent countries in the developing world. Thirdly, it might be possible to define some countries as being both the victims and the perpetrators of exploitation. This is particularly relevant in the case of countries with rapidly growing economies, such as China or South Korea, which once were part of the developing world but whose status in the global economy is now more accurately defined as "emerging" or "developed."

The political rationale is laudable in its intention to provide a theoretical basis upon which affluent governments in the developed world could be persuaded to alleviate suffering by providing support to under-resourced governments in the developing world. If accepted by developed governments, the political rationale would yield overseas aid policies that could have an enormous impact on the well-being of people living in the developing world, and this would undoubtedly be desirable. However, although the political rationale is capable of producing favorable outcomes, its premises necessarily limit its scope. This is probably the most serious objection to it.

The political rationale holds that aid transactions should be seen as compensation for historical malfeasance on the part of developed world governments. But while it is certainly true that there are good reasons for governments in the developed world to adopt this attitude, the political rationale alone cannot provide a sound theoretical basis for the type of aid necessary to alleviate suffering effectively.[8] For example, some suffering has not come about as a result of colonialism or subjugation on the part of countries in the developed world. There are numerous instances in which developing countries have been devastated by natural disasters, civil war, or gross political mismanagement.

While it could be argued that the causes of some of these might actually be traced back to the developed world—climate change or oppressive foreign and economic policies, for instance—the causes of at least some of them are purely local. Earthquakes, tsunamis, volcanic eruptions, civil wars, and failed political systems can all result in extremely poor health conditions and desperate but preventable suffering. But the political rationale states that, unless these conditions are linked to the behavior of developed world governments, there is no justice-based obligation to provide aid or assistance in such circumstances.[9]

The governments of developed countries, according to the political rationale, have an obligation to provide aid to the developing world because of what has caused people's suffering, not simply by virtue of the fact that they are suffering. Those people who are starving as a result of political subjugation or military occupation should be afforded medical aid, but those who are starving because their crops have been obliterated by an earthquake should not. This picture seems incomplete and indicates that the political rationale alone cannot provide a sufficiently plausible theoretical basis for the provision of medical aid to those who need it most. Instead, it requires that injustices should only be addressed when their causes can be traced to the behavior of governments in the developing world. But frequently the circumstances that are arguably most deserving of aid have no such cause.

Moreover, the political rationale fails to offer any kind of guidance for the crucial task of prioritizing health aid. Severe health inequities exist within countries as well as between them. Even in developed countries, there can be vast differences in health outcomes and health conditions between citizens. For example, the average life expectancy at birth of a man living in Kensington, an affluent area in London, is 84.3 years, whereas a man living in Glasgow, also in the UK, can on average expect to live 70.7 years.[10]

Since the central tenet of the political rationale is that governments have an obligation to address the inequities brought about by their behavior, domestic inequities must also be considered. The political rationale offers no guidance on how competing domestic and overseas demands on public funds should be resolved, and therefore it leaves an important policy question unanswered. It is possible that the political rationale could require the prioritization of domestic needs ahead of overseas needs, perhaps even to the outright exclusion of any overseas interventions. It is probably fair to suggest that although the suffering prevalent in developed countries can be serious, and should be addressed, it is rarely as serious as the suffering experienced by those in absolute poverty in the developing world.[11]

The political rationale offers no comprehensive account capable of adequately addressing the problem of global suffering. The scope of the political rationale is far narrower than that which can reasonably be expected of a comprehensive approach to global health ethics. It provides no satisfactory answers to the question of how aid should be prioritized.

The humanitarian rationale, on the other hand, sees individual citizens as the relevant moral agents in obligations to provide overseas aid. At first glance, this approach might seem counterintuitive: Although individuals can and do make contributions to charities, currently the main actors in the provision of global aid are governments. But perhaps this is simply a matter of practicality. The size and complexity of overseas aid payments means that they ought to be decided and negotiated by governments, and the transactions involved should be carried out by governments, but this does not mean that the relevant moral actors are governments. The humanitarian rationale argues this very point and suggests that governments are acting as a necessary proxy for transactions between individual citizens in the countries involved.

According to this logic, when the Australian government makes an aid payment to support a public health initiative in Sudan, for example, this is a manifestation of a payment by the citizens of Australia to the citizens of Sudan. The obligation to provide aid in this scenario does not belong to the Australian government but to the Australian people, and the obligation requires that aid be provided to the people of Sudan, not to the Sudanese government. The fact that the transaction is carried out by governments is merely a matter of expediency.

The humanitarian rationale has at its root the principle of moral equivalence, or "universal undifferentiated moral standing."[12] This principle, simply put, asserts that every person has an equal claim to moral consideration. This thought is at the heart of the liberal tradition and has been central to many civil rights agendas. The humanitarian rationale asserts that in principle each person has a moral relationship with every other person, regardless of nationality or country of residence. This notion is strongly associated with the utilitarian tradition and sees suffering or the prevention of the pursuit of preferences as harmful and therefore as having negative moral value.

We have a moral obligation to relieve suffering or barriers to preference satisfaction whenever doing so does not involve comparable risks to ourselves. When applied to the issue of global suffering, this logic requires that those living in the developed world are morally obliged to prevent harm to those living in the developed world until the point that by doing so they would not cause comparable harm to themselves. However, the present distribution of resources is so distorted that such a tipping point is very unlikely to come about any time soon. Interestingly, some empirical estimates assert that sufficient resources could be diverted to address global poverty without bringing about any appreciable difference to the quality of life of those living in the developed world.[13]

It has been argued that geographical or political borders provide useful and ethically significant demarcations in deciding the boundaries of moral groups.[14] This view is supported by the fact that evolutionary pressure seems to support a preference for assisting members of one's family or one's immediate community over assisting strangers or people living on the other side of the world. However, although there are undoubtedly strong evolutionary reasons for human beings holding this kind of instinctive attitude, it does not stand up to much ethical scrutiny; good ethics does not always conform to our moral instincts but explores them and sometimes requires us to act in opposition to them.

Some of the biggest ethical triumphs in recent history were cases in which the instinct to attribute special moral status to those in our immediate social groups was overcome: the abolition of slavery, universal franchise, and the vast majority of civil rights movements. Our moral group is expanding and becoming more inclusive; people who were historically excluded because of sex, skin color, sexual orientation, or worldview have been gradually admitted to the group. The rationale used for making these changes is applicable to those who as yet are not part of the established moral group. In the case under consideration, it is an argument against exclusion based on geographical location, and it requires that we do not recognize geographical or political borders as having special moral relevance.

Poor access to health resources, prolonged sickness, and premature death are very common phenomena in the developing world, and clearly these involve suffering and are often barriers to preference satisfaction. Furthermore, they constitute important hindrances to economic development. In the developing world, much sickness and premature death is easily preventable. It is caused by treatable conditions, many of which are very effectively contained in the developed world. The question of providing aid to the developing world is therefore largely one of resource allocation: Could the developed world provide medical assistance to the developing world without incurring a comparable risk to itself? We believe that it could.

The political rationale cannot provide a sufficient theoretical basis for the type of interventions required to address global suffering satisfactorily. By reconceptualizing the nature of the moral obligation, however, the humanitarian rationale does not encounter this problem. The humanitarian rationale proposes that inhabitants of the developed world have an obligation to provide aid to the inhabitants of the developing world who are suffering preventable harm regardless of the particular political or economic explanations for the suffering in question.

But the humanitarian rationale must also deal with problems concerning scope. For example, how much aid is the developed world obliged to provide to the developing world? Perhaps this question can be answered by calculating the degree of need in each case: The obligation is to provide as much aid as is necessary to alleviate the problem, so long as doing so does not create a comparable disadvantage to those living in the developed world.

If this model were to become policy in the developed world, it would yield overseas aid interventions on a far larger scale than anything that has been implemented to date. Despite the persuasive case for this type of aggressive redistribution, it is difficult to envisage an immediate radical change to overseas aid. In the case of government spending, for example, even the most generous nations currently allocate only a tiny proportion of their GDP to overseas aid.[15]

INTERNATIONAL FINANCIAL ARRANGEMENTS

Aid payments to the developing world must be considered in the global economic context. Of particular relevance is the system of governmental loans that was implemented in the 1970s and 1980s, ostensibly to help developing world countries to alleviate acute health and wider social problems by investing in their domestic infrastructure. A number of countries in Latin America and the Caribbean took substantial loans from various international financial organizations, such as the World Bank and the International Monetary Fund, for this purpose, but there were specific conditions attached to the loans that affected the ways in which they could be used.

These conditions were primarily concerned with policy reforms in the recipient countries, and it required them to adopt neoliberal economic policies and to implement corresponding political and economic instruments. These conditions attached to the World Bank loans have in many cases crippled clinical and public health services in the recipient countries, and have prevented the kind of reform and investment for which the loans were initially intended; in fact, in some cases the current system is no better than the old system. While it might in some circumstances be desirable to attach such conditions for structural or policy reform to aid payments, these conditions must be sensitive to existing local cultural and political systems.

Perhaps the most damaging consequence of these conditions was the requirement that health services in the recipient countries became privatized. This undid much good work that had previously been done, particularly in containing endemic diseases. Furthermore, recipient governments were required to employ expensive overseas consultants in order to establish and manage the new privatized health systems, which was a particularly inefficient use of the loan. In certain countries, a long-term effect of the privatized health care requirement imposed by the loans has been the emergence of vastly unequal multitiered systems, in which all patients must pay for health care.

In such systems, the rich minority of the population have access to health resources that are far superior to those available to the poor majority. It is difficult to see how such situations—or the policies underpinning the loans that created them—can be ethically justified, although there have been various unsuccessful attempts to do so.[16]

ACCESS TO TREATMENT

While differences in terms of health outcomes and provision exist both between and within countries in both the developing world and the developed world, there is a clear division between even the best-performing developing countries and the worst-performing developed countries. It is possible to make a few general observations about the differences between the two. The average life expectancy of someone living in the developing world is shorter than that of a person living in the developed world.

Moreover, a person living in the developing world is more likely to spend a greater proportion of his or her life in ill health. Medical conditions that are easily treatable in the developed world go untreated in the developing world, and access to vaccines, medicines, and other medical treatment is poor in comparison.

The types of illnesses encountered and the particular social contexts in which they exist make approaches to health policy in the developing world different from approaches in the developed world in significant respects. Preventable diseases such as diarrhea and influenza kill millions of people every year in the developing world. So why are vaccines and medicines not made available to those who need them in the developing world? The answer to this question has two parts.

The first part has to do with affordability. Some treatments are simply too expensive for those living in the developing world. Governments cannot afford to purchase enough drugs for their citizens, and the citizens themselves cannot afford to pay for their own treatment. The second part has to do with logistics: In many cases the health care infrastructure required to distribute medicines and organize mass vaccinations does not exist. Poor people in under-resourced countries either have no access to or cannot afford the simple treatments taken for granted in more affluent countries. Infectious diseases that are controlled or effectively eradicated in the developed world are rampant in the developing world because vaccines are too expensive and vaccination programs are not in place.

The pharmaceutical companies that develop the drugs set drug prices. When a successful drug has been developed, it is protected by a patent preventing the drug from being copied or produced by others. This system means that the company responsible for investing in the research and development of a successful drug can recoup the investment necessary to bring the drug to market and make a profit. For a pharmaceutical company to survive, its profits must at the very least cover the costs of all of its research and development programs, including those that are ultimately unsuccessful.

In fact, it is the incentive of substantial profits that motivates the pharmaceutical companies to undertake expensive research and development in the first place. Predictably, the pharmaceutical industry defends the system of patents and pricing by arguing that it serves the public interest: The development of new and better medical products depends upon commercial incentives for pharmaceutical companies to undertake drug research and development. While this might seem reasonable at first glance, the idea that pharmaceutical companies are motivated by the public interest does not bear much scrutiny. Pharmaceutical companies, which hold patents on new medicines, refuse to supply customers who cannot afford to pay their prices, thus effectively precluding access in much of the developing world.

Furthermore, patent holders frequently refuse to grant licenses to other companies who would produce and supply the same drugs at a reduced cost, and they vehemently pursue legal action against companies who breach patents to do so.[17] The result is usually that a new drug does not become available in the developing world until after the patent has expired, normally ten or more years after it has been granted. The patent holders cannot expect to make much profit from sales in large parts of the developing world while they hold the patent, and they certainly will not do so once the patent has expired.

The profit on new medicine comes almost exclusively from its sale in the developed world, and it is unclear how making patented drugs available in the developing world could harm the profit margins of its developer. Perhaps the pharmaceutical industry could reasonably be concerned that foregoing the patents in the developing world might mean that unlicensed versions of a drug become available in the developed world, thus impacting on profits. However, strict regulation of production and supply could prevent this from occurring. Pharmaceutical companies genuinely motivated by notions of public interest might reasonably be expected to make patented drugs available in the developing world, albeit under strict regulatory conditions.

But it would be unreasonable to expect pharmaceutical companies to act altruistically. It is not clear that shareholders of pharmaceutical companies should subsidize research that, according to both the humanitarian and political models, is the responsibility of all well-off citizens in the developed world. Pharmaceutical companies have fiduciary responsibilities to their shareholders to maximize profits, and to prioritize the public interest ahead of commercial interest might be to overlook these responsibilities. If pharmaceutical companies were concerned more with the public interest than with profits, shareholders might prefer to invest in other industries, thus inhibiting the pharmaceutical industry.

Perhaps we should not expect them to undertake drug research on diseases most prevalent in the developing world unless those diseases are also prevalent in wealthy markets, or unless there are clear advance purchase commitments from motivated buyers. The lesson to be drawn from this analysis is this: If we think medicines ought to be developed for diseases prevalent in the developing world, it is us who should consider paying for it. We cannot expect pharmaceutical companies to undertake this work purely altruistically.

The nature of existing health care infrastructures in many developing countries would make large-scale treatment or vaccination initiatives very difficult, and perhaps in some cases impossible. The establishment of workable health care infrastructures would go some way to allowing the kinds of preventative and reactive treatment programs that could make a significant contribution to addressing the health problems in the developing world. However, some governments in the developing world consistently fail to invest in health care, and often they prioritize military spending ahead of health care spending.

This practice is currently going on in Zimbabwe, North Korea, and Burma, among others. This behavior is sometimes used as an argument against providing medical aid to these countries: If their own governments choose not to prioritize health spending, the developed world should not provide assistance. This point of view is consistent with the political rationale, as described above. However, as we have seen, the obligation to provide aid exists between individuals, and the humanitarian rationale, while justifiably condemning the prioritization of military spending over health spending, would require the developed world to provide health aid to people living in those countries whose governments neglect to do so.

INFECTIOUS DISEASE CONTROL

Infectious diseases pose a threat to individual as well as public health in any given population. In the developed world, health care systems are generally quite efficient in managing and controlling the spread of common infectious diseases. However, in the developing world, with health care systems that are less sophisticated and less comprehensive in their coverage, infectious diseases are much more difficult to control.

HIV/AIDS is a paradigmatic example of this, and we need only compare the infection rates in Western and Central Europe with those in Sub-Saharan Africa to see the extent of this problem.[18] If HIV/AIDS is allowed to continue to spread in the developing world, its already harmful consequences will continue or worsen. The natural spread of HIV/AIDS has been reinforced in some parts of the developed world by unhelpful government interventions, such as the disastrous treatment and education policies of the Mbeki administration in South Africa.[19, 20] In the absence of a preventive vaccine for HIV, any successful initiative to control the disease would involve testing populations, treating those who are HIV positive, and taking measures to prevent further infection.

Incidentally, treating those who are HIV positive with highly active antiretroviral medicines would have another desirable effect: for all intents and purposes they would be rendered noninfectious. AIDS treatment would not only provide them with the care necessary to survive, it would also have effects comparable to a preventive vaccine in terms of the effective protection it provides to the sexual partners of infected people. Such initiatives could potentially require significant infringements on the autonomy of those who are tested. Historically, these violations of autonomy were considered too serious to preclude the option of mandatory HIV testing.

Part of the rationale at the time was that even if those who were affected could have been identified, there was no effective treatment to reduce the fatalities caused by the disease.[21] However, today's treatments for HIV/AIDS are capable of preserving the lives of people with HIV/AIDS and reducing their risk of infecting others. The existence of these treatments casts serious doubt upon the autonomy objection. Identifying those who are infected by HIV/AIDS and treating them could bring about enormous improvements to individual and public health, and this might well be sufficient to override concerns about the potential violation of infected individuals' autonomy.

Let us consider a more complex version of this scenario; namely, the question of whether or not it might be good policy to introduce mandatory HIV testing for pregnant women. There is a 35 percent chance that an infant born to an HIV-positive woman will also be HIV positive. The number of children infected by this process worldwide was estimated to be between 2.1 and 2.8 million in 2004.[22] However, a fairly simple treatment program for the mother and child exists that can produce a reduction in mother-to-child transmission of 67.5 percent.[23]

Unfortunately, in many parts of the world where this type of intervention would be most effective due to a high prevalence of HIV, such as Botswana, being HIV positive carries a stigma that can have fairly severe social consequences. It is conceivable that pregnant women in these circumstances would feel sufficient social pressure that they would avoid attending clinics where they would be mandatorily tested for HIV, thus defeating the purpose of mandatory testing. These social and cultural phenomena might make a policy of mandatory testing difficult, but not impossible, to deliver. For example, a mandatory testing program could aim to guarantee the confidentiality of the HIV status of mothers and newborns in an attempt to minimize such stigmatization and its concomitant negative consequences. Unfortunately, on current treatment modalities it would be difficult for those women who are HIV positive to preserve their anonymity while undergoing treatment.

While such operational challenges are certainly important, there is a prior debate regarding the ethical acceptability of mandatory HIV testing for pregnant women. A rigorous set of conditions have been proposed[24] that must be met in order for mandatory testing to be ethically justifiable. A pregnant woman must first of all have voluntarily decided to carry her fetus to term, in full knowledge of the available alternatives including abortion. A pregnant woman is not morally obliged to carry and deliver a fetus that she does not want. However, when a pregnant woman does voluntarily decide to carry a fetus to term, she arguably accepts an obligation not to injure the fetus and to take reasonable steps to prevent it from being subjected to serious risk of bodily harms such as life-threatening infections. Pregnant women therefore could be seen to have an obligation to ensure that they do not transmit HIV to their fetus, and this would first require the HIV status of the mothers to be ascertained.

Poor health resources and fragmented medical advice and treatment might make such a policy difficult to implement in the developing world. Pregnant women in developing countries might not have sufficient access to alternatives to pregnancy, and therefore a decision to carry a fetus to term might not always be voluntary. The obligations that apply to genuinely voluntary pregnancies would not apply in such cases. Moreover, while abortion can be an ethically acceptable alternative in the early stages of a pregnancy, it is more difficult to justify it for later-stage pregnancies. Substandard health care in the developing world could mean that pregnant women engage with health professionals too late in their pregnancies for abortion to be viable. This, again, might alter the voluntariness of a pregnancy and therefore any obligations that it implies.

The second condition for justifiable mandatory testing is that HIV-positive women who undergo mandatory testing and successfully deliver their children must be given access to life-preserving antiretroviral medication for themselves. This would mean that the mothers would be more likely to be well enough to look after their children, considerably improving the children's chances of survival. Furthermore, it would reduce the pressure on developing societies already struggling to cope with huge numbers of AIDS orphans. However, participation in such an initiative would have to be voluntary, since it would be impractical to enforce or supervise the women's adherence to antiretroviral treatment. Women who undergo some antiretroviral treatment but who do not continue to receive it can develop drug-resistant strains of HIV. This could have serious health consequences not only for the women concerned but also for any future children that they may choose to have and indeed their sexual partners if they practice unsafe sex. Furthermore, there are significant public health implications of introducing drug-resistant strains of HIV.

The third condition is that the anonymity of pregnant women and their children should be maintained throughout and after the pregnancy, for the reasons outlined above. This would be likely to provide a formidable operational challenge to health authorities.

Antiretroviral treatment has the potential to make a significant impact not only on MTCT (mother-to-child transmission of HIV) but also on the overall global spread of HIV/AIDS. Enormous amounts of time and resources have been invested in trying to develop a preventative vaccine for HIV, but to no avail. However, as well as preserving the lives of those who are HIV positive, long-term treatment with modern antiretroviral medications can render them effectively noncontagious.[25] The combination of better health and a reduced chance of infecting others is likely to be a strong incentive for at-risk individuals to seek testing and, for those who are HIV positive, treatment.

This incentive would be stronger still if it was accompanied by changes to the legality of unsafe sex and a shift in the cultural attitudes toward HIV-positive individuals in both the developed and the developing world. By removing these legal and cultural barriers, at-risk individuals would be more willing to be tested. This in turn would allow health care agencies to quantify and track the incidence of HIV/AIDS and to contain it by rigorous treatment with modern antiretroviral medication. Projections published in 2009 suggest that such a policy could have a dramatic impact upon the AIDS epidemic within ten years of implementation, and could reduce the prevalence of HIV in the world's worst affected areas to 1 percent by the middle of this century.[26] However, the price of medications remains a significant obstacle to the implementation of effective control of infectious diseases.

MEDICAL RESEARCH AND CARE FOR RESEARCH PARTICIPANTS

A substantial amount of research into the development of new medical products takes place in the developing world and involves citizens of developing countries as research participants. Such research is almost always carried out by pharmaceutical companies based in the developed world, and the imbalance in wealth between these countries and the communities and individuals involved in research raises a number of ethical concerns about the potential exploitation of research participants in the developing world.

One of the most controversial issues in international research ethics concerns the standard of clinical care that should be afforded to research participants. The central issue is whether participants in the control arms of an international, multicenter trial should be given the same treatment regardless of their geographical location, or whether they should be given the best locally available treatment. This issue triggered more than a decade of heated debate among the international bioethics community, following ACTG 076, an AIDS clinical trial that set out to establish whether an affordable treatment that would reduce the incidence of MTCT could be developed for use in the developing world.

Previous trials in the developed world had demonstrated that pregnant mothers who used a particular treatment regime of the drug Zidovudine were much less likely to pass HIV on to their offspring than those pregnant women who took no antiretroviral medication. At the time of ACTG 076, therefore, the Zidovudine regime was the gold standard in the developed world, but it was unaffordable to most pregnant women in poorer countries. The investigators in ACTG 076 tested a lower, and therefore less expensive, dosage of Zidovudine. The trial sought to find out whether a lower dosage was more effective than no treatment at all, not whether it was more effective than the higher dosage used in the developed world. Those in the treatment arm of the trial received the lower dosage, while those in the control arm received no treatment.

The trial was heavily criticized by medical scholars and ethicists.[27, 28] It directly contravened one of the provisions of the World Medical Association's Declaration of Helsinki,[29] which requires that those in the control arm of biomedical trials be given access to the best available therapeutic and diagnostic techniques. This would require that everyone in the control arm, regardless of their geographical location, should receive the gold standard treatment; only in the absence of a gold standard does a placebo control become acceptable as a means to test the null hypothesis. But some people defended the trial methodology and suggested that the Declaration of Helsinki should in fact be revised to allow this type of trial.

The trial methodology has also been defended by arguing that, since pregnant women in the developing world had no access to Zidovudine or any other antiretroviral therapy, the women in the control arm were no worse off than they would have been if they had not participated in the trial, while those in the treatment arm were likely to be better off. However, this justification is insufficient. It makes little sense in clinical terms, since the purpose of most drug trials is to see how the trial drug performs against the gold standard drug, not poorer treatments.

Critics of the Helsinki Declaration argue that, if it was followed strictly, all new treatments would have to be tested against the best medication available anywhere in the world, even if such a medication was unaffordable for a large proportion of the global population. This would effectively prohibit trials designed to develop treatments that would be affordable in poorer countries. However, both of these defenses rely upon an assumption that drugs are necessarily too expensive for people in the developing world to afford them. The reality is that they are only too expensive because of the high prices demanded by pharmaceutical companies. The distinction between local and global standards of care is artificial, and any argument based upon it is flawed.[30]

A related issue concerns the posttrial clinical care that should be provided to research participants in the developing world. After all, part of the ethical rationale of clinical research in developed countries is that patients, including those in the trial in question, would be afforded access to the drug that was tested successfully in a trial. Due to the cost issues mentioned earlier in this chapter, the same cannot be said for trial participants in the developing world. This raises the possibility of exploitation, as well as the question of whether special provisions ought to be made with regard to posttrial access to medicines.

The Declaration of Helsinki requires that any benefits resulting from clinical research should be made available to the individuals and communities that are involved in the research. This could be taken to mean that research participants should remain on that medication that the trial finds is the most effective, whether it is the trial drug or the best existing alternative. However, it has been argued that such a policy would be unaffordable, and that it might prevent research that is taking place. The economics involved are complicated, but there is reason to believe that this argument is inaccurate.[31]

It perhaps says something about the commercial motivations of the pharmaceutical industry that the debates about standards of care can often—if not always—be reduced to calculations of profitability. But, as we have seen, it would be unreasonable to expect the pharmaceutical industry to stop behaving in accordance with these commercial motivations.

MIGRANT HEALTH WORKERS

The problem of global health inequities is largely one of affordability and resource allocation. Developing world governments usually do not have the fiscal resources to provide health care that is comparable to those countries, such as Canada or the UK, whose public health care systems are able to provide a high standard of health care for their citizens. Sometimes these governments might have the requisite resources, but they prioritize spending in other areas ahead of health care. A significant part of the problem is that developing countries do not have enough health care workers to be able to deliver the requisite services.

One of the biggest contributors to this situation is the widespread migration of health workers from developing countries to developed countries. This cannot be surprising given the economic factors at play. Even the United States does not train a sufficient number of nurses to cover its needs but relies on recruiting nurses from other parts of the world. Nurses, doctors, and other health professionals who train in the developing world frequently go on to spend the majority of their career working in developed countries. Less than one-fifth of the total number of doctors and nurses in the world work in developing countries, and one in five doctors who received their training in the developing world works in the developed world.[32]

The incentives for health care workers are clear: Developed countries promise an overall better standard of life for them and the family members who travel with them, and higher wages mean that they can send a proportion of their salary back home to support their wider family. Furthermore, a large proportion of health spending in the developed world focuses on the control of HIV/AIDS and other infectious diseases, so health care workers whose specialism is not infectious disease have a better chance of finding work overseas than at home. There are also economic advantages for the host countries: a stronger labor market characterized by skilled workers who will accept lower wages and whose training has been provided overseas. But when viewed in a global context, this situation is harmful: It exacerbates rather than addresses the disparities in global health.

One proposed solution to the problem of the migration of health care workers places an obligation on three distinct groups: recruiters and policymakers in the developed world, international medical aid organizations, and health care workers from the developing world themselves.[33] Each of these groups has voluntarily contributed to the problem and is therefore morally responsible for addressing it. The contribution of developed-world governments and policymakers lies both in their willingness to freeload by accepting cheap skilled labor from the developing world and by allowing shortages of health care professionals in their labor markets.

Responsible governments in the developed world should train enough health care professionals to populate their own health care systems, thus removing the need to source labor from the developing world. Arguably, developed world governments should compensate developing nations for the health care workers poached from them; for example, by supporting an educational infrastructure that produces an oversupply of health care workers. While some governments in the developed world recognize this moral responsibility and have taken steps to address it,[34] the problem remains.

The obligation of recruiters in the developing world lies in not contributing to the overall harmful consequences already caused by the migration of health care workers. Responsible recruitment policies would rule out proactively recruiting from countries with critically low numbers of health care professionals. Rather, recruitment should be limited to recruiting individuals only when there is a surfeit of professionals with comparable skills or specialties in their home countries.

To suggest that the health care workers themselves have an obligation not to migrate seems at first glance problematic: It places a moral restriction on their ability to pursue a better life for themselves and their families. However, perhaps migration should be allowed only after health care workers have spent a certain time working in their home countries, giving enough service to pay back the cost of their training. Such policies exist in some countries, such as South Africa, and are similar to those that operate in some European countries whose armed forces pay for the training of doctors in return for a period of military service when they qualify.

A sensible system of migration for health care workers would ensure that there was a net gain, at least in the short and medium terms, to the developing world. It would also incorporate a system of compensation, whereby the countries that benefit from migration provide financial or in-kind reparations to the developing countries that provide the workers. This might include exchange programs for students and early-career professionals, access to equipment, facilities, training, and scholarly resources, and a commitment to direct more research into those medical issues affecting the developing world.

CONCLUSION

This chapter has covered some of the most challenging issues in global health ethics. However, it should not be seen as exhaustive. Space constraints have forced us to omit some very important issues, such as transplant tourism and resource prioritization during global pandemics. We have shown that numerous injustices exist in global health care, and that they are characterized by a clear and consistent recurring division between the resource-poor developing world and the more affluent developed world.

These problems are not simply accidents of nature. They are to a large extent the product of the historical exploitation of developing countries that is reinforced by unfair current global economic policies. This is not to suggest that globalization has not also brought benefits to people living in the developed world. It seems clear, however, that whatever ethical analysis one wishes to avail themselves of, people in the resource-rich parts of the world—and this now includes large numbers of citizens in countries such as India and the People's Republic of China—have moral obligations to assist those in the developing world by providing health aid and, arguably, by restructuring global trade and financial arrangements.

NOTES

1. T. W. Pogge, *World Poverty and Human Rights*, 2nd ed. (Cambridge: Polity, 2008).

2. C. Mathers et al., "Global Patterns of Healthy Life Expectancy in the Year 2002," *BMC Public Health* 4 (66) (2004). doi:10.1186/1471-2458-4-66

3. G. J. Schreiber, P. Gottret, L. K. Fleisher, and A. A. Leive, "Financing Global Health: Mission Unaccomplished," *Health Affairs* 26 (4) (2007): 921–34. doi: 10.1377/hlthaff.26.4.921

4. "Haiti Capital Earthquake Death Toll 'Tops 150,000,'" *BBC News*, January 25, 2010, http://news.bbc.co.uk/2/hi/americas/8477770.stm.

5. P. Farmer, M. C. Smith Fawzi, and P. Nevil, "Unjust Embargo of Aid for Haiti," *The Lancet* 361 (9355) (2003): 420–23.

6. Udo Schüklenk and Christopher Lowry, "Two Models in Global Health Ethics," *Public Health Ethics* 2 (3) (2009): 276–84.

7. Pogge, *World Poverty and Human Rights*.

8. Schüklenk and Lowry, "Two Models in Global Health Ethics."

9. J. Narveson, "We Don't Owe Them a Thing! A Tough-Minded but Soft-Hearted View of Aid to the Faraway Needy," *The Monist* 86 (3) (2003): 419–33.

10. Office for National Statistics, *Interim Life Tables 2006–2008*, Specific statistics from *Big Variation in Life Expectancy*, 2009, http://news.bbc.co.uk/1/hi/health/8317986.stm.

11. P. Singer, *The Life You Can Save: How to Do Your Part to End World Poverty* (London: Picador, 2009), 8.

12. Schüklenk and Lowry, "Two Models in Global Health Ethics."

13. Singer, *The Life You Can Save*, chapter 10.

14. P. Collier, "A New Alms Race to Help the World's Poor," *Observer*, March 15, 2009, http://www.guardian.co.uk/books/2009/mar/15/poverty-life-save-peter-singer.

15. Singer, *The Life You Can Save*, chapter 7.

16. U. Schüklenk, M. Kottow, and P. A. Sy, "Developing World Challenges," in *A Companion to Bioethics*, edited by H. Kuhse and P. Singer, 404–16 (Oxford: Wiley-Blackwell, 2009).

17. G. Anand, "Drug Makers Decry Indian Patent Law," *Wall Street Journal*, February 11, 2010, http://online.wsj.com/article/SB10001424052748703455804575057621354459804.html?mod=WSJ_World_MIDDLENews.

18. UNAIDS, *AIDS Epidemic Update 2009*, Geneva: Joint United Nations Programme on HIV/AIDS (UNAIDS) and World Health Organisation, 2009, http://data.unaids.org/pub/Report/2009/JC1700_Epi_Update_2009_en.pdf.

19. P. Chigwerdre, G. R. Seage III, S. Gruskin, T.-H. Lee, and M. Essex, "Estimating the Lost Benefits of Antiretroviral Drug Use in South Africa," *Journal of Acquired Immune Deficiency Syndromes* 49 (4) (2008): 410–15.

20. U. Schüklenk, "Professional Responsibilities of Biomedical Scientists in Public Discourse," *Journal of Medical Ethics* 30 (2004): 53–60.

21. U. Schüklenk, "AIDS as a Global Health Emergency," In *A Companion to Bioethics*, edited by H. Kuhse and P. Singer, 441–54 (Chichester: Wiley-Blackwell, 2009).

22. UNAIDS, *AIDS Epidemic Update 2005*, Geneva: Joint United Nations Programme on HIV/AIDS (UNAIDS) and World Health Organisation, http://www.unaids.org/epi/2005/doc/EPIupdate2005_pdf_en/epi-update2005_en.pdf.

23. E. M. Connor, R. S. Sealing, and R. Gelber et al., "Reduction of Maternal Infant Transmission of Human Immunodeficiency Virus Type 1 with Zidovudine Treatment," *New England Journal of Medicine* 331 (1994): 1173–80.

24. U. Schüklenk, and A. Kleinsmidt, "Rethinking Mandatory HIV Testing During Pregnancy in High HIV-Prevalence Regions: Ethical and Policy Issues," *American Journal of Public Health* 97 (7) (2007): 1179–83.

25. P. Vernaza, B. Hirschel, E. Bernasconi, and M. Flepp, "Les personnes séropositives ne souffrant d'aucune autre MST et suivant un traitement antiretroviral efficace ne transmettent pas le VIH par voie sexuelle," *Bulletin des Médecins Suisse* 89 (5) (2008): 165–69.

26. R. M. Granich, C. F. Gilks, C. Dye, K. M. De Cock, and B. G. Williams, "Universal Voluntary HIV Testing with Immediate Antiretroviral Therapy as a Strategy for Elimination of HIV Transmission: A Mathematical Model," *Lancet* 373 (2009): 48–57.

27. P. Lurie, and S. M. Wolfe, "Unethical Trials of Interventions to Reduce Perinatal Transmission of the Human Immunodeficiency Virus in Developing Countries," *New England Journal of Medicine* 337 (12) (1997): 853–56.

28. U. Schüklenk, and R. Ashcroft, "International Research Ethics," *Bioethics* 14 (2) (2000): 158–72.

29. World Medical Association, "World Medical Association Declaration of Helsinki," 2008, http://www.wma.net/en/30publications/10policies/b3/17c.pdf.

30. U. Schüklenk, "The Standard of Care Debate: Against the Myth of an 'International Consensus Opinion,'" *Journal of Medical Ethics* 30 (2004): 194–97.

31. Schüklenk, "AIDS as a Global Health Emergency."

32. M. A. Clemens and G. Pettersson, "New Data on African Health Professionals Abroad," *Human Resources for Health* 6 (1) (2008). doi:10.1186/1478-4491-6-1. http://www.human-resources-health.com/content/pdf/1478-4491-6-1.pdf.

33. Schüklenk, Kottow, and Sy, "Developing World Challenges."

34. Department of Health, *Guidance on International Nursing Recruitment* (London: Department of Health, 1999), http://webarchive.nationalarchives.gov.uk/20130107105354/http://www.dh.gov.uk/prod_consum_dh/groups/dh_digitalassets/@dh/@en/documents/digitalasset/dh_4034794.pdf.

2

Global Health Justice

A Perspective from the Global South on a Framework Convention on Global Health*

Lawrence O. Gostin and Ames Dhai

ABSTRACT

This chapter searches for solutions to the most perplexing problems in global health—problems so important that they affect the fate of millions of people, with economic, political, and security ramifications for the world's population. No state, acting alone, can insulate itself from major health hazards. Health threats inexorably spread to neighboring countries, regions, and even continents. It is for this reason that safeguarding the world's population requires cooperation and global governance.

INTRODUCTION

If ameliorating the most common causes of disease, disability, and premature death require global solutions, then the future is demoralizing. The states that bear the disproportionate burden of disease have the least capacity to do anything about it. The states that have the wherewithal are deeply resistant to expending the political capital and economic resources. When rich countries do act, it is often more out of narrow self-interest or humanitarian instinct than a full sense of ethical or legal obligation. The result is a spiraling deterioration of health in the poorest regions, with manifest global consequences and systemic effects on trade, international relations, and security.

This chapter first inquires why global health is a shared responsibility—for the global South and North—and then reconcepualizes the global health enterprise. Second, we examine the compelling issue of global health equity, and ask whether it is fair that people in poor countries suffer such a disproportionate burden of illness and death. Here, we will briefly explore what we call a "theory of human functioning" to support a more robust understanding of the transcending value of health. Third, we describe how the international community focuses on a few high-profile, heartrending issues while largely ignoring deeper, systemic problems in global health. By focusing on "basic survival needs," the international community could fundamentally improve prospects for the world's population. Finally, we explore the value of international law itself, and propose an innovative mechanism for global health reform—a Framework Convention on Global Health (FCGH).

A global coalition of civil society and academics recently launched the Joint Action and Learning Initiative on National and Global Responsibilities for Health (JALI). Following international stakeholder meetings in Oslo, Berlin, Johannesburg, Delhi, and Bellagio, JALI is developing a post-Millennium Development Goal (MDG) framework for global health. JALI's goal is a Framework Convention on Global Health.

In March 2011, the UN General Secretary endorsed the FCGH, calling on the United Nations to adopt it. Moreover, the World Health Organization Director General, Margaret Chan, proposed a "framework" for global health as part of the major reform agenda of the WHO.

Our proposal for a Framework Convention, in a nutshell, is to establish fair terms of international cooperation, with agreed-upon, mutually binding obligations to create enduring health system capacities, meet basic survival needs, and reduce unconscionable inequalities in global health.

RECONCEPTUALIZING "HEALTH AID": FROM "AID" TO GLOBAL JUSTICE

Global health means different things to different people. Often it is used as shorthand for the aggregate of health assistance provided by the affluent to the poor in a donor-recipient relationship as a form of charity, together with the volume and the modalities of this assistance—a concept we will refer to as "health aid."

Framing the global health endeavor as "health aid" provided by the affluent to the poor is fundamentally flawed. This suggests that the world is divided between donors and countries in need. This is too simplistic. Collaboration among countries, both as neighbors and across continents, is also about responding to health risks together and building capacity collaboratively—whether it is through South-South partnerships, gaining access to essential vaccines and medicines, or demanding fair distribution of scarce, lifesaving technologies.

Likewise, the concept of "aid" both presupposes and imposes an inherently unequal relationship in which one side is a benefactor and the other a dependent. This leads affluent states and other donors to believe that they are giving "charity," which means that financial contributions and programs are largely at their discretion. It also means that donors make decisions about how much to give and for what health-related goods and services. The level of financial assistance, therefore, is not predictable, scalable to needs, or sustainable in the long term. These features of health aid could, in turn, mean that host countries might not accept full responsibility for their inhabitants' health, as they can blame the poor state of health on the shortcomings of aid rather than on their own failures.

Conceptualizing international assistance as "aid" masks the greater truth that human health is a globally shared responsibility reflecting common risks and vulnerabilities—an obligation of health justice that demands a fair contribution from everyone—North and South, rich and poor. Global governance for health must be seen as a partnership, with financial and technical assistance understood as an integral component of the common goal of improving global health and reducing health inequalities.

The framework of mutual responsibilities should prove attractive to both the global South and North, creating incentives to develop a far-reaching global health agreement. Southern countries would benefit from increased respect for their strategies; greater and more predictable funding from more coordinated and accountable development partners; reform of politics that harm health, such as those in trade and agriculture; and, most importantly, better health for their populations.

Countries of the North will benefit from increased confidence that development assistance is spent effectively and the prospect of reduced financing needs over time as host countries increase their health spending and build sustainable health systems. All will benefit from lessons on shared health challenges, from economic and educational gains that will come with improved global health, from increased protection from global public health threats—and from mutual goodwill derived from participating in an historic venture to make unprecedented progress toward global health equity.

ARE PROFOUND HEALTH INEQUALITIES FAIR?

Perhaps it does not, or should not, matter if global health serves the interests of the richest countries. After all, there are powerful humanitarian reasons to help the world's least healthy people. But even ethical arguments have failed to capture the full attention of political leaders and the public.

The global burden of disease is not just shouldered by the poor, but disproportionately so, such that health disparities across continents render a person's likelihood of survival drastically different based on where he or she is born. These inequalities have become so extreme and the resultant effects on the poor so dire that health disparities have become an issue no less important than global warming or the other defining problems of our time.

A decade into the twenty-first century, billions of people have yet to benefit from the health advances of the twentieth century. Average life expectancy in Africa is nearly thirty years less than in the Americas or Europe—only two years higher than in the United States a century ago, and twenty-seven years lower than in high-income countries today. Life expectancy in Sierra Leone or Zimbabwe is half that in Japan; a child born in Angola is sixty-five times more likely to die in the first few years of life than a child born in Norway; and a woman giving birth in Sub-Saharan Africa is one hundred times more likely to die in labor than a woman in a rich country.

The yawning health gap cannot be fully understood by using the oversimplified division of the world into the global rich (the North) and the global poor (the South). In fact, 20 percent of the largest fortunes in the world are in so-called poor countries. Even within countries, dramatic health differences exist that are closely linked with degrees of social disadvantage. The poorest people in Europe and North America often have life expectancies equal to those in the least developed countries.

As vividly enunciated by Vicente Navarro, "It is not the North versus the South, it is not globalization, it is not the scarcity of resources—it is the power differentials between and among classes in these countries and their influence over the state that are at the root of the poverty [and health] problem" (Navarro 2009).

ETHICAL UNDERPINNINGS FOR
GLOBAL HEALTH JUSTICE

Human instinct tells us that it is unjust for large populations to have such poor prospects for good health and long life simply by happenstance of where they live. Although almost everyone believes it is unfair that the poor live miserable and short lives, there is little consensus about whether there is an ethical, let alone legal, obligation to help the downtrodden. What do wealthier societies owe as a matter of *justice* to the poor in other parts of the world?

Perhaps the strongest claim that health disparities are unethical is based on what we call a theory of human functioning. Health has special meaning and importance to individuals and the community as a whole. Health is necessary for much of the joy, creativity, and productivity that a person derives from life. Individuals with physical and mental health recreate, socialize, work, and engage in family and social activities that bring meaning and happiness to their lives. Perhaps not as obvious, health also is essential for the functioning of populations. Without minimum levels of health, people cannot fully engage in social interactions, participate in the political process, exercise rights of citizenship, generate wealth, create art, and provide for the common security.

Amartya Sen famously theorized that the capability to avoid starvation, preventable morbidity, and early mortality is a substantive freedom that enriches human life. Depriving people of this capability strips them of their freedom to be who they want to be and "to do things that a person has reason to value." Other ethicists have expanded on this theory, claiming that health, specifically, is important to the ability to live a life one values—one cannot function when one is barely alive. Under a theory of human functioning, health deprivations are unethical because they unnecessarily reduce one's ability to function and the capacity for human agency. Health, among all the other forms of disadvantage, is special and foundational, in that its effects on human capacities impact one's opportunities in the world and, therefore, health must be preserved to ensure equality of opportunity.

But Sen's theory does not answer the harder question about who has the corresponding obligation to do something about global inequalities. Even liberal egalitarians who believe in just distribution, such as Nagel, Rawls, and Walzer, frame their claims narrowly and rarely extend them to international obligations of justice. Their theories of justice are "relational" and apply to a fundamental social structure that people share. States may owe their citizens basic health protection by reason of a social compact. But positing such a relationship among different countries and regions is much more difficult.

BASIC SURVIVAL NEEDS: AMELIORATING SUFFERING AND EARLY DEATH

Most development assistance is driven by high-profile events that evoke public sympathy, such as a natural disaster in the form of a hurricane, tsunami, drought, or famine; or an enduring catastrophe such as AIDS; or politicians may lurch from one frightening disease to the next, irrespective of the level of risk, ranging from anthrax and smallpox to SARS, novel influenza strains (H5N1 and H1N1), and bioterrorism.

What is truly needed, and what richer countries instinctively (although not always adequately) do for their own citizens, is to meet what we call "basic survival needs." By focusing on the major determinants of health, the international community could dramatically improve prospects for good health. Basic survival needs include sanitation and sewage, pest control, clean air and water, tobacco reduction, diet and nutrition, essential medicines and vaccines, and well-functioning health systems.

Meeting everyday survival needs may lack the glamour of high-technology medicine or dramatic rescue, but what they lack in excitement they gain in their potential impact on health, precisely because they deal with the major causes of common disease and disabilities across the globe. Mobilizing the public and private sectors to meet basic survival needs could radically transform prospects for good health among the world's poorest populations.

Meeting basic survival needs can be disarmingly simple and inexpensive, if only it could rise on the agendas of the world's most powerful countries. It does not take advanced biomedical research, huge financial investments, or complex programs. Consequently, what poor countries need is not foreign aid workers parachuting in to rescue them. Nor do they need foreign-run state-of-the-art facilities. Rather, they need to gain the capacity to provide basic health services themselves.

GLOBAL GOVERNANCE FOR HEALTH: A PROPOSAL FOR A FRAMEWORK CONVENTION ON GLOBAL HEALTH

If law is to play a constructive role, innovative models are essential, and here we make the case for a Framework Convention on Global Health. We are proposing a global governance-for-health scheme incorporating a bottom-up strategy that strives to:

- build health system capacity
- set priorities to meet basic survival needs
- engage stakeholders to bring to bear their resources and expertise
- harmonize the activities among the proliferating number of actors operating around the world
- evaluate and monitor progress so that goals are met and promises kept

The framework convention approach is becoming an essential strategy of powerful transnational social movements to safeguard health and the environment. A series of international environmental treaties serve as models for global health governance, culminating in the 1997 Kyoto Protocol to the UN Framework Convention on Climate Change. Although the United States failed to ratify, and highly polluting transitional states such as China and India are largely exempt, the Kyoto Protocol represents a nascent attempt at global cooperative governance to reduce global climate change. But even this approach can be painstakingly difficult, as the stalled climate change negotiations make clear.

The Framework Convention on Tobacco Control, one of only two treaties negotiated under the WHO's constitutional authority, was modeled on environmental framework conventions, notably the UNFCCC. It, too, has inventive governance approaches to tobacco control that include: *demand reduction*—price and tax measures, as well as nonprice measures; *supply reduction*—control of illicit trade and sales to minors, as well as creation of economically viable alternatives to tobacco production; and, most controversially, *tort litigation*—international cooperation on tort actions and criminal prosecutions, such as information exchange and legal assistance.

THE KEY MODALITIES OF AN FCGH

An FCGH would represent a historical shift in global health, with a broadly imagined global governance regime. The initial framework would establish the key modalities, with a strategy for subsequent protocols on each of the most important governance parameters. It is not necessary, or perhaps even wise, to specify in detail the substance of an initial FCGH, but it may be helpful to state the broad principles:

- FCGH mission—convention parties seek innovative solutions for the most pressing health problems facing the world in partnership with non-state actors and civil society, with particular emphasis on the most disadvantaged populations.
- FCGH objectives—establish fair terms of international cooperation, with agreed-upon, mutually binding obligations to create enduring health system capacities, meet basic survival needs, and reduce global health disparities.
- Engagement and coordination—finding common purposes and process among a wide variety of state and non-state actors, setting priorities, and coordinating activities to achieve the mission of the FCGH.
- State party and other stakeholder obligations—incentives, forms of assistance (e.g., financial aid, debt relief, technical support, subsidies, taxation, tradeable credits), and levels of assistance, with differentiated responsibility for developed, developing, and least developed countries.
- Institutional structures—conference of parties, secretariat, technical advisory body, and a financing mechanism, with integral involvement of non-state actors and civil society.
- Empirical monitoring—data gathering, benchmarks, and leading health indicators, such as maternal, infant, and child survival.
- Enforcement mechanisms—inducements, sanctions, mediation, and dispute resolution.
- Ongoing scientific analysis—processes for ongoing scientific research and evaluation on cost-effective health interventions, such as the creation of an Intergovernmental Panel on Global Health, comprised of prominent medical and public health experts.
- Guidance for subsequent lawmaking process—content, methods, and timetables to meet framework convention goals.

STRENGTHS OF THE FRAMEWORK CONVENTION PROTOCOL APPROACH

Facilitating global consensus. The framework convention protocol approach can galvanize a global consensus as states and stakeholders negotiate the treaty. The incremental nature of the governance strategy allows the international community to focus on a problem in a stepwise manner, avoiding potential political bottlenecks over contentious elements.

Facilitating a shared humanitarian instinct. The creation of international norms and institutions provides an ongoing and structured forum for states and stakeholders to develop a shared humanitarian instinct on global health. A high-profile forum for normative discussion can help educate and persuade parties, and influence public opinion, in favor of decisive action. And it can create internal pressure for governments and others to actively participate in the framework dialogue. The imperatives of global health have to be framed not just as a series of isolated problems in far-off places but as a common concern of humankind.

Building factual and scientific consensus. The framework convention protocol approach can be used to build international consensus about the essential facts of global health, such as the causes of extremely poor health and stark disparities, as well as the most cost-effective solutions. The FCTC process, for example, facilitated discussion about the harm of tobacco and the role of the industry, which was vital to the treaty's adoption.

Transcending shifts in political will. An ongoing diplomatic forum can also help to transcend the inevitable ebbs and flows of interest in international cooperation around global health. As political environments change, governments can become more or less interested in creating new international obligations, or complying with existing obligations. One of the strengths of an FCGH is that it can serve as a lasting entity that is resistant to temporary shifts in political will.

Engaging multiple actors and stakeholders. The really interesting and vital aspect of an FCGH is not merely how it governs interstate responsibilities. The critical challenge is how to make it do the really hard work of mobilizing the diverse drivers of health, including NGOs, private industry, foundations, public/private hybrids, researchers, and the media. It is essential to harness the ingenuity and resources of these non-state actors. The FCGH, therefore, should actively engage major stakeholders in the process of negotiation, debate, and information exchange.

An FCGH offers an intriguing approach, but it faces enormous social, political, and economic barriers. But given the dismal nature of extant global health governance, an FCGH is a risk worth taking. It will, at a minimum, identify the truly important problems in global health. Solutions will not be found solely in increased resources, although that is important. Rather, an FCGH can demonstrate the imperative of targeting the major determinants of health, prioritizing and coordinating currently fragmented activities, and engaging a broad range of stakeholders. It will also provide a needed forum to raise visibility of one of the most pressing problems facing humankind. An FCGH would represent a historical shift in global health, with a broadly imagined global governance regime.

A TIPPING POINT

We have sought to demonstrate why politically and economically powerful countries should care about the world's least healthy people. Although no single argument may be definitive in itself, the cumulative weight of the evidence is now overwhelmingly persuasive. Perhaps we are coming to a tipping point in which the status quo is no longer acceptable and it is time to take bold action. Global health, like global climate change, may soon become a matter so important to the world's future that it demands international attention, and no state can escape the responsibility to act.

If that were the case, states would need an innovative international mechanism to bind themselves, and others, to take an effective course of action. Amelioration of the enduring and complex problems of global health is virtually impossible without a collective response. If all states and stakeholders voluntarily accepted fair terms of cooperation, then it could dramatically improve life prospects for millions of people. But it would do more than that. Cooperative action for global health, like global warming, benefits everyone by diminishing our collective vulnerabilities.

The alternative to fair terms of cooperation is that everyone would be worse off, particularly those who suffer compounding disadvantages. Even if the economically and politically powerful escaped major health hazards, they would still have to avert their eyes from the mounting suffering among the poor. And they would have to live with their consciences knowing that much of this physical and mental anguish is preventable.

What is most important is that if the global community does not accept fair terms of cooperation on global health soon, there is every reason to believe that affluent states, philanthropists, and celebrities simply will move on to another cause. And when they do, the vicious cycle of poverty and endemic disease among the world's least healthy people will continue unabated. That is a consequence that none of us should be willing to tolerate.

REFERENCES

Arias, E. 2010. "United States Life Tables 2006." *National Vital Statistics Reports* 58 (21): 140. http://www.cdc.gov/nchs/data/nvsr/nvsr58/nvsr58_21.pdf.

Daniels, N. 2001. "Justice, Health, and Healthcare." *American Journal of Bioethics* 1 (2): 1526–61.

Gostin, L. O. 2008. "Meeting Basic Survival Needs of the World's Least Healthy People: Toward a Framework Convention on Global Health." *Georgetown Law Journal* 96:331–92. http://ssrn.com/ abstract=1014082.

———. 2010a. "The Unconscionable Health Gap: A Global Plan for Justice." *Lancet* 375:1504–5. http://ssrn.com/abstract=1635902.

———. 2010b. "Redressing the Unconscionable Health Gap: A Global Plan for Justice. *Harvard Law & Policy Review* 4:271–94. http://ssrn.com/ab stract=1635895.

Gostin, L. O., E. A. Friedman, and G. Ooms et al. 2011. "The Joint Action and Learning Initiative: Towards a Global Agreement on National and Global Responsibilities for Health." *PLoS Medicine* 8 (5): e100–31.

Navarro, V. 2009. "What We Mean by Social Determinants of Health." *International Journal of Health Services* 39 (3): 423–41, at 430.

Sen, A. 1999. *Development as Freedom*. Oxford: Oxford University Press, 1999.

UN Secretary General. 2011. "Uniting for Universal Access: Towards Zero New HIV Infections, Zero Discrimination and Zero AIDS-Related Deaths: Report of the Secretary General." UN Doc A/65/979 (March 2011), at para. 73. http://reliefweb.int/report/world/uniting-universal-access-towards-zero-new-hiv-infections-zero-discrimination-and-zero.

UNICEF. 2007. "The State of the World's Children 2007." http://www.unicef.org/sowc07/.

———. 2008. "Progress for Children: A Report Card on Maternal Mortality 2008." http://www.childinfo.org/files/progress_for_children_maternalmortality.pdf.

World Health Organization. 2009. World Health Statistics (2009) (reporting that average life expectancy at birth in Africa is fifty-two years compared with seventy-six years in the Americas. The gap between rich and poor is still higher when measured by the number of years of healthy life (i.e., life without significant illness or disability). http://www.who.int/ whosis/whostat/EN_WHS09_Table1.pdf.

————. 2011. "Reform for a Healthy Future: An Overview, 20 July 2011 (Proposing a Charter or Framework for Global Health Governance as a Key Output)." WHO Reforms for a Healthy Future: Report by the Director General, EBSS/2/2, 15 October 2011 (proposing a framework, code, or charter to guide all global health stakeholders, with agreed targets and indicators or rights and responsibilities). http://apps.who.int/gb/ebwha/pdf_files/EBSS/ EBSS2_2-en.pdf.

* Printed with permission of the authors. Previously published in *South African Journal for Bioethics and Law* 5 (1) (June 2012) and Creative Commons. An expanded version of this paper was published in the *Georgetown Law Journal* in 2008.

3

A Virtuous Reading of Health Equity under the Affordable Care Act

Peter Tan

ABSTRACT

Health equity stands as one of the most contentious issues, raising questions about how best to access health resources and who should bear the cost. The United States has historically been of two minds: one approach stressed the inherent equality present in a universally accessible system of health care, the other the freedom from governmental overreach by developing insurance based on the free market. Instead of favoring one over the other, the Affordable Care Act (ACA) has chosen a hybrid route that features elements of both in order to maximize access to health. This balanced development of the ACA suggests a virtue ethics formulation, where health equity itself becomes the excellence in question. But this virtuous approach can also be used to critique the ACA itself. This is not a universal single payer system, so health care will not be accessible to all—a strike against both the mandate of health equity and the eudaimonism of virtue ethics. This makes the ACA vulnerable to the performative inconsistency of not living up to its own standard of excellence. But since the virtues are unique to societies, they must be seen in the context of that society's values. If health care is to be universal, social policies will have to reflect that value.

INTRODUCTION

With the passage of H.R. 3590, the Patient Protection and Affordable Care Act of 2010, better known as "Obamacare" but henceforth known as the Affordable Care Act (ACA), the United States came closer to solving the century-old challenge of how to provide better health care to more people at a lower cost. It was framed in the language of health equity and spurred by economic necessity. Since its enactment, more recent statistics indicate a greater need on both fronts: as of 2012, 20 percent of all Americans above sixty-five are uninsured,[1] and by 2020, health care costs are estimated to rise to 20 percent of the gross domestic product (GDP).[2]

The result of this lack of access and expense is that Americans' life expectancy is twenty-fourth among thirty members of the Organization for Economic Co-operation and Development (OECD) countries.[3] While it is too early to assess its outcomes, it is possible to do the next best thing, which is to assess what the ACA is itself. What exactly is included in it? What is it meant to reform, and how does it plan on such reform? How is it justified? Is it a form of universal health care? Why has it been so misunderstood? I will argue that while falling short of its goal of health equity, the ACA is the best health insurance system America can realistically expect at the moment.

This chapter is a critical analysis of the ACA by way of its historical development and its projected goals. It is not a critique based on outcomes, but on how the ACA has been *structured* to address the biggest obstacles to health care in America. I will base my analysis on virtue ethics. From its historical antecedents to its present development, the entire arc of the ACA has been informed by an appeal to the national character of the United States. The question of who we want to be as a nation is at the heart of the type of health care that we have.

HEALTH EQUITY

The debate surrounding a national health plan has centered on access, but whereas it originally began with an appeal to a governmental duty to offer compulsory health care, the emphasis now has shifted toward human rights. This approach analyzes how best to guarantee the average person's right to access health care, which has been formalized by the concept of health equity. Not coincidentally, the immediate precursor to the ACA was formally known as the Health Equity and Access Reform Today Act of 1993.

"Health equity" is simple by definition and yet surprisingly difficult to fully comprehend. This is due to its intentional vagueness. "Health" refers not just to a lack of disease, but more holistically as the general well-being of any given individual; "equity" is the impartial and fair distribution of goods.

In 1985, the World Health Organization (WHO) defined it as an *ideal* where "everyone should have a fair opportunity to attain their full health potential and, more pragmatically, that no one should be disadvantaged from achieving this potential if it can be avoided."[4] When WHO revisited the question fifteen years later, it referred to health equity as a type of transparency of access to the health system, free from the "differences, which are unnecessary and avoidable but, in addition, are also considered unfair and unjust."[5] Health equity is thus linked to a type of social justice rooted in the tradition of distributive justice. It has also left it open to a great deal of interpretation.

Because of its open-endedness, health equity is often better understood as a negative concept. Braveman and Gruskin (2003) refer to it as "the absence of systematic disparities in health (or in the major social determinants of health) between groups with different levels of underlying social advantage/disadvantage." Importantly, "health disparity" does not refer to just any difference in health: It is a specific type of difference wherein certain social groups experience persistent discrimination of disadvantage. This, too, is vague. When do disparities become systematic? What counts as persistent? Who and what determine these levels of advantage/disadvantage? These are not easily parsed out and agreed upon.

But health equity defined as such is not meant to offer guidance on such a granular level. It is above all a normative value—it is not a direct quantity. There is a value in being able to access health care. And like any value *that* there should be equal access to such care is not by itself measureable, although the attainment of that value by the general public *can* be empirically derived from real-world data. To put it another way, the need for access to health care is a qualitative claim, but whether that goal has been achieved is subject to quantitative analysis. Disparities in health can be culled from hospital or civic or NGO records; social advantage/disadvantage can be measured by geography, age, proximity to disease vectors, income levels, population density, and more.

This is why health equity is not health *equality*. "Equality" refers to a quantifiable relationship between things, and not all health inequalities reflect health inequities. Heart disease is more prevalent in men than women; there are in all probability more incidents of frostbite in Alaska than Hawaii, and so on. Those are all unequal distributions of health concerns. But they do not reflect an inequity.

It should also be emphasized that health equity refers to access to health care, not to health insurance. Even if someone does have health insurance, because of deductibles or lack of resources, health care may still be unaffordable or unavailable. Indeed, that is one of the inequities the ACA seeks to reverse.

Health equity is thus achieved by eliminating health inequities until access to health care is assured. The wording used by WHO makes it an ongoing project. Thus the purpose of health equity is to act as the ACA's regulative ideal, a telos that can guide social projects to realize the ultimate aim of adequate and fair access to health care. Without it, a health care system would not know what to measure and for what purpose.

HISTORY OF THE ACA

A full understanding of the ACA requires an appreciation of the century-old debate regarding how best to let the public access health services. There are two major approaches to achieving this end. First is to make it the responsibility of the federal government to offer such health care. This is the universal health care approach, also known as compulsory health insurance. The second approach is to limit the role of the federal government in favor of private and voluntary programs.

These competing versions of health care access are the poles that have defined the issue. The early twentieth-century Progressivist advocates of universal health care modeled their program after Germany's successful 1883 compulsory sickness insurance as an attempt to improve the living conditions of workers. Backed by labor and initially by the AMA, momentum for it had grown to the point that its passage in 1916 seemed but a formality. "At present the United States has the unenviable distinction of being the only great industrial nation without compulsory health insurance," claimed social campaigner Irving Fisher (1917). "Within another six months, it will be a burning question."[6] Efforts to achieve true universal health coverage has since then been frustrated, but its prospect has propelled the health care debate in America—and not just from Democrats.

Economists have cited America's private insurance model as cumbersome and inefficient, an increasing burden on (rather than a danger to) free enterprise,[7] with significantly poorer health outcomes compared to universal systems (Sood et al. 2007). It has also been a bipartisan goal. Indeed, presidents Roosevelt (both Theodore and Franklin), Truman, Johnson, Nixon, and Clinton all called for universal health coverage during their administrations. The closest America has come to universal health coverage is with the Medicare and Medicaid program of 1965.

Like many other universal plans, they operate on a single-payer system of health care access.[8] But unlike a true universal plan that insures every citizen, they are available only to the elderly, the poor, and those with certain disabilities. In 1997 under the Children's Health Insurance Program (CHIP), the U.S. government also included children of families with incomes too high for Medicaid but too low to afford private insurance.

The opponents of compulsory health care amply spell out the limitations on the role of government in health care. Traditionally made up of private enterprise and those suspicious of governmental overreach, this second approach to health equity is based on how Americans accessed health throughout the nineteenth century. This depended on either out-of-pocket fee-for-service health spending, or private insurance firms for coverage, which is seen as a health care system that best served American individualism. In a rebuttal to the nationalized health care plan floated by Democrats in 1915, the vice president of Prudential Insurance, Dr. Frederick Hoffman (1917), claimed that "the propaganda for compulsory health insurance . . . represents rather the plans and purposes of the international socialist movement than the aims and ideals of the overwhelming majority of American wage-earners."

In the midst of World War 1, universal health care was derided as "the Prussian menace,"[9] and after the Russian Revolution in 1917, it was aligned with socialism and communism. Universal health care has since then had to address the false specter of anti-Americanism. By 1919, the AMA reversed itself and warned of the Bolshevism of compulsory health care such that, in 1932, the editor of the *Journal of the American Medical Association* opined outright that the issue of universal health care hinged on the "question of Americanism versus Sovietism for the American people."

The question of how the majority of Americans would access health was thus answered by holding to the status quo of employer-based benefits and private insurance companies.[10] And yet the history of health care in the United States is marked by a steady move toward the universalization of health services. The main driver of better access to health was the rapid rise in health care costs as treatment, medicine, and antibiotics increased life spans, and with that, medical expenses. In 1900, the average life expectancy was forty-seven years,[11] and "the cost of health care treatment was considered a minor problem compared to the loss of wages due to sickness for most workers."[12]

By 1960 life expectancy was sixty-seven years, and spending on health was 5.2 percent of GDP; by 2010, those numbers were seventy-nine years and 17.9 percent,[13] or twice the average percentage of OECD countries.[14] Saddled with an increasingly inefficient health care delivery system, private insurance companies and businesses faced economic pressure to find creative ways to insure the workforce. This led to prepaid medical plans such as Blue Cross in 1929, and the precursors to HMOs such as Kaiser Permanente in 1938.

The dependence on private insurance makes it easy to forget that, despite the rejection of any government-based universal health care, the government was in fact responsible for creating the conditions that made those advances in private insurance possible. This was done by giving tax credits to individuals receiving and companies offering insurance as part of employment benefits. In 2006, Massachusetts introduced a further refinement of the private insurance model, albeit on the state level. In order to broaden the risk pool and make health care affordable to more people, the state mandated that individuals had to purchase health insurance. A state-run exchange was then created to help people compare and purchase privately run health insurance.

This blend of mandated coverage using private insurance means—a key element in the ACA—was first proposed in 1989 by the conservative Heritage Foundation as a way to address health equity using market-based solutions instead of a single-payer universal health plan advocated by the Clinton administration (Butler 1989). The ACA added to the Heritage plan a requirement for insurance companies to accept new subscribers regardless of past medical history. This was done in order to subscribe even more people, ensuring the broadest possible risk pool.

The health care debate in America has been informed by polar opposite approaches to health care. And, as it turns out, a good way to understand the structure of the ACA is to see it as a finalized product of this hybrid health care system. It is at once universal in scope but uses private insurance markets to realize its claim. It is best understood as a response to make as much of universal health care a possibility given the limitations of American culture and politics—or, what amounts to the same thing viewed from the other side, to make the traditional private insurance market as efficient as possible by making health insurance universally compulsory.

ELEMENTS OF THE ACA

The health care reforms set out by the ACA are widespread and far-reaching. It is worth pointing out that its reforms will not directly affect how the majority of Americans access health care. As of 2010, a full 55 percent of Americans are covered under employer-based health plans (U.S. Census 2010). The ACA does not address current employee-based insurance benefits. It is meant to address the other 45 percent, thereby broadening the risk pool and making health care access more affordable.

The result is a 906-page document that contains ten titles necessary for reform.[15] The general approach of the ACA is to unify the two historical approaches to accessing health care in order to create a hybrid that achieves health equity better than the separate approaches working on their own. Separateness definitely increased inequity. Working apart, they shared the overlapping end of issuing access to health care, assuring inefficiencies in cost. Moreover, on their own, both government programs and private insurance faced fundamental problems.

For government-issued care, the problem was that, despite being single payer and therefore having the hallmark of a universal health plan, it was not universal. Indeed, it was meant to cover only those who qualified according to age, economic status, or disability. And yet both Medicare and Medicaid have controlled costs and per-enrollee spending growth better than private insurance has (Holohan and McMorrow 2012). This means that the most efficient way to distribute health care is also the one that by design limited who was covered.

The problem for private insurance is even more vexing. People who need health insurance the most are often those who are most expensive to insure, while healthy people who are inexpensive to insure oftentimes forego insurance because they have not had health complications that needed insurance. Private insurance thus faced the prospect of an ever-shrinking risk pool made up of high-risk subscribers.[16] Part of the reason for the rapidly escalating cost of health insurance was not just because of the increased dependence on technologies or biomedical research or even the layers of bureaucracy; it was systemic to the very model of private insurance itself.

The ACA's hybrid approach seeks to address these inherent shortcomings by combining the strengths of both to counter the inefficiencies of any one. In general the strategy is to expand and protect government-sponsored insurance plans and to make private programs gain federal oversight but also coordination.

On the public side, Medicaid and CHIP would be extended and preserved, and closing coverage gaps for medication would protect Medicare. Medicare spending will be cut to Medicare Advantage plans that are administered through private insurance companies. Medicaid would be expanded for subscribers with incomes at 133 percent of the poverty level, although in 2012, the Supreme Court struck down the mandatory expansion of Medicaid and left it to individual states to decide whether to expand their Medicaid rolls.

Much more is done to bolster the private side. Not only are tax credits and subsidies given to make insurance more affordable, but also the government now mandates individuals to either be insured or face penalties. This essentially gives private insurance companies greater business opportunity by opening competition for market share. Protections have been put in place to stop the practice of medical underwriting or denying coverage according to preexisting medical conditions. The net effect of the ACA is to broaden the risk pool and bring economies of scale into health care that would offset its cost. Over the next ten years, the ACA is expected to save slightly more than its $1.17 trillion in cost (U.S. Congressional Budget Office 2013).

There are other mechanisms that address health equity. The ACA has provisions to increase the health care workforce; it trims long-term costs by focusing on the prevention and reduction of preventable disease and the promotion of well-being; and it addresses long-term health care services if disability does strike. The ACA creates pathways for generic versions of medicine, and an entire section is devoted to the modernization of the Indian health care system. Considered separately, these different titles of the ACA make it seem scattershot and unfocused. But taken as a whole, they anticipate what health care services must look like if the public and private sectors are united.

THE VIRTUE OF THE ACA

The ACA is unique in that nowhere else does the concept of health equity create so much national angst because nowhere else is the question of equal access to health care answered by two very different appeals to national character. Is the United States founded on justice (which argues for the primacy of equal access with a compulsory system)? Or is it the land of the free (which argues for an individual's trust in the free market)?

Descriptively, how the ACA chooses to answer this question, with its hybrid public-private system of health coverage, is by compromise. This suggests that the best way to critique the ACA is by first analyzing how closely its development mirrors a robust virtue ethics. It can in fact be seen as one of the most public applications of virtue ethics.

This virtuous structure can be difficult to grasp because it does not come naturally to those of us who conceive of public projects in terms of obligations and rights. Contemporary virtue theory repudiates what Anscombe (1958) calls the "law conception of ethics," where every issue can be resolved by relying on universally applicable principles.

Current virtue ethicists, while differing in detail and emphases, make variations on the same claim: Enlightenment moral theory has bequeathed a totalizing ethical landscape where, on the one hand, there is the universally derived duty or rule, and, on the other, there is irrational moral action. Moral excellence is determined by how closely those obligations (deontologically or consequentially derived) are observed. Moral vice occurs when those obligations have been violated. This familiar ethical schema—it is, after all, the system behind academic grades and performance/satisfaction ratings—understands excellence vertically. That which adheres closer to ethical rationality is ranked higher, so on the top there is excellence and on the bottom vice.

The way the ACA has been created to address health equity suggests a different understanding of the relationship between excellence and vice. The model of compromise means that the excellent decision is that which finds common ground between seemingly disparate approaches. This is at heart a very Aristotelian approach. When, in Book 2 of the *Nicomachean Ethics*, Aristotle defines virtue (excellence) as the balance between two extremes, he is anticipating the structure of how the ACA has been formed.

To Aristotle, the virtue of courage lies between the vices of cowardice and arrogance. To the question of health care, the ACA's approach lies between the negative vice of private health insurance models that cover fewer people at rapidly escalating rates and the positive vice of covering everyone at the expense of respect for individual choice. With the moral focus shifted from rational absolutism to the balanced life, the hybrid that looked like mere compromise is now actually an excellence.

Excellence according to virtue theory has no opposite. There is no other side to a point in the middle. Additionally, what is excellent is not defined by what the vice is not. That is true only for deontological or consequentialist ethics. Virtue is what happens when both vices, positive and negative, are operative *at the same time*. Virtue is not virtue *without* its vices. Aristotle's courageous person must know fear but must be willing to act rashly despite this knowledge. Analogously, the ACA's hybrid approach requires respect for individual preferences while allowing as much universal access to health services that such respect would allow.

Recasting the ACA as a virtue supplants the modern insistence of pitting the duties of the government against the liberty rights of individuals. Left to modern modes of ethical debate, that conversation has gone nowhere. The ACA's complex interweaving of public and private is more than a rationalized concept calculated to bring universalizable assent: character is not obligation, and virtue is not a right. Taken together, they are something far deeper. It represents a way of being that defines who we are as a nation. The argument here isn't just that the ACA is the right thing to do—it is the right thing to do because overcoming health inequity is the right way to be.

The defense of the ACA's virtue is thus informed entirely by the telos of health equity. In the context of health care, it is the goal of equal access to health services that justifies the ACA. It helps realize the full potential of the nation, assures its well-being, and allows for the further flourishing of its citizens.

The descriptive parallels between the development of the ACA and virtue theory are hard to ignore. But this relationship has another side; namely, how virtue theory can be used to critically assess the ACA itself. Given that health equity has been identified as that which justifies its virtue, how well does the ACA address health inequalities? This is problematic for the ACA. By design it does not give true universal access to health care, even though the public parts of it operate on a single-payer model. And while it is set to extend health care coverage to twenty-six million people, it will also leave thirty million uninsured.[17] By 2019, the ACA is estimated to cover 93 percent of the population,[18] a number significantly greater than the 83 percent if the ACA were not enacted, but it is still not by any means universal.

The ACA thus seems to be guilty of not being truly excellent by its own ethical justification. There is still unequal access to health care services, which goes against the mandate of health equity and the eudaimonism of virtue ethics. The ACA is, in other words, vulnerable to the performative inconsistency of practicing the excellence that it has identified. What does this mean for the ACA's virtue?

One way to address this issue is by using some contemporary developments in virtue theory. Slote's (1992) agent-based formulation argues that actions (or in this case laws) are ethical according to the virtuous intent of the agent, which in this case is the ACA. This is distinguished from the Aristotelian agent-focused formulation, where virtue is measured by the virtuous inner dispositions of any one agent. Indeed, because the agent is here not a single person but a law, it is difficult to know just how to apply an agent-focused approach. While a law's intent can be discerned, nothing can be said about its inner disposition inasmuch as a law cannot be said to even have one. Given this, that the ACA's intent is to decrease health inequalities, is enough to count the ACA as virtuous in its approach.

There is, however, an even deeper problem. At the same time that the ACA is descriptively applying a virtuous ethical framework to health care, its deliberation exposes the reservations many have with virtue theory. The lack of a universal virtue is more than theoretically problematic—it introduces a procedural difficulty that frustrates attempts to establish real-world standards that span cultural values. Excellence is relative to what has been determined to be vices, and so, while virtue theory is particularly adept at determining an excellence given a set of extreme positions, absent those vices the theory is often silent as to what is actually an excellence *qua* excellence. Excellence is, in other words, relative not just to culture, but also to the procedural structure of virtue theory itself.

In the case of the ACA, health equity has been identified as the telos that should guide any attempt to deliver health care services. Statistically and comparatively speaking, however, health equity is best realized with some true form of universal health coverage (Davis, Schoen, and Stremikis 2010). But the ACA cannot argue for such type of coverage, because universal health insurance has already been identified as a vice—which is to say, an extreme. There is no way for virtue theory to claim it as a point of balance.

Measured with health equity in mind, it is clear that, while health inequities will decrease with the ACA, there still will be health inequity. Agent-based theories may claim that the intent is enough to make it virtuous, but the practical effect is hard to ignore. The ACA will not cover tens of millions of people, and if that counts as excellence, then it is an excellence only in reference to America's particular culture. Simply put, the ACA is the best that America can do at this particular time. But it isn't the best that can be done, and what *is* best can't be done because the ACA has been defined by cultural parameters not of its making.

CONCLUDING REMARKS: THE ACA AS AMERICA'S MORALITY PLAY

In this sense the ACA is the leading edge of a proxy war between competing cultural values that America has been fighting for over a century. Caught in between progressive campaigns for universal health coverage through compulsory insurance and conservative rebuttals that feared the loss of liberty through expanded government programs, the development and purpose of the ACA is reminiscent of a morality play acted on a national level. The ACA's deft negotiation between cultural extremes creates a unique health insurance scheme that realizes the goal of health equity using America's peculiar political and cultural capital.

The challenge of the ACA is to not just respond to values beyond its control but to actually form social values based on health equity. This is more difficult than may appear: Virtue theory's character-driven ethics demands that these newly created values exist, not just on the level of abstract rights or duties or social utilities, but on the deeper level of dispositions. The ACA may now be law, but for it to be truly effective, it has to become a habit.

This is where the other deeply held character trait of rendering issues in economic terms can actually help in the United States. The reason to adopt the ACA was primarily an economic argument. No country can be globally competitive when spending a fifth of its GDP on health-related cost. Competing countries offer better coverage with better outcomes for less than half the per-enrollee cost, and no nation can afford to lose a workforce because of uninsured health issues. As such, the ACA is essentially an economic argument that happens to be more humane than what came before it. What is needed is a humanitarian argument to make more economic sense than the ACA. For that to happen, what we value as a nation first needs to change. There is, of course, a virtuous argument for doing so.

NOTES

1. Congressional Budget Office, July 2012, http://www.cbo.gov/sites/default/files/cbofiles/attachments/43472-07-24-2012-CoverageEstimates.pdf.

2. Centers for Medicare and Medicaid Services, http://www.cms.gov/Research-Statistics-Data-and-Systems/Statistics-Trends-and-Reports/NationalHealthExpendData/NationalHealthAccountsProjected.html.

3. OECD 2010, "Health Care Systems: Getting More Value for Money," OECD Economics Department Policy Notes, No. 2.

4. World Health Organization, http://www.who.int/hia/about/glos/en/index.html.

5. Margaret Whitehead, "The Concepts and Principles of Equity in Health," *World Health Organization Regional Office for Europe*, Copenhagen, 2000, 5, http://salud.ciee.flacso.org.ar/flacso/optativas/equity_and_health.pdf.

6. Irving Fisher, "The Need for Health Insurance," *New York State Journal of Medicine* 17 (1917): 81.

7. Neeraj Sood, Arkadipta Ghosh, and Jose Escarse, "Final Report: The Effect of Health Care Cost Growth on the U.S. Economy," http://aspe.hhs.gov/health/reports/08/healthcarecost/report.html.

8. The single-payer system features the government serving as the administrator to collect all insurance fees, which are used to directly pay private medical institutions for services. It is not socialized medicine. It is socialized insurance. This is the system used by Taiwan, Denmark, and Canada, among others.

9. "A Brief History: Universal Health Care Efforts in the US," http://www.pnhp.org/facts/a-brief-history-universal-health-care-efforts-in-the-us.

10. While it is easy to make this a debate between the working class and Big Business, the reality was not anywhere near as binary.

11. http://demog.berkeley.edu/~andrew/1918/figure2.html.

12. Paul Starr, *The Social Transformation of American Medicine* (New York: Basic Books, 1982), 258.

13. See http://demog.berkeley.edu/~andrew/1918/figure2.html for life expectancy statistics; and http://www.cdc.gov/nchs/data/hus/2011/125.pdf for percent GDP statistics.

14. http://www.oecd.org/health/health-systems/oecdhealthdata.htm.

15. A fine summary of the ACA is available at the Department of Health and Human Service's website, http://www.hhs.gov/healthcare/rights/law/index.html.

16. This is known as the "death spiral," where insurance companies have to raise rates to its increasingly high-risk subscribers until the rates become too prohibitive to attract other subscribers.

17. http://healthaffairs.org/blog/2013/06/06/the-uninsured-after-implementation-of-the-affordable-care-act-a-demographic-and-geographic-analysis/.

18. https://www.cms.gov/Research-Statistics-Data-and-Systems/Research/ActuarialStudies/downloads/PPACA_2010-04-22.pdf.

REFERENCES

Anscombe, G. E. M. "Modern Moral Philosophy," *Philosophy*, Vol. 33, no. 124 (January, 1958).

Aristotle. *Nicomachean Ethics*, Terence Irwin, trans. Indianapolis, IN: Hackett Publishing Company, 1985.

Braveman, Paula, and Gruskin, Sofia. "Defining Equity in Health." *Journal of Epidemiology and Community Health*, 2003, Vol. 57, no. 4:254–58.

Butler, Stuart. "Assuring Affordable Health Care for All Americans." (October 1, 1989). http://www.heritage.org/research/lecture/assuring-affordable-health-care-for-all-americans.

Davis, Karen, Schoen, Cathy, Gruskin, Kristof, and Kristof Stremikis. "Mirror, Mirror on the Wall: How the Performance of the US Health Care System Compares Internationally-a 2010 Update," *The Commonwealth Fund*, http://www.commonwealthfund.org/~/media/Files/Publications/Fund%20Report/2010/Jun/1400_Davis_Mirror_Mirror_on_the_wall_2010.pdf.

Hoffman, Frederick L. *Facts and Fallacies of Compulsory Health Insurance*. Newark, NJ: Prudential Press, 1917.

Holohan, John, and McMorrow, Stacey. "Medicare and Medicaid Spending Trends and the Deficit Debate." *The New England Journal of Medicine*, August 2, 2012, no. 367: 393–95. http://www.nejm.org/doi/full/10.1056/NEJMp1204899.

Slote, Michael. *From Morality to Virtue*. Oxford, UK: Oxford University Press, 1922.

U.S. Census, *Census 2010*, http://www.census.gov/2010census/.

World Health Organization. "Glossary of Terms Used." http://www.who.int/hia/about/glos/en/index.html.

4

Global Perspectives on Long-Term Care for the Elderly[1]

Rosemarie Tong

ABSTRACT

Global aging will increase the burden of long-term care worldwide. Social critics have raised serious questions about whether it is *primarily* the responsibility of governments, individuals, or families to provide for the long-term care needs of elderly people. In this chapter, I speculate that families will increasingly be asked to care for their elderly members. This situation would be less worrisome if, contrary to fact, most countries were not tempted to turn to women to meet their need for more family caregivers. Because asking women to leave the paid workforce to do family care work will probably weaken women's recent economic and social gains, I propose another solution to the family care problem; namely, a thorough deconstruction of ingrained notions about who should work (men) and who should care (women).

INTRODUCTION: THE GLOBAL PHENOMENON OF AGING

Aging is a global phenomenon. People are living longer in both developed countries and developing countries. Worldwide, approximately five hundred million people were at or above age sixty-five in 2006. This number will increase to one billion or about 16 percent of the world's population in 2030 (Department of State 2007: 2). In the United States, 20 percent of the population will be sixty-five years or older by 2030 (Daniels 2006: 27), and, by 2040, the number of U.S. octogenarians will exceed the number of U.S. preschool children (Daniels 2006: 27). The situation will be even grayer in many developed European countries.

By 2050, half of northern Europe will be nearly fifty (Daniels 2006: 27), and the populations of Italy and Spain will be closer to sixty than fifty (Weisman 2005:

A01). Moreover, many developing countries (Albert and Cattell 1994: 39) are aging at a faster rate than developed countries. It took the United States sixty-nine years to increase the size of its over-age-sixty-five population from 7 percent to 14 percent (Department of State 2007: 15), but Singapore accomplished this same feat in only nineteen years (Department of State 2007: 7). Particularly significant is the fact that by 2050 the population of adults over age sixty-five years will be larger than the population of children under five years for the first time in human history (Department of State 2007: 6).

The primary reasons for global aging are twofold. First, fertility rates are decreasing in all countries whether they are developed or developing. Since 1960 the fertility rate worldwide has gone down from 5 to 2.7, and, in the world's developed countries, it has plummeted to 1.5, a number lower than the replacement rate required for a stable population size (Global Aging Initiative 2008: 2). Japan's replacement rate of 1.3 is dramatically low (AsiaSource 2003), but other countries, including Russia, Ukraine, Germany, Italy, Poland, Romania, Bulgaria, and Spain also have very low fertility rates (McAdams 2006). In Latin America and Southeast Asia as well as Europe and North America, an increasing number of women say they prefer active engagement in the paid workforce to bearing and rearing a large number of children (Department of State 2007: 14). What is more, opting to be entirely childless is a growing trend, particularly in some European countries where studies of young women indicate that from 12 to 16 percent of them plan to remain childless (Shorto 2008: 39).

The other primary cause of global aging is the simple fact that people are living longer. Between 1960 and 2000, life expectancy at birth grew from 50.4 to 71 in East Asia (Shrestha 2000: 207), from 56.8 to 70.4 in Latin America and the Caribbean (Shrestha 2000: 207), and from 69.7 to 76.9 in the United Sates (Arias 2002: 33). Even more noteworthy is Japan's current life expectancy at birth: an amazing eighty-two years (Department of State 2007: 8).

On the face of it, increased life expectancy and lower fertility rates would seem to be an occasion for global celebration (Montgomery, Borgatta, and Borgatta 2000: 37–39). But when human beings fail to produce enough children at the very same time they begin to live far longer lives than before, a crisis situation can be produced relatively rapidly. First, there is the most obvious problem: How do young people support elderly people, if the number of elderly people significantly exceeds the number of young people?

For example, in 1940 there were one hundred U.S. workers available to support every eleven U.S. retirees (Voice of America 2005: 2). By 2050, that same number of U.S. workers will need to support forty to fifty U.S. retirees (Voice of America 2005: 2). Moreover, also by 2050, in the seven most developed European countries, there will be only two workers for every one retiree in need of support (Department of State 2007: 3).

Throughout the world, there will be a "great-grandparent boom" (Department of State 2007: 11). People will find themselves simultaneously responsible for supporting their children, their retired parents, *and* their retired grandparents. In China, this state of affairs is termed the "1-2-4" problem: As the first cohort of China's one-child policy reach adulthood, they find themselves singly responsible for both their parents' and grandparents' long-term care (Kaneda 2006: 2). There has even been alarmist talk in China about the "1-2-4-8" problem: one Chinese child responsible for the care of two elderly parents, four elderly grandparents, and eight elderly great-grandparents (Liu 2008: 29).

Second, the costs of caring for large numbers of elderly people are probably greater than the costs of caring for large numbers of young people. Increasingly, chronic diseases such as diabetes, hypertension, cardiovascular disease, arthritis, and senile dementia account for a higher percentage of the overall global disease burden.

According to the Global Burden of Disease Project, in 2002 "non-communicable diseases accounted for 85% of the burden of disease in high-income countries and a surprising 44% of the burden of disease in low- and middle-income countries" (Department of State 2007: 12). Cardiovascular disease and cancer are currently the "two top killers" (Benderly 2007: 1) in developing countries such as Brazil and China as well as in developed countries such as France and the United States.

In India, where the battle against deaths from diarrhea, malaria, pneumonia, and other infectious diseases continues, cardiovascular disease is, nonetheless, the number-one killer (Benderly 2007: 1). Moreover, India has more people with diabetes than any other nation in the world, and Asian nations are projected to bear the brunt of Alzheimer's disease by 2050, with nearly 59 percent of the world's Alzheimer population living within their boundaries (Benderly 2007: 2).

Third, and related to the growing population of elderly people with costly chronic diseases, is the fact that, worldwide, there are not nearly enough health care workers, let alone health care workers who specialize in geriatrics (Benderly 2007: 1). In the United States, for example, where nurses and nurse aides do the bulk of elder care (Mion 2003: 4), there was a 6 percent shortage of skilled nurses in 2005, and that percentage is expected to rise to 29 percent by 2020 (Herman 2006). Compounding this growing problem is the fact that nurse aide turnover in the United States averages 71 percent annually, and nearly 90 percent of home health aides quit their jobs within their first two years of employment (Schmid 2008).

Not surprisingly, developed countries like the United States have sought to secure extra health care workers from primarily, though not exclusively, developing nations (Hochchild 2002: 17). Between 2000 and 2002, the United Kingdom alone imported thirteen thousand nurses and four thousand physicians, most of them from developing countries (Deeming 2004: 775–92). As developed countries lure foreign health care workers to their shores, developing countries are left with bare-bones staffs to meet the health care needs of their own people.

This situation often forces many developing countries to choose between meeting the health care needs of their young as opposed to their old (Engelman and Johnson 2007: 17–18). In many African countries, over 50 percent of physician and nurse positions are vacant (Daniels 2006: 30). A particularly disconcerting statistic is one reporting that "some seven thousand expatriate South African nurses work in OECD countries, while there are thirty-two thousand nursing vacancies in the public sector in South Africa" (Daniels 2006: 30).

GOVERNMENT AS PRIMARY
LONG-TERM CARE PROVIDER

Given the state of affairs sketched above, people may think their respective governments should have the primary responsibility for providing individuals with long-term care. Yet an increasing number of governments are unwilling and/or unable to shoulder this financial burden. Although many communitarian and socialist countries subsidized health care costs for their entire population in the past, it is doubtful that they will be able to do so as generously in the future. Indeed, government-subsidized health care is but a memory in the former Union of Soviet Socialist Republics (McAdams 2006: 1).

Similarly, it is a thing of the past in the People's Republic of China (Kaneda 2006: 2), where, by the way, it was always assumed that families would meet most of their elderly members' long-term care needs (Liu 2008: 29). Just as significantly, many European countries, including some of those that have been most loudly lauded for the health care benefits they provide to their citizens (Walker 2000: 83), now wonder whether their public programs can be sustained as their populations gray. Retrenchments in long-term care are noticeable in Belgium, France, Greece, Italy, Portugal, Luxembourg, Germany, the Netherlands, and the United Kingdom (Walker 2000: 83).

Only a few European countries have resisted the urge to provide fewer health care benefits to elderly people. For example, Norway and Denmark remain exceptionally committed to providing publicly subsidized, long-term care to their citizens, for two reasons: (1) their populations are still willing to pay very high taxes for social welfare programs (Blackman 2001: 184–8); and (2) their populations are decidedly opposed to marginalizing care work (Williams 2000: 57–58). Indeed, the Danish state "is based on an explicit principle of social inclusion for both older people and women of working age, who are relieved of any duty to provide unpaid care work" (Blackman 2001: 184). Other countries that make publicly subsidized, long-term care a priority are Japan and Israel.

In 1996, the Japanese Ministry of Health and Welfare proposed and subsequently passed a publicly subsidized, long-term care plan for all of its elderly people (Hong and Liu 2000: 221). In 1988, Israel made long-term care in the *home* a *legal* right (Schmid 2005: 191). Israel provides for two levels of benefits: (1) a 100 percent disability allowance for people who are *highly* dependent on help from others to carry out most activities of daily living; and (2) up to a 150 percent disability allowance for people who are *completely* dependent on others to carry out most activities of daily living (Schmid 2005: 192). Eligibility is means-tested, but not in the stringent ways it is tested in the United States, for example.

Unlike some of the European countries described above, the United States offers its people only modest, long-term care social benefits. Established in 1965, the U.S. Medicare program provides elderly U.S. people over the age of sixty-five with in-patient hospital costs, outpatient hospital costs, physicians' fees, some medical supplies, some surgical services, some diagnostic tests, and, most recently, a limited prescription drug benefit. It offers very little in the way of long-term care, however. In fact, Medicare pays for no more than one hundred days of care in a skilled nursing home following a hospitalization, provided the services are related to acute health conditions or to hospice care at the end of life (Wilson 1995: 45).

Because Medicare does not provide funds to assist elderly U.S. people with activities of daily living such as toileting, bathing, dressing, getting in and out of bed, money managing, meal preparing, shopping, and house cleaning, elderly U.S. people who need this type of help must pay for it out-of-pocket, get family members or friends to provide it, or qualify for the U.S. Medicaid program.

Established in 1964, the U.S. Medicaid program pays for the health care needs of indigent U.S. people. To become qualified for long-term care provided at home or, more likely, in a nursing home, a single individual can have no more than $13,050 in total assets. If the individual is married to someone who is living in the community, the spouse can keep between $74,824 and $104,400 in assets plus a home and car (Repko 2008). Because poverty is the entry condition into the Medicaid program, some elderly U.S. people try to hide their assets in protected investments or to give them to family members surreptitiously.

This practice is surely morally indefensible because these individuals "take advantage of a program for the poor [Medicaid] without actually being poor themselves" (Binstock 1998: 10). Therefore, the U.S. government now prevents individuals who transfer substantial assets within five years of applying to Medicaid from becoming eligible for Medicaid benefits (Lankford 2002: 100).

INDIVIDUALS AS PRIMARY LONG-TERM CARE PROVIDERS

As governments struggle either to maintain public programs or to avoid inaugurating them, they have targeted individuals as having the primary responsibility to provide for their own long-term care needs. Conversations about individuals' responsibility to subsidize their own long-term care needs are particularly loud in the United States (Callahan 1991: 280–93) and a growing number of European countries. However, they can also be heard in Hong Kong (Chan and Pang 2007), Beijing (Zhai and Qiu 2007), and South Korea (Fan 2007), places where individuals used to look forward to being pampered in their old age.

In the United States, health-care-industry representatives routinely exhort individuals either to save funds for their long-term care needs or to purchase long-term care insurance for themselves. A decade ago, two million U.S. citizens had private long-term care insurance. Now over seven million U.S. citizens have it (Edlund, Lufkin, and Franklin 2003: 3). An increasing number of people in the United States fear that the Medicare and Medicaid programs will fail them just when they need them most (Zhang 2009). They have legitimate fears about running out of money for long-term care several years before they die. The average rate for a private room in a U.S. skilled nursing home in 2002 was $168 per day or $61,320 per annum (Edlund, Lufkin, and Franklin 2003: 2).

By 2017 or so, that same room will cost around $336 per day or $122,640 per annum (Edlund, Lufkin, and Franklin 2003: 2). Moreover, home health care—the kind of care most people prefer worldwide—is not necessarily less expensive than care delivered in an institutional environment. In fact, it can be considerably more expensive than institutional care. In 2002, professionally delivered home health care in the United States averaged $432 per day or $157,680 per annum, over twice as much as 2002 skilled nursing home care (Edlund, Lufkin, and Franklin 2003: 2).

Slowly, the U.S. population, like populations throughout the world, is being educated about the high cost of long-term care and the fact that the government may lack sufficient funds to pay for it. Specifically, the U.S. government may require U.S. workers to labor until they are seventy before receiving the first one of their Social Security checks. "Inaugurating this small change in Social Security alone would add an estimated $13 trillion to the U.S. economy by 2025" (Lohr 2008: 3).

Other countries, particularly the United Kingdom and the member countries of the European Union, have similar plans. No longer will their people be able to take early retirement with full benefits in their early sixties or even late fifties. In particular, Italians can expect some changes. In 2008, the median retirement age for Italian men was less than fifty-nine years of age, which meant that Italian men were spending about twenty-one years living in retirement (Engardio and Matlack 2005: 44–47).

The belief that individuals should finance their own long-term care is growing not only in Western countries but also in Eastern countries (Tao, Wah, Chan, and Fan 2007; Chan and Pang 2007; Zhai and Qiu 2007; Boisaubin, Chu, and Catalano 2007; Tao and Wah 2007; Agich 2007; Fan 2007; and Engelhardt 2007). For example, a sample study of Hong Kong families, health care professionals, and administrators showed much support for the view that individuals should either save funds for their own long-term care voluntarily or be required by the government to do so (Chan and Pang 2007: 422). In a similar study conducted in Beijing, there was also support for compulsory saving for long-term care (Zhai and Qiu 2007: 442). Moreover, Singapore already requires individuals to save for their own long-term care needs (Engelhardt 2007: 520).

The claim that individuals have the main responsibility to pay for their own long-term care is supported by several plausible arguments. Philosopher Tristram Engelhardt Jr. has claimed that imposing such a responsibility on individuals reduces: (1) the *moral hazard* of "over-expending" public funds (supposedly, people are more frugal with their own money than the government's); (2) the *political hazard* of politicians who promise citizens long-term care benefits that the government cannot realistically fund; (3) the *demographic hazard* of expecting young people to pay the long-term care bills of old people, be they strangers or relatives; (4) the *personal and family ties hazard* of viewing the state rather than one's kin as one's main source of support; and (5) the *bureaucratic hazard* of administrating costly paperwork to secure needed public funds (Engelhardt 2007: 523–24).

However persuasive Engelhardt's arguments may be in the abstract, they seem to weaken in the concrete. Requiring people to work longer to finance their own long-term care needs is reasonable, provided the people in question are relatively healthy. Similarly, requiring people to save money to finance their own long-term care needs is reasonable, provided they can do so without jeopardizing their ability to meet their current basic needs.

In this connection, consider a 2003 U.S. study conducted by the Employee Benefits and Retirement Institute (EBRI), which concluded that U.S. workers would have to increase their savings by a factor of 5 percent to 25 percent in order to meet their own long-term care needs (Fronstin and Salisbury 2003).

Demanding, as a matter of law, that U.S. workers save this percentage of their earnings would require Herculean efforts on the part of some individuals. Specifically, U.S. women in the lowest economic quintile of the U.S. population would have to save more than 25 percent of their take-home pay, a saving that would be extremely difficult given these women's low incomes (VanDerhei and Copeland 2003). It is one thing to require well-to-do individuals to save a substantial percentage of their take-home pay for future long-term care needs but quite another to require individuals living from paycheck to paycheck to do so.

FAMILIES AS PRIMARY LONG-TERM CARE PROVIDERS

Given that many individuals—particularly women and people in developing countries—may not be able to save enough funds to meet their own long-term care needs, governments may ask and, in some instances, even require families to financially assist them (Parker and Dickenson 2001: 247). But, as noted above, there is some question about families' willingness and/or ability to help support their elderly members.

Young people in the East as well as the West are starting to publicly raise the question whether it is fair for elderly people to expect young people to make considerable sacrifices for them. With respect to this sensitive issue, U.S. health care ethicist Daniel Callahan (1991) had this to say over fifteen years ago:

> [I]t is an old and hard moral question to know what we should make of demands for self-sacrifice. Most moral rules have common sense and practicality to commend them.
>
>   Murder, lying, and theft ordinarily have tangibly bad consequences for those who commit such acts. Even our self-interest commends us to avoid them. Matters are otherwise when we are morally asked to give up our lives, or personal hopes, for the sake of another.

Only under special circumstances can that seem to make any sense at all from the viewpoint of self-interest, even of the most benign sort. It is not for nothing that almost all Western moralities have been careful to distinguish between duty and supererogation. They all recognize that a morality designed to apply to a whole community cannot require that everyone be a saint or a selfless paragon of altruism. The notion that we might as a matter of social policy burden families with the heroic duty of caring for the chronically ill or those in need of a course of rehabilitation that may fail and render them chronically ill or disabled ought at least to raise a red flag of warning. (157–58)

To be sure, questioning young people's obligations to elderly people is disconcerting. If people worldwide believe that parents have the primary responsibility to care for their young children, then, why should there be any question about whether adult children should have the primary responsibility to care for their elderly parents? Why should a child who takes care of an elderly parent view himself as a "hero" or "saint" rather than simply someone who is discharging a duty?

In addressing this question, it is important to stress that although all cultures explain children's obligations to elderly parents in terms of some duty or affection for them, some cultures emphasize duty and others emphasize affection. For example, in Asian countries with an intact Confucian tradition, all children, but especially the oldest son, still believe it is their non-negotiable moral duty to take care of their elderly parents (Li 1994: 71–72).

Because parents give life to their children and take care of them until they are adults, children reason that they owe their parents a debt of gratitude. Therefore, not to take care of one's elderly parents in their years of need is shameful and enough to warrant society's condemnation (Hong and Liu 2000: 165–82; Liu 2000: 183–99; Koyano 2000: 200–23; Hu and Chou 2000: 224–48; Lee, Lee, Yu, Sun, and Liu 2000: 269–296; Wong 2000: 297–321; Yu, Shihlong, Zehuai, and Liu 2000: 322–38).

The need to reciprocate one's parents for the gift of life and more is felt by most adult children in the West, although the emphasis seems to be on affection rather than duty. In fact, philosopher Jane English (1991) has claimed that affection, not duty, is the primary basis for adult children's obligations to parents. She comments that:

Although I agree that there are many things that children *ought* to do for their parents, I will argue that it is inappropriate and misleading to describe them as things "owed." I will maintain that parents' voluntary sacrifices, rather than creating "debts" to be "repaid," tend to create love or "friendship." The duties of grown children are those of friends, and result from love between them and their parents, rather than being things owed in repayment for the parents' earlier sacrifices. . . . Seen in this light, parental requests for children to write home, visit, and offer them a reasonable amount of emotional and financial support in life's crises are well founded, so long as a friendship still exists. (147; 152–53).

But whether filial obligation is based mostly on duty or mostly on affection, worrisome issues still remain. For example, who has the responsibility to care for individuals who have no children or who are totally estranged from the children they do have? In modern societies, about 20 percent of women do not give birth, and this percentage is growing more rapidly than previously expected (Department of State 2007: 16). In addition, many women and men are childless because they lose their children to disease or war. Childless single men and women are particularly vulnerable in their old age if they are poor (Lee, Lee, Yu, Sun, and Liu 2000: 292). Another issue is the only child issue, alluded to previously.

Is it fair that an only child should have to shoulder the entire burden of caring for one or two elderly parents, whereas a child with siblings can share this duty? Similarly, is it fair for siblings to expect whichever one of them feels most obligated to help their parents to do so? Why should the most generous sibling be burdened in ways that his or her ungenerous siblings escape? Finally, is it fair to ask children in their sixties who have looked forward to their retirement as a responsibility-free time to become the primary caregivers for their elderly parents? (Montgomery, Borgatta, and Borgatta 2000: 33–35)

Emphasizing that caring for one's elderly parents is burdensome is troubling. Yet it is not necessarily wrong for adult children not to want to be directly responsible for their parent's long-term care. As it stands, most families usually negotiate among themselves about who will be their elderly parent's primary caregiver. For example, in a recent study of 688 primary family caregivers, over 70 percent surveyed assumed major responsibility for the long-term care of elderly relatives by *default*. Because no other family member was willing and/or able to take on this responsibility, they agreed to accept it.

Other factors that played a role in selecting an individual as the primary family caregiver were: family history (24 percent), proximity to parent(s) (21 percent), no competing obligations (15 percent), and access to resources (15 percent). Interestingly, gender was mentioned by only 11.2 percent of the study participants, despite the fact that all of the study participants were *female* (Albert and Cattell 1994: 132–33).

The fact that so few of the women surveyed thought that gender played a significant role in their consenting to be their parent's primary caregiver is rather surprising. In my estimation, this fact speaks to just how deeply ingrained our gender system is. Women, more than men, still feel it is they who should sacrifice—personally and/or professionally—to care for needy family members.

Reflecting on this state of affairs, economist Carroll Estes stresses that women should think carefully before leaving their jobs to care for a family member. Importantly, she notes that elderly U.S. women, for example, are not nearly as well off as elderly U.S. men because U.S. benefits for the elderly are gender-biased against women in at least three ways. Specifically, Estes (2006) observes that:

1. Retirement income is linked to waged labor, which is itself gendered;
2. Nonwaged reproductive labor, performed predominantly by women, is not recognized or counted under state policy as labor; and
3. Retirement policy is based on a model of family status as married with male bread-winner (and with marital status as permanent rather than transient) (88–89).

Because of these three factors, says Estes, state policy "sustains the subordination of women by imposing a normative and preferential view of a particular family form with a male breadwinner and a dependent wife that is inherently disadvantageous to the majority of older women (the majority of whom are not married, especially among women of color and the very old)." In sum, elderly U.S. women are often poorer than elderly U.S. men largely because they have not worked long enough in the paid workforce instead devoting their energies to unpaid family work (Estes 2006: 89).

CONCLUSION

As the world's population ages, new arrangements will need to be made between the government, individuals, and families to meet elderly people's long-term care requirements. No matter how the responsibilities for elderly people's long-term care are allocated, however, families will probably be called on for major help.

To be sure, many elderly people will not need much in the way of family-provided long-term care. They will remain healthy enough to care for themselves (Choi and Dinse 1998: 159) or wealthy enough to hire nonfamilial caregivers (Rosen 2007: 13). Moreover, a good measure of elderly people will find government-provided long-term care benefits sufficient to meet their needs.

But there will still be millions of elderly people who will look to their families or family-like persons (close friends, charitable individuals/groups, people who share the same plight) for help to meet their long-term care needs, and many societies will automatically call on women to provide this help. For example, after decades of sex-selecting males for their one and only child, a practice that has resulted in a dramatic sex-ratio imbalance of 119.6 males for every 100 females in China (Hudson and Boer 2008: 186), the Chinese are now starting to sex-select for girls (Liu 2008: 28).

Apparently many young Chinese couples are increasingly of the opinion that daughters are more likely than sons to minister to them in their old age. Moreover, some elderly Chinese couples that do not have a daughter or are childless are trying to acquire a daughter through a process akin to adoption. Advertisements for "daughters" now appear in Chinese newspapers, some of them promising ample rewards to the women who answer them (Liu 2008: 29).

But what happens if women refuse to be society's caregivers for fear they will reach old age poorer and sicker if they leave the paid workforce to care for family members (Fields 2008: A17)? As a first response to this question, consider a recent article on long-term care in Japan. Beginning in 1963, various rounds of the Japanese National Survey on Family Planning asked the question: "What is your opinion about children caring for their elderly parents?"

Surveyed individuals could choose one of the following responses: "good custom," "natural duty," "unavoidable," and "not a good custom." Between 1963 and 1996, the number of married Japanese women of reproductive age who answered either "good custom" or "natural duty" fell from 80 percent to 47 percent (Ogawa and

Retherford 1997: 87–88). During approximately the same period of time "expectations of old-age support from one's own children" declined from 65 percent to 13 percent (Ogawa and Retherford 1997: 89).

The article concluded with the observation that in view of Japanese women's growing reluctance to be caregivers, "the [Japanese] government's efforts to shift some of the responsibility for caring for the elderly from the social security system back to families will not be very successful" (Ogawa and Retherford 1997: 91).

Clearly, unless developed and developing countries explode the gender system that captures their collective imaginations, they will run the risk of not having enough caregivers to meet their needs. The challenges of global aging present a unique opportunity to weaken the two norms that uphold the world's gender systems; namely, the ideal worker norm, theorized by Joan Williams (Williams 2000: 1), and the ideal careworker norm, alternately celebrated and criticized by feminist care ethicists (Gilligan 1982, Held 2006, Kittay 1999, Noddings 1984).

Williams (2000) reasons that "domesticity" is a rigid gender system that separates market work from family work and then structures market work "around the ideal of a worker who works full time and overtime and takes little or no time off for childbearing or child rearing." As Williams sees it, "Though the ideal worker norm does not define all jobs today, it defines the good ones: full-time blue-collar jobs in the working-class context, and high-level executive and professional jobs for the middle class and above" (1).

Structured in this way, market work has no patience for caregivers who are distracted by family work. Workers who put their families above their work commitments are punished with marginalization in the workforce. But this state of affairs has negative consequences for caregivers. Their marginalization disqualifies them from the rewards of market work, including not only "responsibility and authority" but also the extra money they need to care for themselves and others. The only way to change this inequitable state of affairs, argues Williams, is to make the workplace conform to the family rather than the family to the workplace. The ideal worker would then become someone who has time for both family and work and is able to care because of the way the workplace is structured.

Eradicating the ideal worker norm is no easy matter, however. For example, in the United States, many feminists have tried for over a quarter of a century to persuade men and women to be equally involved in both work life and family life. Although this style of life would prevent either men or women from being full-time workers or full-time family caregivers, it would result in greater gender equality (Tong 2009: 11–47). Yet to this day, relatively few U.S. men and U.S. women have had the resolve to restructure their lives in the way recommended.

A *New York Times* article in 2008 detailed just how much resistance that one well-salaried U.S. couple met trying to get work schedules that would provide them with additional time for their children. After two years of haggling with their employers, they got their preferred schedules, but not without having to accept a 10 percent salary cut. The couple stated that they were willing to take the pay cut, fully "understanding that [such] . . . an option [is] available only to those who can make ends meet in the first place" (Belkin 2008: 49).

If affluent U.S. couples have trouble negotiating family-friendly schedules, it stands to reason that less affluent U.S. couples and individuals will probably have even more trouble doing so. Moreover, chances are that if one is a man rather than a woman, a request for more family time may be met with a particularly high level of resistance. For example, U.S. men who make their commitments to their families too widely known at the workplace are still viewed with suspicion as uncommitted workers or as "oddballs" (Press 2007: 41).

Countries that are really serious about gender equity realize that the only way not to marginalize care work is to destroy both the ideal careworker norm and the ideal worker norm. These countries do not aim to pull women out of the paid workforce so men can stay in it. Instead, they contemplate requiring men to take time off for family matters. For example, in Norway there is currently a debate to make paternity leave mandatory so that women can return to work for that period of time. The Norwegian government guarantees about fifty-four weeks of maternity leave and six weeks of paternity leave at 80 percent of salary (Shorto 2008: 40).

Significantly, most workplace family-care leave and benefit policies still emphasize childcare leaves. But, in the future, they will probably have to emphasize eldercare leaves just as much, if not more. This shift in emphasis from childcare to elder care may, in my estimation, present new opportunities for society to view men as just as able as women to deliver care. Because women give birth to children, they were assigned the duty to rear them (Tong 2009: 85–86). But there is no equivalent "natural" reason for women to care for elderly people, and so the rationale for men not caring for elderly people is not as plausible as the rationale for men not taking care of infants and children. Perhaps this state of affairs is why men were given official responsibility for caring for elderly parents in so many societies.

To be sure, most men did not actually do the care work assigned to them. Their wives, sisters, and daughters did it for them. But in the face of a burgeoning aging population, now may be the ideal time to ask men to develop their caregiving skills. There are too many elderly people with too many needs. Women cannot be expected to meet all of the world's increasing caregiving needs. Men will have to help women care for elderly people or elderly people will need to fend for themselves.

Men have started to care for children more than in the past. There is simply no compelling reason why they cannot also care for elderly family members' needs (Belkin 2008). To be sure, elder care may be particularly frightening for men. The bodies of elderly people speak of diminishment, disintegration, and death— threats to the autonomous self who charts the course of *his* destiny. They speak of nature, materiality, and that which cannot be controlled but must instead be accepted.

But it is precisely by coming to terms with the reality of enfleshment that men could join with women to overcome the dichotomies that are at the root of job segregation and gender inequity. Vulnerability is our common fate as human beings.

We need to construct our workplaces and families in ways that acknowledge our dependence on each other. In order for us to be properly autonomous, men as well as women need to do care work. Only then will women's old age be as good as men's (Dodds 2007: 500–10).

NOTE

1. This chapter shares some material from an article titled "Long-Term Care for the Elderly: Whose Responsibility Is It?" previously published in *International Journal of Feminist Approaches to Bioethics* (IJFAB) 2 (2): 2009. Used with permission.

REFERENCES

Agich, G. J. 2007. "Reflections on the Function of Dignity in the Context of Caring for Old People." *Journal of Medicine and Philosophy* 32 (5): 483–94.

Albert, S. M., and M. G. Cattell. 1994. *Old Age in Global Perspective: Cross-Cultural and Cross National Views*. New York: G. K. Hall & Co.

Arias, E. 2002. "National Vital Statistics Reports: United States Life Tables, 2000." *National Center for Health Statistics* 51 (3): 33.

AsiaSource. 2003. "Japan's Aging Population: A Challenge for Its Economy and Society." *AsiaTODAY*. http://www.asiasource.org/news/at_mp_02.cfm?newsid=102450.

Belkin, L. 2008. "When Mom and Dad Share It All." *New York Times Magazine*, June 15, 2008, 44–78.

Benderly, B. L. 2007. "Grow Old Along with Me—and 690 Million Other People by 2030." Disease Control Priorities Project. http://www.dcp2.org/features/56/grow-old-along-with-meand-690-million-other-people-by-2030.

Binstock, R. H. 1998. "The Financing and Organization of Long-Term Care." In *Public and Private Responsibilities in Long-Term Care*, edited by L. C. Walker, E. H. Bradley, and T. Wetle. Baltimore: Johns Hopkins University Press.

Blackman, T. 2001. "Conclusion: Issues and Solutions." In *Social Care and Social Exclusion*, edited by T. Blackman, S. Brodhurst, and J. Convery. New York: Palgrave Publishers.

Boisaubin, E. V., A. Chu, and J. M. Catalano. 2007. "Perceptions of Long-Term Care, Autonomy, and Dignity, by Residents, Family, and Care-Givers: The Houston Experience." *Journal of Medicine and Philosophy* 32 (5): 447–64.

Callahan, D. 1991. "Families as Caregivers: *The Limits of Morality*." In *Aging and Ethics: Philosophical Problems in Gerontology*, edited by N. S. Jecker. Totowa, NJ: Humana.

Chan, H. M., and S. Pang. 2007. "Long-Term Care: Dignity, Autonomy, Family Integrity, and Social Sustainability: The Hong Kong Experience." *Journal of Medicine and Philosophy* 32 (5): 401–24.

Choi, N. G., and S. Dinse. 1998. "Challenges and Opportunities of the Aging Population: Social Work Education and Practice for Productive Aging." *Educational Gerontology* 24 (2): 159–74.

Daniels, N. 2006. "Equity and Population Health: Toward a Broader Bioethics Agenda." *Hastings Center Report* 36 (4): 22–35.

Deeming, C. 2004. "Policy Targets and Ethical Tensions: UK Nurse Recruitment," *Social Policy and Administration*, December, Vol. 38, no. 7: 775–92.

Department of State and the Department of Health and Human Services, National Institute on Aging, National Institutes of Health. 2007. *Why Population Aging Matters: A Global Perspective*. U.S. Department of State.

Dodds, S. 2007. "Depending on Care: Recognition of Vulnerability and the Social Contribution of Care Provision." *Bioethics* 21 (9): 500–510.

Edlund, B., S. Lufkin, and B. Franklin. 2003. "Long-Term Care Planning for Baby Boomers: Addressing an Uncertain Future." *Online Journal of Issues in Nursing* 8 (2): 2.

Engardio, P. and C. Matlack. 2005. "Now, the Geezer Glut: Global Aging." *Business Week*, January 30.

Engelhardt, H. T. Jr. 2007. "Long-Term Care: The Family, Post-Modernity, and Conflicting Moral Life-Worlds." *Journal of Medicine and Philosophy* 32 (5): 519–36.

Engelman, M., and S. Johnson. 2007. "Population Aging and International Development: Addressing Competing Claims of Distributive Justice." *Developing World Bioethics* 7 (1): 8–18.

English, J. 1991. "What Do Grown Children Owe Their Parents?" In *Aging and Ethics: Philosophical Problems in Gerontology*, edited by N. S. Jecker. Totowa, NJ: Humana.

Estes, C. 2006. "Critical Feminist Perspectives, Aging, and Social Policy." In *Aging, Globalization and Inequality: The New Critical Gerontology*, edited by J. Baars, D. Dannefer, C. Phillipson, and A. Walker. Amityville, NY: Baywood Publishing Co., Inc.

Fan, R. 2007. "Which Care? Whose Responsibility? And Why Family? A Confucian Account of Long-Term Care for the Elderly." *Journal of Medicine and Philosophy* 32 (5): 495–518.

Fields, S. 2008. "Death, Be Not Proud." *Washington Times*, June 19, A17.

Fronstin, and D. Salisbury. 2003. "Retiree Health Benefits: Savings Needed to Fund Health Care in Retirement." *Employee Benefits and Retirement Institute*. EBRI Issue Brief #254, February 2003.

Gilligan, C. 1982. *In a Different Voice*. Cambridge: Harvard University Press.

Global Aging Initiative. 2008. "Global Aging Initiative." Center for Strategic and International Studies. http://www.csis.org/gai/.

Held, V. 2006. *The Ethics of Care: Personal, Political and Global*. New York: Oxford University Press.

Herman, C. 2006. "U.S. Unprepared for Impact of Aging Population on Health Workforce according to UAlbany Center for Health Workforce Studies." http://www.albany.edu/news/releases/2006/apr2006/aging_impact_chws.shtml.

Hochchild, A. R. 2002. "Love and Gold." In *Global Women: Nannies, Maids, and Sex Workers in the Global Economy*, edited by B. Ehrenreich and A. R. Hochchild. New York: Henry Holt and Company.

Hong, Y., & W. T. Liu. 2000. "The Social Psychological Perspective of Elderly Care." In *Who Should Care for the Elderly?*, edited by W. T. Liu and H. Kendig. Singapore: Singapore University Press.

Hu, Y., and Y. Chou. 2000. "The Cultural Politics of the Asian Family Care Model: Missing Language and Facts." In *Who Should Care for the Elderly?*, edited by W. T. Liu and H. Kendig. Singapore: Singapore University Press.

Hudson, V. M., and A. D. Boer. 2008. "China's Security, China's Demographics: Aging, Masculinization, and Fertility Policy." *Brown Journal of World Affairs* 14 (2) (Spring/Summer): 185–200.

Kaneda, T. 2006. *China's Concern over Population Aging and Health*. Washington, DC: Population Reference Bureau.

Kittay, E. F. 1999. *Love's Labor: Essays on Women, Equality, and Dependency*. New York: Routledge.

Koyano, W. 2000. "Filial Piety, Co-Residence, and Intergenerational Solidarity in Japan." In *Who Should Care for the Elderly?*, edited by W. T. Liu and H. Kendig. Singapore: Singapore University Press.

Lankford, K. 2002. "Look Back Doesn't Equal Take Back." *Kiplinger's Personal Finance* 56 (4): 100.

Lee, R. P. L., J. Lee, E. S. H. Yu, S. Sun, and W. T. Liu. 2000. "Living Arrangements and Elderly Care: The Case of Hong Kong." In *Who Should Care for the Elderly?*, edited by W. T. Liu and H. Kendig. Singapore: Singapore University Press.

Li, C. 1994. "The Confucian Concept of Jen and the Feminist Ethics of Care: A Comparative Study." *Hypatia* 9 (1): 70–89.

Liu, M. 2008. "Playing with the Old Blood Rules." *Newsweek*, March 17, 27–29.

Liu, W. T. 2000. "Values and Caregiving Burden: The Significance of Filial Piety in Elder Care." In *Who Should Care for the Elderly?*, edited by W. T. Liu and H. Kendig. Singapore: Singapore University Press.

Lohr, S. 2008. "For a Good Retirement, Find Work. Good Luck." *New York Times*, June 22.

McAdams, L. 2006. "Russia Losing Battle in Population Growth to Disease, Low Birth Rates." *Voice of America.* http://www.voanews.com/content/a-13-2006-03-08-voa29/312403.html.

Mion, L. C. 2003. "Care Provision for Older Adults: Who Will Provide?" *Online Journal of Issues in Nursing* 8 (2): 2.

Montgomery, R. J. V., E. F. Borgatta, and M. L. Borgatta. 2000. "Societal and Family Change in the Burden of Care." In *Who Should Care for the Elderly?*, edited by W. T. Liu and H. Kendig. Singapore: Singapore University Press.

Noddings, N. 1984. *Caring: A Feminine Approach to Ethics and Moral Education.* Berkeley: University of California Press.

Ogawa, N., and R. D. Retherford. 1997. "Shifting Costs of Caring for the Elderly Back to Families in Japan: Will It Work?" *Population and Development Review* 23 (1): 59–94.

Parker, M., and D. Dickenson. 2001. "Resource Allocation." In *The Cambridge Medical Ethics Workbook: Case Studies Commentaries and Activities*, edited by M. Parker and D. Dickenson. Cambridge, UK: Cambridge University Press.

Press, E. 2007. "Do Workers Have a Fundamental Right to Care for Their Families? The Front in the Job-Discrimination Battle." *New York Times Magazine*, June 29, 41.

Repko, M. 2008. "Medicaid Puts Greater Responsibility on Families for Nursing Home Payments." *Buffalo News.* http://www.buffalonews.com/home/story/406684.html.

Rosen, R. 2007. "The Care Crisis." *Nation* 284 (10): 11–16.

Schmid, H. 2005. "The Israeli Long-Term Care Insurance Law: Selected Issues in Providing Home Care Services to the Frail Elderly." *Health and Social Care in the Community* 13 (3): 191–200.

Schmid, R. E. 2008. "Medical Care System Not Ready for Aging Baby Boomers." *AARP Bulletin Today.* http://bulletin.aarp.org/yourhealth/policy/articles/medical_care_system_not_ready_for_mass_of_aging_baby_boomers_study_says1.html.

Shorto, R. 2008, June 29. ¿No hay bebés? Keine kinder? Nessun bambino? No babies? *New York Times Magazine*, June 29, 34–41; 68–71.

Shrestha, Laura B. 2000. "Population Aging in Developing Countries." *Health Affairs* 19 (3): 207.

Tao, J., and L. P. Wah. 2007. "Dignity in Long-Term Care for Older Persons: A Confucian Perspective." *Journal of Medicine and Philosophy* 32 (5): 465–82.

Tao, J., L. P. Wah, H. M. Chan, and R. Fan. 2007. "Exploring the Bioethics of Long-Term Care." *Journal of Medicine and Philosophy* 32 (5): 395–400.

Tong, R. 2009. *Feminist Thought: A More Comprehensive Introduction*, 3rd ed. Boulder, CO: Westview.

VanDerhei, J., and C. Copeland. 2003. *Can America Afford Tomorrow's Retirees: Results from the EBRIERF Retirement Security Projection Model.* EBRI Issue Brief Number 263: Washington, DC.

Voice of America. 2005. "Populations Are Aging Worldwide." *Voice of America News* 2.

Walker, A. 2000. "Sharing Long-Term Care between the Family and the State—A European Perspective." In *Who Should Care for the Elderly?*, edited by W. T. Liu and H. Kendig. Singapore: Singapore University Press.

Weisman, J. 2005. "Aging Population Poses Global Challenges." *Washington Post*, February 2, A01.

Williams, J. 2000. *Unbending Gender: Why Family and Work Conflict and What to Do about It.* New York: Oxford University Press.

Wilson, N. 1995. "Long-Term Care in the United States: An Overview of the Current System." In *Long-Term Care Decisions: Ethical and Conceptual Dimensions*, edited by L. B. McCullough and N. L. Wilson. Baltimore: Johns Hopkins University Press.

Wong, O. M. H. 2000. "Children and Children-in-Law as Primary Caregivers: Issues and Perspectives." In *Who Should Care for the Elderly?*, edited by W. T. Liu and H. Kendig. Singapore: Singapore University Press.

Yu, E. S. H., L. Shihlong, W. Zehuai, and W. T. Liu. 2000. "Caregiving Survey in Guangzhou: A Preliminary Report." In *Who Should Care for the Elderly?*, edited by W. T. Liu and H. Kendig. Singapore: Singapore University Press.

Zhai, X., and R. Z. Qiu. 2007. "Perceptions of Long-Term Care, Autonomy, and Dignity, by Residents, Family, and Caregivers: The Beijing Experience." *Journal of Medicine and Philosophy* 32 (5): 425–46.

Zhang, J. 2009. "Panel Lists Ways to Rein in Medicare Costs." *Wall Street Journal.* June 16. http://online.wsj.com/article/SB124510124035616413.html.

5

Safety and Public Health

Evaluating Acceptable Risk

Michael Boylan

ABSTRACT

Calculations of risk assessment for public health often require adjudicating tradeoffs of various public goods. One essential element in such a calculation is the concept of public safety. Safety is a condition to which all would aspire. However, what is really meant by safety? There are negative and positive senses, both of which have to do with the loss or acquisition of particular goods of agency. The worldview of the practitioner is also key to her understanding of just what constitutes safety. This chapter outlines an understanding of safety within a context of various fallacies in risk assessment and then suggests a positive direction to public policy.

INTRODUCTION

Ladies and Gentlemen, because of a clear and present danger from terrorism, it is hereby declared that from this moment forward civil liberties will be severely reduced so that we might be able to create a safe and peaceful society—free from violence where we might be able to go about our business without interference.

Various political leaders have delivered this fictive declaration to their citizens throughout history (Woodward 2008, Gordon and Trainor 2007, Suskind 2008, Draper 2008, Mayer 2008). The rationale that leaders generally give for this (if they are forthcoming) is that the country is under siege by foreign enemies who seek to change life (as the citizens have been accustomed). All of this is given in the name of defending the country. This good flows from "protection from unwarranted bodily harm," which I have argued elsewhere is a legitimate category of public health (Boylan 2004b: introduction; Boylan 2011).

356

However, the cost of acquiring this good of agency is the loss of human rights that also constitute a category of public health (Hessler 2008). How does one go about a risk assessment in which some tradeoff will occur? This chapter will suggest that the concept of public safety (as discussed here) will be a good starting point. Thus, this chapter seeks to explore the place of safety within our lives. Three common forms of ignorance that lead to improper risk assessment will be examined and some brief recommendations will follow on how public policy should proceed through proper risk assessment.

DEFECTIVE RISK ASSESSMENT DUE TO THREE FORMS OF IGNORANCE

This section will contend that there are three forms of ignorance that lead to defective risk assessment in public health policy: goods myopia, money/power, and the externalist/internalist conflict. In order to put these into context, let us begin with safety. Safety is of primary concern to us all. I hold it to be a fundamental requirement for action. Without safety (to some degree) we cannot act. This is why its protection is cogent to public health. Let's unpack this.

"Safety" has several meanings (a few of which will be developed later). At this point it must be clear that one common understanding of "safety" is "safe from losing such and such." In this way "safety" is transitive in nature. It requires objects from which we are safe from losing. Presumably these are most especially the key goods that we hold to be important. But what are these goods? And how do we rank them in importance? I contend that the goods of agency can be ranked in the following hierarchy.

Thus, in this context one *should* be more concerned about losing basic food, water, sanitation, clothing, shelter, and protection from unwarranted bodily harm (including access to basic health care) than she is from losing her summer vacation in Sienna. This is because the former goods are first-level basic goods while the latter is a third-level secondary good.

It is my conjecture, in any case, that there are many who fail to distinguish these sorts of gradations. These individuals do not properly assess risk because of this failure. I believe that this is especially true among those who possess goods in all the categories (the affluent). In some respects I believe it to be true that some individuals in this category are blind to the relative worth of their various goods and may even value level-three secondary goods on a par with their basic goods.

THE TABLE OF EMBEDDEDNESS[1]

Basic Goods

Level One: *Most Deeply Embedded*[2] (that which is absolutely necessary for human action): food, water, sanitation, clothing, shelter, and protection from unwarranted bodily harm (including access to basic health care)

Level Two: *Deeply Embedded* (that which is necessary for effective basic action within any given society).

- Literacy in the language of the country
- Basic mathematical skills
- Other fundamental skills necessary to be an effective agent in that country; for example, in the United States some computer literacy is necessary
- Some familiarity with the culture and history of the country in which one lives
- The assurance that those you interact with are not lying to promote their own interests
- The assurance that those you interact with will recognize your human dignity (as per above) and not exploit you as a means only
- Basic human rights such as those listed in the U.S. Bill of Rights and the UN Universal Declaration of Human Rights

Secondary Goods

Level One: *Life Enhancing* (medium to high-medium on embeddedness)

- Basic societal respect
- Equal opportunity to compete for the prudential goods of society
- Ability to pursue a life plan according to the Personal Worldview Imperative
- Ability to participate equally as an agent in the Shared Community Worldview Imperative

Level Two: *Useful* (medium to low-medium embeddedness)

- Ability to use one's real and portable property in the manner she chooses
- Ability to gain from and exploit the consequences of one's labor regardless of the starting point
- Ability to pursue goods that are generally owned by most citizens; for example, in the United States today a telephone, television, and automobile would fit into this class

Level Three: *Luxurious* (low embeddedness)

- Ability to pursue goods that are pleasant even though they are far removed from action and from the expectations of most citizens within a given country; for example, in the United States today a European vacation would fit into this class
- Ability to exert one's will so that she might extract a disproportionate share of society's resources for her own use

One example to illustrate what I mean occurred in the wake of the Enron disaster. I heard the wife of a top executive at one of the nation's largest failed companies break down in tears about their impending personal "bankruptcy" and the severe straits they would now have to live under as she compared her lot to those of the many employees who had lost their life savings in the company's stock-funded 401k retirement plan.

However, the so-called personal bankruptcy was part of a well-orchestrated plan by her husband to shield over $250 million in assets (all in strict accordance with the bankruptcy laws). Bankruptcy would shield them from lawsuits beyond the directors and officers' liability suits (largely covered by insurance). As a result of the company's collapse, this executive couple would be "bankrupt," but he and his wife would still have more than $10 million a year for the rest of their life (and more if interest rates go up)!

I'm sure that the wife of the executive really thought it might be tough to struggle by on only a few million dollars a year. This is because the meaning of "tough" here is merely to have fewer luxury goods at her disposal. However, to compare her plight to those company employees who lost everything in company stock that her husband was pumping employees to buy and hold in their retirement and investment accounts is to see the loss of any goods of agency as "on a par."

If I have to sell my house and move into a one-bedroom apartment, or if I have to "un-retire" and get a job at 70-plus in order to insure that there is bread on the table, my hardship is far greater than that of someone who now must make do with only two homes instead of seven. And yet, if the person on the radio was speaking her heart (and I believe she was), then she saw *no difference* in her plight and that of the company employees who were likewise *ruined*.

Individuals like the aforementioned executive's wife will be termed "goods myopic." These individuals, because of their near-sighted attention on what is closest at hand (the negative change in luxury goods), fail to judge the broader relationship of all the various goods of agency: recognizing the goods that are logically primary to action per se. Perhaps because the origins of action (from a monetary point of view) have been fulfilled for so long—perhaps their entire lives—they don't give it another thought. Perhaps they view all discomfort on a par: X's discomfort at no longer having the money to buy her prescription drugs for her arthritis condition and Y's discomfort at having to sell her back-up jet (the one with the pretty art deco wet bar). It is difficult to say, but goods myopia is symptomatic of those who have not critically thought about questions of goods allocation in the society: distributive justice.[3]

Another example of goods myopia concerns universal health coverage. In the United States there is no universal health coverage. This is largely because the wealthy Americans in the top quintile of income see their potential loss of level-two and level-three secondary goods (via necessary taxes) as being on a par with the acquisition of health coverage by those in the lowest three tiers. The Table of Embeddedness suggests that primary health care is a level-one basic good. A level-one basic good trumps a level-two or three secondary good.

Thus, the Table of Embeddedness demands that the rights claims of those without health care supervenes those affluent Americans' claims for their excess money to purchase level-two or level-three secondary goods. At the writing of this chapter around forty-seven million Americans or 15 percent of our population do not have assured access to health care. Thus, the condition of goods myopia (if I am correct in my assessment) is contributing to a major public health disaster in the United States: lack of access to primary health care. In 2010 the Afforable Health Care Act was passed by Congress and signed by the president. Its strategy is to require everyone to purchase private health insurance. If people cannot afford the premiums, there are some proposed subsidies. However, detractors to the plan are so vehment in their anger at covering thirty-seven million of the forty-seven million that they have set out several lawsuits against the plan (which fully began in 2014). Then in June 2012 the U.S. Supreme court affirmed the constitutional-ity of the law in a 5–4 decision with Chief Justice Roberts writing the opinion for the majority. However, this did not stop the naysayers. Those opponents of the bill in the House of Representatives used the power of originating the budget to shutdown the government.

The reason given for this antipathy to providing government-assisted health care is that purchasing health insurance is seen on a par as purchasing a new car. Both are nice to have, but only if you have the money to afford it. Detractors say that the Afforable Health Care Act is tantamount to the government buying everyone a car!

Goods myopia is really a form of ignorance—causing improper risk assessment. The Table of Embeddedness sets out my vision of the proper ordering. Though some might quibble here and there with what goods are on which level, it has been my experience that, for the most part, there is general consensus that this hierarchy cor-rectly represents the embeddedness of goods vis-à-vis the primary conditions neces-sary for action. To fail to recognize this and to view all goods on a par is to exhibit moral ignorance.[4] Obviously, this sort of ignorance is important.

If one is gauging her safety and views all goods on a par, then the amount of goods that need protection is rather large. It may be analogous to a computer user who fails to distinguish between various types of document and graphic files in her computer memory management. One must have a system of priority that is based upon a de-fensible standard. If the public is expected to protect the goods of its citizens, then there are two choices (given scarcity of resources): (a) protect and supply the goods of agency according to the hierarchy of embeddedness (proximity to action as per the Table of Embeddedness) or (b) protect all goods as on a par with the sorting mecha-nism being one's ability to influence government. In case (a) the government would end up showing concern to the poorest in society *before* less embedded claims are met (this is analogous to the medical concept of *triage*). In case (b) those with influ-ence would be protected while those less powerful would have to fend for themselves or die. There would be no recognition of need (triage). The result of choosing this option is that the many must sacrifice for the good of the few (assuming a standard bell curve wealth distribution). Such a strategy would cause great disruption among those who are already less well off.

If the Table of Embeddedness is the blueprint for a system of moral allocation of goods in society, then only case (a) is acceptable. In the United States and in most other Occidental regimes, case (b) is more often the ruling principle. Since case (b) is based upon moral ignorance and since case (b) may require extraordinary measures to protect itself, case (b) may illegitimately create conditions under which the many may have to rearrange their lives to a great degree in order to protect the most affluent in society (contra to the dictums of ethically based distributive justice). Joseph Stiglitz has written recently that this sort of trend toward economic inequality actually threatens democracy because it creates an oligarchy of the super-rich who have the resources to disproportionately influence legislation and public policy (Stiglitz 2012).

The *second* basic cause of improper risk assessment is due to an ignorance that stems from lusting after money and/or power. The most common venues for this defect lie within the business community or within the political arena.

In each case there arises a distraction that distorts proper assessment by introducing a new factor (money/power) that is not relevant to the mission of the institution. In the case of business this distraction is generally built around increasing profits. The drive to profits is what makes business tick. However, there can be some difficulties when the interests of the directors and officers are not in line with the shareholders.

In the 2008 subprime mortgage crisis in the United States, various firms such as Bear Sterns, Fannie Mae and Freddie Mac, Lehman Brothers, AIG, and Merrill Lynch (among others) did not follow established mortgage and financial practice in order that they might garner extra profits among borrowers tagged "subprime" (meaning that they do not fit into the established categories of eligibility for loans). This pool of people (aka the poor) has traditionally been very profitable for business from the food industry to the insurance industry because this population is charged extra fees and conditions against a risk pool that has few options (Boylan 2008c).

The temptation is to enter this market to exploit the poor who have few options and are not generally in contact with lawyers who might protect their interests. These businesses enter this lucrative market on explotitative terms, and to protect their risk they create insurance and exotic derivative investment vehicles. The conjecture is that by spreading the risk, if something went wrong, it would have a ripple effect everywhere and so dissipate into a series of small events.

The problem was that what was thought to be (in the jargon of probability theory) a series of independent events (whose risk is only additive) became a dependent series whose events are multiplied.[5] This was a major mistake in risk assessment. The risk was put into the wrong category type. The cause was that the businesses really *wanted* it to work because they could make so much more money than the traditional loan methodology.

This same sort of reasoning occurs in government as well. For example, in government the prize is maximizing power. It is often dressed in a finery of politics that says that it is acting for the public good (and sometimes this is true). However, when one assesses the threat to the general populace, then the risk/reward calculus must be based upon sound, verifiable, externalist criteria (Boylan 2004a: chapter 6). For example, then-president George W. Bush started a war of choice (preemptively) based on faulty intelligence that cost thousands of lives (Roberts et al. 2006). Surely, this is a public health disaster. It was caused by ignorance induced by the fallacy of money/power that distorted prudent risk assessment. The president had a Republican Congress and could effectively do what he wanted. Because he was in such a powerful position, and because "from the very beginning, there was a conviction that Saddam Hussein was a bad person and that he needed to go," O'Neill told CBS, "for me, the notion of pre-emption, that the U.S. has the unilateral right to do whatever we decide to do, is a really huge leap" (CNN Politics 2004).

Because we had the power to topple Saddam Hussein, all other checks and balances were minimized. Because there was no tax raised to pay for the war meant that the president thought that he had plenty of money to do whatever he wanted. The money/power faction moved the United States to create a public health disaster in the Middle East. It is the second form of ignorance that hampers risk assessment.

The *third* form of ignorance that hampers assessment of risk is the externalist/internalist conflict. It is my opinion that issues of morality and justice should rely upon externalist criteria (as much as possible, Boylan 2004a: chapter 5). This is because morality and politics exist within the community realm. As public policy, their operations should be transparent for all to see and to give input. However, often the internalist perspective ends up winning the day. To put this into perspective, let us return to the concept of safety. "Safety" comes from the Latin, *salvus*, meaning "uninjured, entire, and healthy."

The first of these criteria is negative. One is safe if he is in the state of *not* being injured. The second two are positive and indicate an aspect of safety that can be tied to peace and social justice (represented here via the Table of Embeddedness). Let us return, then, to the first criteria of being uninjured. "Uninjured" can mean both lack of *actual* injury (interpreted in this chapter as having been deprived of some good of agency), and *potential* injury (interpreted in this chapter as being at risk for losing some good of agency).

When we are threatened or *feel* threatened, we seek to form some strategy of protection. For example, New Orleans and Texas in the United States often face terrible hurricanes during September. When a potential category-3 storm (or higher) is detected, the potential threat to public safety must be addressed by effective preventative measures. This derives both from a description of some state of affairs along with an interpretation of that description. The description should be empirically based, and the possible outcome assessments should be grounded in data informed by precautionary reason and invoking, where appropriate, the rule to rescue (Beyleveld and Pattinson 2000, Cranor 2004, Sheehan 2007, Cookson et al. 2008).

When Hurricane Katrina was approaching New Orleans in 2005, many in FEMA (the Federal Emergency Management Agency) projected a model of the best possible outcome instead of a precautionary model that would expect the worst reasonably calculated fate.[6] Other instances of public health threat—such as the avian flu or the new outbreaks of tuberculosis, should be treated with the same precautionary reason model. This is not a prescription for alarmism. Some use the motto of precautionary reason based upon biased personal fear or other such internalist criteria to create highly inappropriate social/political responses (Beyleveld and Pattinson 2000, Cranor 2004).

In philosophy, we often talk in inductive logic about inference to the best empirically based explanation. This isn't perfect since statistically based conjecture on future events is never certain. But it is the best externalist model for public consumption. The difference between threat perceived by internalist and externalist criteria is significant.

An illustration of this sort of failure comes from a personal example. Padraig (not his real name), my relative, wanted to visit me. However, because I was residing in the inner city for a time, Padraig got a motel room outside the city and insisted that I travel to see him in the suburbs because they were so much safer. Padraig could have stayed with me and saved the cost of a motel room and all the extra meals he had to eat because he was so far away from me. I should mention that though I was residing in the inner city, I did *not* live in one of the highest crime areas, nor did I live in the safest section of the city. The worldview that supported Padraig's position was something like the following:

1. There is a great amount of crime and violence in the inner city.
2. The criminals can detect a country boy by sight.
3. The bandits will immediately ravage detected country boys.
4. Padraig didn't carry a gun and was not a good fighter.
5. Padraig wanted to visit me, but he didn't want to do so at the peril of his life.

There are a great many Padraigs in this world who base their fears upon unacknowledged racism. I have walked with people who visibly stiffen when they see people of a different race (or otherwise "other") approaching on the same sidewalk. These people are not wielding knives, chains, or submachine guns. They are just walking.

President Obama related a personal example (before he became president) of being a black man walking down the street and hearing the sound of car doors locking as the occupants sought to protect themselves from the possibility of attack by the "other."[7]

Why is it that Padraig and others have this fear of the inner city? Perhaps it is television or the movies or the scuttlebutt around the water cooler at work. But the fear is unfounded based upon externalist criteria. The murder rate in the inner city at that time was 7.1 per 100,000, while that in suburbs and other venues was 6.1 per 100,000.[8] Statistically this is not a great difference (a net difference of 1.0 per 100,000). One is *virtually* as safe in the inner city as he is in the suburban motels, sidewalks, and the restaurants where I had to meet him.

Not only that, but Padraig came to visit me by automobile via the interstate highway system, which has a fatality rate of 15.26 per 100,000.[9] Padraig was willing to undergo exposure to a risk of 15.26 (per 100,000) to drive to the suburban environs, but he was unwilling to expose himself to a marginal differential of 1.0 per 100,000 to see me where I lived. Given these statistics, Padraig's attitude is irrational based upon externalist criteria.[10] There had to be something else driving his concern for safety.

From the Table of Embeddedness it is clear that the goods of agency that we are afraid of losing do not come in "one size fits all." There is an absolute right for people to be concerned with losing the level-one basic goods of agency *if* this fear is grounded in reasonable judgments about the facts. In the case of Padraig, his fears were *not* grounded in such reasonable judgments. The mortality statistics show that Padraig was opening himself up to more harm by driving his car on the interstate to see me than he would have been in coming to see me on the street where I lived. Yet Padraig chose to have me meet him in the suburbs. Why was this? For safety reasons, of course. When I confronted him with my conviction that there was no justifiable safety reason for me to meet him in the suburbs, he said that safety considerations were an intuitive thing and not subject to rational scrutiny. He wasn't going to act in a manner that made him feel "uncomfortable."

I can understand Padraig's defense of internalist-based intuitionism as a reason for his decision, but I cannot agree with it. For one thing one need merely turn to examples such as those in the 1950s not feeling comfortable eating at a lunch counter at which African Americans are allowed to eat (à la pre-1964 U.S. Civil Rights law). If I were to confront some person (call him Mel) who didn't want to have lunch with me at a resturant that served African Americans because he was "uncomfortable eating around those sort of people"—based upon Mel's internalist intuitions about safety, then I'd say that the origin of his "discomfort" was not rational but instead was based upon prejudice.

But what of this prejudice? Where does it come from? It is my opinion that it arises from attitudes that have been uncritically assimilated from one's family, friends, and larger society. It is *rhizomic* (to use the terminology of Deleuze and Guattari) in that it grows like a fungus in wild and often unconnected directions (Deleuze and Guattari 1987). Thus, the prejudice against African Americans, for example, had such bizarre exemplifications as an aversion to allow African Americans to swim in public swimming pools frequented by European Americans.[11] There is no scientific basis for this fear. There is no known "germ" to be caught from contact between the races or ethnic groups. Thus, this intuitive inclination is irrational.[12]

Sometimes these internalist-based fears cause parents to forego vaccinations that can prevent serious, potentially fatal diseases—from DPT to vaccinations against human papilloma virus (HPV)—and there is developing a culture of vaccination phobia that is not externalist supported and threatens the public health.[13]

If much of the average American's (and others) sense of safety is not based upon the externally based fear of absolute loss of the basic goods of agency (using precautionary reason) but internally based intuitions grounded in ill-founded prejudice, then we must attribute it to a psychological disposition that is the fruit of an unreflective, chaotic worldview. Because unreflective, chaotic worldviews are not to be trusted or followed, they should be given no credence in the formulation of public policy regarding risk assessment of safety.

We should not create public policy just to make the general public "feel good" (if "feel good" means to feed unreflective, chaotic worldviews). Unfortunately, the democratic process (in practice) seems to do just that. When situations of uncertainty arise among the general population, there is therefore an inclination to listen to a *strong voice* who claims he will "take care of everything." This is reinforced by repetition.[14] Thus, the consequence of people with unreflective, chaotic worldviews is to create a rush to judgment with a mob mentality that has little to do with a reasoned approach to how we are to achieve safety.

In fact, it is likely to produce the opposite effect. When we waste resources fighting imaginary pseudoproblems, there is less left to address real needs. This leaves uncovered other more pressing difficulties that might threaten public health safety. For example, one might imagine spending billions to fight potential enemies (national and terrorist threats) far beyond the point of diminishing returns with the effect of not having enough money to protect against real and immanent public health threats such as avian flu, drug-resistant tuberculosis, or the antibiotic-resistant bacteria that are at the heart of the hospital sepsis crisis. It is no small mistake to follow the example of Padraig and pay extravagantly to protect against imaginary internalist-based risks in the name of safety.

EVALUATING ACCEPTABLE RISK

In my book, *A Just Society*, I contend that policy considerations must be created within a context of public discourse informed by a common body of knowledge (Boylan 2004a: chapter 5). The common body of knowledge is a repository of the received facts and values from the community perspective. Any social dialogue depends upon this (Pöder 2009). The model of social dialogue that I would put forth for evaluating acceptable risk begins by the avoidance of the three fallacies mentioned above (goods myopia, money/power, and the externalist/internalist conflict).

In order to show the way this process should work in a positive way, I will turn to Rosemarie Tong's essay about her experience on a task force for preventative strategies and policies concerning avian flu (Tong 2008). Tong shows how a discussion of the relative value of public goods should be evaluated. What the task force (sponsored by the North Carolina Institute of Medicine/North Carolina Department of Public Health) did was to obtain representatives from important segments of the community and to create a process of social discourse that clarified for everyone just what the shared community worldview actually was.

This examination included not only the panel members but also input from the larger community including various sorts of health care professionals as well as volunteers. Establishing such a common base at the outset allowed profitable discussion to ensue. For example, when should a public health official be allowed to quarantine an area? This largely is due to the competing goods involved. Losses of level-one basic goods to the population tell more strongly than losses of economic goods to big business (because of the Table of Embeddedness). By making recourse to the common body of knowledge, some closure beyond mere legal rights was possible. Also important was establishing a list of best practices based upon the experience of Canada's response to the SARS epidemic.

And what of the politicians? By acting beforehand to shape policy, the panel preempted politicians and special interest groups who might intervene in a crisis with the force of their money and power to alter events to their own interests (rather than the public's, aka the shared community worldview). Strategic planning can most effectively proceed within the context of a well-established common body of knowledge. Thus the first important component in effective public risk assessment is to act before crises when the problem might not be skewed by special interests of money/power that are also subject to goods myopia.

The second important ingredient in these recommendations is not allowing passionate, internalist-based criteria to override the externalist-based inference to the most likely explanation. An example of this can be found in the recent scare about childhood inoculations possibly causing autism (in rare cases). Children in the United States have a .6 percent chance of becoming autistic. If significant numbers of children were not inoculated, then we might approach various other underdeveloped countries whose rates for childhood mortality due to preventable disease approaches 26 percent.

Thus indulging in the internalist fears concerning a possible link between childhood vaccinations and autism and not vaccinating one's child could result in markedly higher risks of mortality due to the diseases prevented in the vaccination. The differential (in the extreme) could be as much as forty-three times! Is it worth it to put our children at such higher risks due to the unproven risks (by externalist standards) in order to placate internalist fears and superstitions? Definitely not!

Societies cannot allow themselves to be so blackmailed––especially since all the externalist data we do have points in the opposite direction (Wallace et al. 2008, Schafer et al. 2008, Hettinger et al. 2008). Public health risk analysis must not take precautionary reason to the extreme of indulging in every scare tactic that special interest groups happen to dream up. Instead, we must foster a culture that honors decision making based upon inference to the best externalist information (scientific research).

CONCLUSION

The way forward in evaluating public health risk is to:

1. Avoid the three common fallacies—(a) goods myopia, (b) money/power, and (c) the externalist/internalist conflict.

2. Convene task forces in order to study impending public health problems *before* they occur and to garner a wide range of opinions from the community in order to shape a common body of knowledge that will be useful in creating a strategic plan of contingent action.

3. Study best practices of others who have had analogous problems.

4. Insist that the community publicly commit to externalist evidence over internalist fears and superstitions. It may be true that when there is a crisis that our reflective reasoning capacities are impaired or shut down. Regardless, if communities, countries, and the world adopted these guidelines for public health risk assessment, we would live in a safer and healthier world.

NOTES

1. I have argued for the ordering of these goods in Boylan 2004a, cf. Alvarez 2007. The argument recognizing the Table of Embeddedness comes from an analysis of the grounds of human action:

The Argument for the Moral Status of Basic Goods

1. All people, by nature, desire to be good—Assertion
2. In order to become good, one must be able to act—Fact
3. All people, by nature, desire to act—1, 2
4. People value what is natural to them—Assertion
5. What people value they wish to protect—Assertion
6. All people wish to protect their ability to act—3–5
7. Fundamental interpersonal "oughts" are expressed via our highest value systems: morality, aesthetics, and religion—Assertion
8. All people must agree, upon pain of logical contradiction, that what is natural and desirable to them individually is natural and desirable to everyone collectively and individually—Assertion
9. Everyone must seek personal protection for her own ability to act via religion, morality, and/or aesthetics—6, 7
10. Everyone upon pain of logical contradiction must admit that all other humans will seek personal protection of their ability to act via religion, morality, and/or aesthetics—8, 9
11. All people must agree, upon pain of logical contradiction, that since the attribution of the Basic Goods of agency are predicated generally, that it is inconsistent to assert idiosyncratic preferences—Fact
12. Goods that are claimed through generic predication apply equally to each agent, and everyone has a stake in their protection—10, 11
13. Rights and duties are correlative—Assertion
14. Everyone has at least a moral right to the Basic Goods of Agency, and others in the society have a duty to provide those goods to all—12, 13

2. "Embedded" in this context means the relative fundamental nature of the good for action. A more deeply embedded good is one that is more primary to action.

3. For a discussion of my views in the context of theories of distributive justice, see Gordon 2009.

4. Of course, I am not considering here those who recognize the relative embeddedness of the goods of agency and act anyway to elevate their personal claims for less embedded goods over another's claim for basic goods. For a discussion of some of these issues, see Kirsch (2011).

5. The classic case in probability texts is taking out black or white balls from a sack. If one replaces his selection after each try, the events are independent. However, if one does not replace the ball, then the next event is dependent upon the entire action sequence.

6. For a brief overview of the public health failures of the FEMA response to Hurricane Katrina, see Brinkley 2007, Van Heerden and Bryan 2006, and Horne 2008.

7. "Obama Recalls Being Followed, People Locking Doors on Him—In Other Words, Being a Black Man in America," http://www.huffingtonpost.com/2013/07/19/obama-racial-profiling_n_3624881.html.

8. *Crime in the United States: 1999*, 190. This data is based upon the *Uniform Crime Reports* that is submitted to the FBI and interpreted by statisticians.

9. *Traffic Fatalities and Fatality Rates: 1999.*

10. Another example is the Washington, D.C., sniper killer of 2002. Two of his six victims were killed as they pumped gasoline. I was appalled when attending a cub scout leaders meeting for my son's pack that several of the committee members were refusing to go to gasoline stations themselves because they feared getting shot. There are many thousands of gas stations in the region. There were two fatalities. The odds of the next one being *you* are very low. But these individuals decided to pay people to gas their cars for them rather than "take the risk." Considering the much higher risks they take every day, this is irrational based upon the externalist criteria.

11. One example of this phenomenon is the amusement park at Glen Echo, Maryland. It wasn't until the late 1960s that African Americans were allowed to swim in the public swimming pool. Some say that the controversy about interracial swimming caused the amusement park to close. On the other hand, the YMCA integrated its swimming facilities in the 1940s. The irrationally bizarre reasons behind swimming pool segregation are beyond the scope of this chapter except as they offer good reasons for not solely trusting "gut feelings" when it comes to matters of ethics and social philosophy.

12. One poignant example of this exact example comes from Michele Norris's "The Race Card Project," http://theracecardproject.com/: A white nine-year old child from the north is visiting relatives in Montgomery, Alabama, and innocently drinks from the "blacks only" drinking fountain. When her relative admonishes her the little girl says, "It didn't taste any different to me." This site is filled with short, pithy statements like these.

13. David Shenk, "The New Pandemic of Vaccine Phobia," http://www.theatlantic.com/national/archive/2009/10/the-new-pandemic-of-vaccine-phobia/28703/.

14. In the second edition of my informal logic text, *Critical Inquiry: The Process of Argument* (Boulder, CO: Westview, 2009), I have added a new logical fallacy: the fallacy of repetition—"The truth of a proposition is not affected by the number of times it is asserted—even though repetition may psychologically make it seem plausible to the audience. Each assertion of a proposition is an independent event and must be evaluated as such."

REFERENCES

Andorno, R. 2002. "Biomedicine and International Human Rights Law: In Search of a Global Consensus." *Bulletin of the World Health Organization* 80 (12): 959–63.

Audi, R., and N. Wolterstorff. 1997. *Religion in the Public Square*. Lanham, MD: Rowman & Littlefield.

Beauchamp, T., and J. Childress. 2009. *Principles of Biomedical Ethics*, 6th ed. New York: Oxford University Press.

Daniels, N. 2008. "Reflective Equilibrium." *The Stanford Encyclopedia of Philosophy*, Fall 2008 edition, ed. Edward N. Zalta. http://plato.stanford.edu/archives/fall2008/entries/reflective-equilibrium/.

Faunce, T. A. 2005. "Will International Human Rights Subsume Medical Ethics? Intersections in the UNESCO Universal Bioethics Declaration." *Journal of Medical Ethics* 31:173–78.

Harris, J. 2003. "Consent and End of Life Decisions." *Journal of Medical Ethics* 29:10–15.

Holm, S. 2009. "Global Concerns and Local Arguments: How a Localized Bioethics May Perpetuate Injustice." In *The Philosophy of Public Health*, edited by A. Dawson, 63–72. Farnham: Ashgate.

Kant, I. 1985. *Fundamental Principles of the Metaphysics of Morals*. Translated by Thomas Kingsmill Abbott. http://en.wikisource.org/wiki/Groundwork_of_the_Metaphysics_of_Morals.

Luther, E. 1986. *Ethik in der Medizin*. Halle: Martin Luther Universität.

Macklin, R. 1998. *Against Relativism: Cultural Diversity and the Search for Ethical Universals in Medicine*. New York: Oxford University Press.

Mann, J. M. 1997. "Medicine and Public Health, Ethics and Human Rights." *The Hastings Center Report* 27 (3): 6–13.

Rawls, J. 1996. *Political Liberalism (With a New Introduction and the "Reply to Habermas")*. New York: Columbia University Press.

6

Toward Green Bioethics and Health Rights

Lessons from Bhopal and Fukushima

Sanghamitra Padhy

ABSTRACT

Environmental disasters impinge on human health in a myriad of ways; in some cases it has an immediate effect and in some, it has a prolonged impact. The challenge for ethics and policy in the case of disaster has been to respond to issues of due care and protection from harm and risk of harms and promotion of health of individuals and communities. In biomedical ethics, the questions are usually posed as a health versus environment issue, where health is prioritized as a more urgent issue and environmental concerns are relegated to a secondary position. Whereas there are dangers posed to health by human interactions with the environment such as climate change, air and water pollution reveal a strong linkage between health, the environment, and justice. I argue for a biomedical approach that advances from a health care context to an ethics that includes the natural environment since how we treat our natural environment has important bearing on the health of individuals and communities.

INTRODUCTION

How often do we consider the ecological footprints of corporations and its implication for human health?[1] Consider the Union Carbide disastrous gas leak in Bhopal in 1984, and the nuclear meltdown at Chernobyl in 1986 and Fukushima in 2011. All three reveal the failure of corporations and the government to protect people from harm. This is seen not only in the impact on human life and environment but also in the presence of toxic pollution months and years after. In the case of Bhopal, there is also a failure to properly clean up the site.[2]

The three disasters are a call for precaution and a holistic disaster response plan. They point to a need for public policy to attend to the due care to victims, protection from harm and risks of harms, and promotion of health and environment of those affected. The lessons of Bhopal and environmental and health disasters in Chernobyl and Fukushima suggest that we need a deeper understanding of the connection between environmental and health ethics. It is important to ask: What should be the moral obligation of states and private actors toward protection and prevention of harm to the health of individuals and communities? Would a moral claim to health alone provide remedy to Bhopal and Fukushima victims, or should the boundaries of responsibility be extended to the care of the environment?

To answer such questions, I want to draw lessons from Beauchamp and Childress's framework of Principlism. They propose four principles: nonmalfeasance, beneficence, autonomy, and justice, to evaluate ethical responsibility due to individuals and communities. These principles draw from a framework of common morality, a set of shared judgments on morality, and hence are applicable to all persons and all places.[3] However, as some scholars argue, the theory is abstract, and its general clinical approach does not lend itself to all empirical data and hence suggests a case-based approach.[4]

While case studies are important for determining ethical violations, these are specific and do not provide a rubric to assess moral reasoning across cultures. And hence, what is needed, as John-Stewart Gordon claims, is a method of specification and balancing, based on empirical data.[5] This method has been found to be particularly useful to prioritize health rights of individuals and communities in varied cultural contexts, and it can be developed to determine moral obligations toward nature, individuals, and communities.

Mainstream debates in bioethics have thus far missed the inclusion of environment as a factor in health considerations—and the discipline as well. It is perceived that human health has a higher priority over the natural environment, and hence the treatment of health is disconnected from its natural contexts. Taking Bhopal as my case study and drawing a few lessons from Fukushima, I will suggest ways through which balance between environment and health can be attained through the expansion of a common morality framework.

This necessitates a revisit to Union Carbide's legacy in India and in Fukushima to determine moral principles regarding the responsibility of state and private actors to protect the health of victims in the case of such disasters.

THE TRAGEDY AT BHOPAL AND FUKUSHIMA

The tragedy began in Bhopal, India. Forty tons of methyl isocyanide leaked from Union Carbide Corporation's fertilizer and pesticide plant on December 3, 1984.[6] The gas from the explosion killed about three thousand people in the first week of the accident, approximately thirty thousand more in the twenty-six years since, and it caused physical and psychological impairments to an additional fifty thousand people.[7] Survivors suffer from varied health damages such as ocular, respiratory, skin and blood ailments, miscarriages, cancer, and psychological traumas.

While corporate and state entities dismiss Bhopal as a one-time incident or accident, it represents an ongoing crisis. The victims continue to suffer from various respiratory and skin ailments, and children of victims have had vision, respiratory, and physical disabilities. To the post-Bhopal generation, contaminants left at the toxic site continue to harm, as chemicals have seeped into the water supply, posing environmental and health risks. Residents in resettlement camps complain of stomach ailments from consuming contaminated water.

Fukushima was assessed as a meltdown in the Daiichi nuclear plant triggered by the Japanese earthquake and tsunami, although as evidence shows it was an avoidable disaster.[8] Its radioactive materials contaminated neighboring land, water, and agricultural produce, and clean-up operations at the site may take decades. Further, it portends health risks in the future. While there has been an immediate outpour of public support for victims of Fukushima, the challenge of continuous medical support remains a vital need.

THE FOUR-PRINCIPLE APPROACH

Bioethics concerns itself with the protection and promotion of the health of individuals and communities. Bioethics provides a set of moral norms to guide state's obligations toward protection and promotion of health, which is recognized as a common morality of societies. The extent of obligations may vary depending upon the resources of the state, but minimally it recognizes that the protection of the health of populations involves an obligation not to inflict harm and redress victims in case of injuries to health. While limiting harm is a fundamental goal of ethics, there are differences with respect to assessing harm and how obligations of agents and entitlements of victims are determined.

In ethics the rights and obligations to health are defended through two main frameworks: consequentialism holds that the rightness and wrongness of actions are to be determined by their good and bad consequences; and deontology, which judges the rightness of an action based on duty and moral obligations.

In their founding principles, Beauchamp and Childress explore morality and obligations toward health not as an absolute criterion as many deontologists would claim, but as standard principles to guide responsibility toward the protection of health. These principles are guides to public policy, and its postulates are: nonmaleficence, which is the obligation not to inflict harm on others; beneficence, which is the positive obligation to promote the health of those harmed or are at risk of being harmed; and autonomy and justice.[9]

Even so, these principles primarily define the relationship between doctor and patient; their emphasis on the responsibilities due to patients with regard to their health care and life of dignity. These tools not only provide specificity to policies but also balance the conflicting positions on how human health is to be assessed. For instance, should imposing risks or harm on populations exclude restrictions on liberty posed during public health emergencies? As a practical tool to assess ethics of decisions, Principlism demarcates how harm is to be assessed in the Bhopal case and what should be the due care to patients.

Even so, Principlism promises flexibility in analyzing how health care can be improved. It is limited in its inclusion of factors such as the environment that may impact health. This questions the conventional divide of clinical health and the environment as separate issues. Contemporary issues such as climate change demonstrate that health and environment have a deep and complex relationship.[10] David B. Resnik and Christopher J. Portier argue that access to natural resources and exposure to environmental hazards has a definite impact on health. Further, assessments of justice in terms of vulnerable groups are limited to manifested health impacts, omitting potential harms due to the environment.

The question, then, is whether justice should only be limited to humans—or extend to the natural world?[11] While Principlism provides fundamental values through which health-related decisions can be assessed, its scope needs to be expanded to include the social and natural aspects of individuals' and communities' worldviews.

In human rights law, health is recognized as a fundamental human right that obligates states to ensure the protection and promotion of health of all individuals in its jurisdiction. Health and human rights enjoy a unique, symbiotic relationship; health worsens when human rights are ignored, and human rights abuses impact health.[12] Jonathan Mann, former head of WHO's AIDs program, compares this reciprocal relationship of human rights and health to natural allies; human rights is considered a formidable tool for advancing health standards in the world.[13]

International Human rights law recognizes the importance of health to human rights in several treaties and covenants. Article 12 of the Internationl Covenant on Economic, Social, and Cultural Rights (ICESCR) guarantees the right to health to all individuals and communities.[14] As a human right, health is recognized as an obligation of the state, and governmental responsibilities include: 1) respecting rights, meaning the state cannot violate rights directly, 2) protecting rights through the prevention of the violation of rights by non-state actors, and provision of redress to people in case of violation, and 3) fulfilling rights through its various apparatuses.

This suggests that the right to health is not only a negative right, where the state protects individual rights from violation, but is also a positive right requiring the state to adopt measures to promote the health of its people.[15] The human right status guarantees health rights equal protection under the law, whereby different treatment must be based on objective and reasonable criteria. This is an important safeguard that human rights provide to ensure justice in health rights.

Another corollary of a human rights perspective to health is the inclusion of the participative element. Nobel Laureate Amartya Sen observes, "Freedom from avoidable ill health and from escapable mortality" are the most important freedoms, and this can be best insured through participatory politics in which people are not mere patients but agents of change.[16] He emphasizes that health rights are integral to human freedom. The right to health includes two other derivatives: scientific progress and the environment.

While the dissemination of scientific knowledge and progress is considered a fundamental human right, the environment has yet to gain a formal status in human rights law. The next section will evaluate the concept of harm and risks of harm principles to elucidate how ethics and law can integrate health and environment.

THE CONCEPT OF HARM

Harm, normatively speaking, is an act of wronging or adversely affecting another party's interests. Wrongdoing, as Beauchamp and Childress note, is caused by the violation of a right, whereas harm can be caused irrespective of a wrong act, say a natural disaster.[17] They define harm as actions that may thwart, defeat, or set back some party's interest and specifically with causing pain, suffering, and death.

Harms are distinguished between ones caused by natural factors and those caused by agents. To environmentalists, the question is how to separate natural factors from unnatural ones. Climate change has made it clear that human actions are responsible for the degradation of nature and unnatural weather patterns.

From an environmentalist standpoint, there are three important claims made about the relation between harm and nature.[18] The first view held by the deep ecology school is that only naturally occurring states possess moral value, and this should be weighed in public policy and technology policymaking.[19] An important critique of their work extends to technological interventions such as genetically modified organisms as human attempts to create nature. A second view (a variant of deep ecology) holds that the integrity of our ecosystem needs to be maintained and that all things have an intrinsic moral worth warranting protection.

Some scholars have expanded on this notion of moral worth to moral ways of dealing with nature. Christopher Stone claims that the environment needs to be treated with sensitivity, as it transforms us into better human beings.[20] He contends that the human-nature relationship is also about the inescapable construction of ideal human character.[21] A third view is that there needs to be protections from human interventions that deteriorate the environmental quality, including protecting the environment for human health and social well-being.

At a more general level, this debate suggests that the principle of harm needs to shift from the traditional divide of natural and agents to a more expansive notion of human interventions. Hence, technological interventions need to be assessed not only for the value or benefits its adds but also for the human, social, and environmental costs.

HARM, OBLIGATION, AND DUE CARE

The obligations of the actors involve an avoidance of harm and the risks of harm. Hence, actions by individuals and other parties are supposed to refrain from malicious or harmful intent and avoid harm and risk of harm.[22] This concept can be expanded to determine the state's obligations to human health. If these are extended to the realm of actions that arise from industrial accidents, production of dangerous chemicals in residential areas could be considered a public harm.

The obligation not to impose harm also includes taking steps to prevent harm from being imposed. In the case of environmental hazards, state negligence to take precautionary measures exposes people to harm and risks of harm. For example, the construction of a pesticide plant in Bhopal within city limits placed citizens at risk, even if the state did not knowingly or intentionally cause the harm. Nuclear technology discourse in Japan points to a similar trajectory as the political agenda of crafting a strong national identity has subsumed all opposition to nuclear energy, and this has resulted in policies favoring the industry.[23]

In India, as a promise of a green revolution, Union Carbide was allowed to set up a fertilizer and pesticide plant in 1969 in Bhopal, a one-thousand-year-old town with little infrastructural capacity for growth. The municipal government's protests regarding the production of methyl isocyanite were overruled by the central and state governments' keenness on UCC's continued presence because it provided employment opportunities to thousands of people.[24]

The operation of a fertilizer plant in the midst of a bustling city and the lack of communication about the plant to residents is itself an act of harm. This disaster changed the contour of how we define industrial risk by making us realize the potency of the industry to cause mass death, injury, illness, and loss beyond the parameters of the industry's boundary.[25] Prior to this time, the notion of industrial risk focused on the workforce and the workplace.

However, the definition of harm should incorporate immediate and evidential impact on health. To the environmentalist, this is especially problematic, as environmental impact assessments tend to be based on short-term studies and the ecological loss to community life is rarely estimated. For instance, reports on the aftermath of Fukushima showed deep psychological trauma, especially for the elderly.[26] Sugimoto et al. have given accounts of farmers saying, "For generations, my family has lived in a close relationship with this land. I will feel accursed for losing the lands that my ancestors passed down to me . . . watching my cattle die is like witnessing the killing of my own children."[27]

In addition, the challenge of cleanup adds up to the risk of exposure and harm. Cleanup at the Fukushima site, given the nature of radioactive materials, will take decades, and hence exposure to harm remains an unknown factor. In Bhopal, it is evident in the denial game of both the state and the corporation to clean up the Bhopal site. There is evidence that toxics left at the site have contaminated groundwater quality in the vicinity of the abandoned site, and those living in resettlement colonies have had ongoing health issues.[28]

As Beauchamp and Childress argue, harm also involves a standard of due care by the agents as demanded of a reasonable and prudent person.[29] The claim to due care determines whether the agent who is causally responsible for the risk is legally or morally responsible to take sufficient and appropriate care to avoid causing harm. In the case of Fukushima, Chernobyl, and Bhopal, agents have not done enough—imposing unreasonable risks of harm to the human population.

The notion of due care also draws attention to the social and cultural context, as treatment of patients and how resources are distributed can be detrimental to the community sense of justice. In the case of Bhopal, miscarriage has deleterious effects in the Indian social context, and this has been overlooked by medical practice. There are many social stigmas attached to women who cannot bear children—she is looked down upon by members of her family, her husband, and by society at large.[30] Furthermore, the triage concept used to assess beneficiaries of medical help was not a fruitful exercise, as cultural beliefs such as respect for the elderly prioritized how families took care of the patients.

Overall, Bhopal suggests a failure to assess risks and protect citizens. While ethical and legal theory has pointed out these responsibilities, they have also been limited in assessing the environmental costs of the tragedy. The assessment of justice tends to focus only on manifested health impacts, not potential harms to the environment. In the narrow sense, justice is an instrument for human well-being and respects individuals and the community's sense of relationship with the natural world.[31] Our sense of justice needs to be expanded to include the social and natural aspects of individuals' and communities' worldviews.

REVISITING BHOPAL

In the 1960s, India began to modernize its economy and society through scientific and technological interventions in the agricultural sector. This brought about increased use of pesticides and insecticides and intensive farming.

The Green Revolution, as it was called, promised self-sufficiency in food supplies. Union Carbide's Bhopal fertilizer plant was an integral component of the vision of the Green Revolution;[32] it was designed to manufacture pesticides and fertilizers in

India. The establishment of UCC in India was celebrated as a profitable venture; to the manufacturer it meant low operating cost, cheap labor, and exclusive access to the Indian market, and to the consumer it seemed less expensive to have the plant in India than to import fertilizers and the Indian state gained from the capital investment.

The vision of the Green Revolution was considered so perfect that neither the state nor the corporation took measures to assess the risk factors. Nor did they inform people of the hazards of a toxic industry within city limits. There was a complete lack of preparedness, as revealed in the growth of residential settlements near the factory and in cost-cutting initiatives by the company. The company's desire for and the state's overemphasis on economic growth contributed to the worst toxic disaster in history. It was a preventable catastrophe.

On the night of December 2, 1984, what resulted from the leakage was[33] the transformation of the bustling town of Bhopal to ghostly one. Dead bodies and animal carcasses littered the streets, people ran in panic, and many gasped for life.[34] The city had no disaster response plan, and the administrators were caught unaware and were ignorant as to evacuation procedures. The city lacked the medical infrastructure to cope with the injured. Hospitals and clinics accounted for a total of 1,800 hospital beds and three hundred doctors. In the first week ten thousand people were admitted to the largest government hospital, equipped with only three hundred beds. The lack of infrastructure and the inability of the state to handle the crisis created a dialogue of inaction and inability to respond to people's needs.

Since there was also the ignorance of the exact nature of the chemical that caused the injuries, there was no immediate available treatment for patients. UCC doctors claimed that the gas was only a nonlethal gas and that the mild irritation and breathlessness caused by it was short term. Hence, only symptomatic treatment with the help of eye drops and steroids was given to the patients in the initial few weeks. But these symptoms posed a greater health issue than was perceived at that time.

The crisis and the response to it give rise to ethical and human rights questions about corporate and state responsibility toward health. The violation of the zoning law, allowance of a hazardous industry in a residential area, and denial of health care to victims is against the principle of nonmaleficence; it also violates individuals' right to health through denial of information to them about the site, and the state did not make any attempts to protect people's rights from violation by the corporation.

RESPONSIBILITY OF DUE CARE

The remedial measures attempted by the state and corporation further violated ethical norms of justice for the vulnerable, which continues even now, as the state has allowed the polluters to escape liability for cleaning the toxic site. In the process, the state poses risks of harm to post-Bhopal generations.

The relief and rehabilitation measures instituted by the state were harmful and discriminatory. There was no accurate information given to the people about the number of deaths, the gas leak, the reasons for their clinical symptoms, and their appropriate treatment. Shrivastava notes in his study that there was no one account of the number of deaths that occurred in the first week itself; figures varied from 1,754, as stated by the government in the lawsuit filed in New York, to 2,000 by newspapers, to 3,000 by voluntary organizations, to 6,000 by the local people.[35] One reason for this range is that all available medical help was directed toward caring for the engaged, hence few resources were available to register the dead, perform autopsies, issue death certificates, and systematically cremate or bury the bodies.

Treatment offered to victims was even more lackadaisical. The few autopsies that were conducted in the first week detected some form of cyanide poisoning to be the main cause of death,[36] but medical treatment to patients for cyanide poisoning became a controversial issue, one, because doctors were unaware of the long-term impact of cyanide poisoning, and two, because the government did not allow medical professionals to use sodium thiosulphate, the sole antidote to cyanide poisoning.

Complaints of victims were various, such as breathlessness, dry cough, chest pains, restrictive lung diseases, dry eyes, miscarriages, and still births. Some of these symptoms were related to cyanide poisoning.[37] The fact that the government had allowed the production of cyanide in the Carbide plant without safety procedures helped Union Carbide with regard to liability.

The Madhya Pradesh relief operations claimed that the effects of the 1984 disaster were not long lasting and the case could be closed. On the contrary, studies by the International Medical Commission on Bhopal demonstrate that Bhopal Syndrome has long-term health effects on multiple body systems.[38] Studies showed evidence of chromosomal disorders, as shown by disabilities in children of victims who were exposed to the gas.[39] This evidence demands a policy that would not approach Bhopal as one "incident" or "accident" to be settled through compensation, but a tragedy that has impacted people at several levels and is a continued issue.[40]

ECOLOGICAL ISSUES

There are primarily two kinds of ecological issues here: 1) the immediate ecological loss and 2) the toxic chemicals left at the site. The ecological damage such as animal and plant loss caused by the accident was treated as a secondary issue, given the demand for resources for human damages.

While this was a big footprint, it was ignored, and there was neither any scientific study on the effects of MIC on plant and animal life nor monitoring of plant and animal health. The case of continued pollution left at the site is far more controversial, as the factory remains contaminated with thousands of tons of highly toxic chemicals in sheds, storerooms, and solar evaporation ponds, and they pose health hazards. Greenpeace reports of 1999 and 2002 document the presence of chloroform, lead, mercury, and a series of other chemicals in the breast milk of nursing women who live near the factory.[41] Yet Union Carbide, and, as of 2001, Dow Chemicals, refuse any liability for cleaning up the site.

The *New York Times* cites an e-mail by Scott Wheeler, a company spokesman, on Dow's liability to clean up: "As there was never any ownership, there is no responsibility and no liability—for the Bhopal tragedy or its aftermath," and he made it clear that Dow could not finance cleaning up the site because it could potentially open up the company's liabilities. The blame game of cleanup that has ensued as a result is one of a corporate refusal to own up to its responsibilities and of a state more interested in economic development and financial investment in India than protecting human health from harm and risks of harm.[42]

In a letter to the Indian ambassador to the United States in 2006, the Dow chairman, Andrew N. Liveris, sought assurance that it would not be held liable for the mess on the old factory site "in your efforts to ensure that we have the appropriate investment climate." A recent report by *Frontline* has a call by Ratan Tata, one of India's big industrialists, to open a consortium of industrial volunteers to clean up the site, which in the process legitimized Dow's refusal to remediation. Liabilities aside, even the steps taken to clean up the toxins are questionable.

What is striking in this market-technology-state partnership is that human health and the environment were not worthy considerations in the debate. The cause of the Bhopal tragedy and the remedial actions both by the corporate agent and the state have failed to protect people from harm and have exposed them to greater health risks.

A recent ruling of the Madhya Pradesh District Court sentenced the responsible agents to prison for two years, similar to the penalty imposed in road accidents. This needs to be revisited, especially since the factors of the UCC gas leak case point to the fact that this was neither an incident nor an accident, but an act of negligence and a failure to take appropriate safety measures.

Compensation is an even murkier issue—not only because of the numbers that have been accounted for but also the process of determining the beneficiaries of compensation.[43] For the corporation, in its varied lawsuits filed first in New York and then in India, it was a case of comparing an Indian life to an American life. The state simply underestimated the figure of the population affected by the gas.

Initially it attempted to hold Union Carbide liable in the American courts through class action lawsuits, but this failed. The result was a 1994 out-of-court settlement mediated by the Indian Supreme Court and Union Carbide, promising a $470-million-package to victims—which would compensate five hundred thousand people an average of $550 per person.

The procedures for compensation also fell short. The application process divides claims based on a six-step process: A for no damage, B for those who recovered fully after treatment, C for permanent damage after treatment, D for temporary partial disablement, E for permanent partial disablement, and F for permanent total disablement. What these criteria emphasize are only some clinical aspects of the disease, and hence did not take into account the social definition of disabilities. For instance, there has been no initiative to take gender into account or stress-related illness. Sterility in women was not merely a clinical problem, as sterility was a ground for exclusion from social processes.

The tragedy thus raises questions of not only how to protect people's health but also how to prevent future health issues, as the toxins remain at the site. Legally it remains a question of liability and compensation to the victims; socially it remains a question of how to deal with the pressures on the community due to deaths, disabilities, and loss of labor; economically, it remains a question of how to deal with the various damages financially. These questions point to the larger issue of the structures of domination and subordination in society and the particular use of reason to subjugate nature.

The International Medical Commission on Bhopal (ICMB) in its recommendations of 1994 emphasizes that relief and rehabilitation in Bhopal needs to broaden its understanding of the challenges of health damages.[44] It has stressed that health practitioners and the Bhopal government need to do the following:

1. Reorganize the health system to establish a network of community-based primary care clinics.
2. The gas-related disease categories need to be broadened to include central nervous system and psychological (post-traumatic stress disorder) injury.
3. Rehabilitation medicine, including both Western and Indian expertise, needs to be developed.
4. Health data collected by various government research teams such as the Indian Council of Medical Research needs to be published and available for the general population. This is not only important in the case of Bhopal but will provide the knowledge base for future policies.
5. Gas victims to have the right of access to their medical records.
6. Criteria for compensation should include medical, economic, and social damage to the victims.

The only recommendation that has been accepted so far has been the creation of community-based primary health clinics. These smaller clinics have been able to attend to the holistic sense of health care and resettlement better than government-run centers. It is here the state ought to integrate both Western notions and Islamic and Hindu notions of what constitutes good health.

The tragedy caused the victims to extend these familiar notions of duty and right action to comprehend the loss of family members, their suffering, and the loss of the immediate environment. Hence, an understanding of the victims' worldview is necessary to achieve redress for the injustices suffered and to represent the victim's point of view.

Along with the social factors, ecology needs to be added as a relief and compensatory measure of evaluations, and in terms of the larger worldview of locals. The quintessential relation between society, health, and the environment needs to be recognized by practitioners and policymakers. The human right to health can be protected based on the social relationship people have with the natural world.

In the case of Bhopal and Fukushima, or any other case of industrial pollution, the concept of health needs to include the environment for three reasons: one, the environment is an instrument to good health, and that the ecological footprints of Union Carbide, TEPCO, the gas/radioactive leak and the toxic wastes at the site pose health hazards to people living in the vicinity. Hence, ecological costs of technological risks need to be assessed to protect the health of the population.

Two, our interaction with nature is guided by our moral and cultural values; hence when nature is destroyed, it presents as an imbalance in our personal being. Three, since environment is a borrowed property from the future,[45] humans have responsibility to protect the environment not only for the needs of this generation but also for the health of future generations.

Borrowing from this notion of ecological stewardship, one can argue that technological practices with potential to impact human health need to be evaluated from this perspective of what we owe to the future. Hence, the moral and legal considerations of health needs to be expanded to include not only societal and patient health but also how the natural surroundings enable the exercise of health rights by communities and individuals.

NOTES

1. This is probably true when a corporate action causes public health hazards, but even so these are limited to considerations of immediate health injuries and rarely are factors such as long-term health injuries, environmental damages, and social costs taken into account.

2. It is estimated that there is still about 350 tons of toxic waste in the site. The government has finally decided to incinerate these toxics in some facilities of the government in cities such as Nagpur and Indore. However, locals in these cities are against the initiative, as they are apprehensive of another disaster like Bhopal. See "Bhopal Gas Victims Oppose Disposal of Waste in Nagpur," *Times of India*, July 17, 2011.

3. Ibid.

4. See Albert R. Jonsen and Stephen E. Toulmin, *The Abuse of Casuistry* (Berkeley: University of California Press, 1988).

5. Jochen Vollman, John-Stewart Gordon, and Oliver Rauprich, "Applying the Four-Principle Approach," in *Bioethics* 25 (6) (2011): 293–300.

6. For Union Carbide, this accident was only a technical malfunction and failure of employees in India. In fact, right after the disaster Warren Anderson clarified to his stockholders that this case would have no financial impact on their stock options.

7. It must be noted that there is no accurate estimate of the death toll; government reports put the death toll at 1,754, whereas media reports based on the scene assessment place it at about 3,000. Local residents claim around 6,000 deaths. See Paul Shrivastava, *Bhopal: Anatomy of a Crisis* (Cambridge, MA: Ballinger Publishing Company, 1987).

8. Lincoln L Davies, "Beyond Fukushima: Disasters, Nuclear Energy and Energy Law," *Brigham Young University Law Review* 6 (2011): 1937.

9. *Supra* note 3.

10. See David B. Resnik and Christopher J. Portier, "Environment and Health," in Mary Crowley, ed., *From Birth to Death and Bench to Clinic: The Hastings Center Bioethics Briefing Book for Journalists, Policymakers, and Campaigns* (Garrison, NY: The Hastings Center, 2008), 59–62, http://www.thehastingscenter.org/Publications/BriefingBook/Detail.aspx?id=2170&t erms=resnik+and+%23filename+*.html.

11. Ramachandra Guha, *Social Ecology* (New Delhi: Oxford University Press, 1994).

12. Sofia Gruskin, Michael A. Grodin, George J. Annas, and Stephen P. Marks, ed., *Perspectives on Health and Human Rights* (New York: Routledge, 2005).

13. Jonathan M. Mann, Lawrence Gostin, Sofia Gruskin, Troyan Brennan, Zita Lazzarini, and Harvey Fineberg, "Health and Human Rights," in *Health and Human Rights: A Reader*, edited by Jonathan M. Mann, Sofia Gruskin, Michael A. Grodin, and George J. Annas (New York: Routledge, 1999).

14. ICESCR (International Covenant of Civil and Political Rights). 1966 GA Resolution 2200 (XXI), UN GAOR, 21st Session, Supplement No. 16, at 49, UN document A/6316 UN, Geneva.

15. Human rights law does, however, recognize that resource and other constraints can impose limits on how states take measures to promote health. In practical terms, this means that the right to health is more than just passing a law.

16. Amartya Sen, "Health and Development," *Bulletin of the World Health Organization* 77 (1999): 619.

17. Tom L. Beauchamp and James F. Childress, *Principles of Biomedical Ethics* (New York: Oxford University Press, 2009).

18. Gregory E. Kaebnick, "Nature, Human Nature, and Biotechnology," in *From Birth to Death and Bench to Clinic*, edited by Mary Crowley (Garrison, NY: The Hastings Center, 2008), 117–20.

19. Alexander Gillespie, *International Environmental Law, Policy and Ethics* (Oxford: Clarendron Press, 1997).

20. Christopher Stone, "Ethics and International Environmental Law," in *Oxford Handbook of International Environmental Law*, edited by Daniel Bodansky, Jutta Brunnée, and Ellen Hey (Oxford: Oxford University Press, 2007), 291–314.

21. Alexander Gillespie, *International Environmental Law, Policy and Ethics* (Oxford: Clarendron Press, 1997).

22. Beauchamp and Childress, *Principles of Biomedical Ethics*.

23. Sebastian M. Pfotenhauer, Christopher F Jones, Krishanu Saha, and Sheila Jasanoff, "Learning From Fukushima," *Issues in Science and Technology* 28 (3) (Spring 2012): 79–84.

24. Town and Country Planning Department, *Bhopal Development Plan* (Bhopal: Municipal Corporation, 1975).

25. Usha Ramanathan, "Communities at Risk: Industrial Risk in Indian Law," *Economic and Political Weekly*, October 9, 2004, 4521–27.

26. A. Sugimoto, S. Krull, S. Nomura, T. Morita, and M. Tsubokura, "Perspectives: Lessons from the Fukushima Nuclear Crisis," World Health Organization, *Bulletin of the World Health Organization* 90 (8) (August 2012): 629–30.

27. Ibid.

28. Ruth Stringer, Iryna Labunska, Kevin Brigden, and David Santillo, "Chemical Stockpiles at Union Carbide in Bhopal: An Investigation," Greenpeace Research Laboratories Technical Note 12/2002, November 2002.

29. Beauchamp and Childress, *Principles of Biomedical Ethics*.

30. "Gas Disaster Results in 400 Abortions," *MP Chronicle*, October 4, 1985.

31. Guha, *Social Ecology*.

32. Prior to this, UCC was mainly a battery manufacturing plant.

33. MIC gas leaked into the water storage tank, and an operator at the Union Carbide plant noticed a small leak of methyl isocyanate (MIC) gas and increasing pressure inside a storage tank. A faulty valve allowed a ton of water used for cleaning internal pipes to mix with forty tons of MIC. Despite efforts, this could not be checked, as the safety measures in place had not been in use in the plant for several weeks to cut down costs. As a result, the small leak of MIC gas could not be contained, and in a couple of hours the safety valve gave way and sent a plume of poisonous MIC gas into the air in Bhopal.

34. One person living near the plant in a slum hut said, "I sleep with my mouth open, and so I was the first to awaken around 1:00 am. I was coughing badly and my eyes were burning. I ran outside to see what was happening. And I found people were running in all directions, all at once. I woke up my wife and we just ran away, wherever we could go." Cited in K. S. Dhillon, "Bhopal's Deadliest Night—A Case Study," *Bhopal Post*, June 23, 2010.

35. Paul Shrivastava, *Bhopal: Anatomy of a Crisis* (Cambridge: Ballinger Publishing Company, 1987), 65.

36. Union Carbide Corporation, *Bhopal Methyl Isocyanate Incident Investigation Team Report* (Danbury, CT: Union Carbide Corporation, March 1985).

37. "The Bhopal Disaster Aftermath: An Epidemiological and Socio-Medical Survey," Bangalore: Medico Friends Circle, 1985.

38. Beauchamp and Childress, *Principles of Biomedical Ethics*.

39. See "Methyl Isocyanate Exposure and Growth Patterns of Adolescents in Bhopal," 290 (14) (October 8, 2003), http://jama.ama-assn.org/cgi/content/full/290/14/1856.

40. As Paul Shivastava notes, Bhopal has meant different things to different stakeholders. To the industry it is an incident, to the state it is an accident, to local people a disaster or tragedy. While the event may be the same, the definitions suggest the meaning of Bhopal to each of these stakeholders.

41. Stringer, Labunska, Brigden, and Santillo, "Chemical Stockpiles at Union Carbide in Bhopal: An Investigation."

42. Somini Sengupta, "Decades Later, Toxic Sludge Torments Bhopal," *New York Times*, July 7, 2008, http://www.nytimes.com/2008/07/07/world/asia/07bhopal.html?pagewanted=1&_r=2&ref=Bhopal.

43. A report published in the *Washington Post* in 1994 revealed that only twenty-six thousand claims had been settled by 1994, and most of these were in the better-off thirty-six city wards affected by the gas.

44. "Bhopal Disaster and the BP Oil Spill," *The Hindu*, August 4, 2010, http://www.thehindu.com/opinion/op-ed/article550062.ece.

45. See World Commission on Environment and Development, *Our Common Future* (Oxford: Oxford University Press, 1987).

Discussion Topics: Part IV

Wanda Teays

1. What do you believe are the most pressing health care issues we face? What should be our priorities as a society?
2. What should we do to achieve justice in health care? Set out four steps that could be taken to address some of the major health inequities (e.g., as noted in the first three chapters of this section).
3. Ralph de la Torre, chairman and chief executive officer of Steward Health Care System, says he's created the ultimate business model for the age of Obamacare: a national chain of no-frills hospitals:

   De la Torre said that Steward would deliver low-cost, state-of-the-art care through the use of advanced electronic medical records systems, new preventive medicine approaches, and the standardizing of everything throughout the chain, from billing to emergency room procedures. . . . Under the Affordable Care Act, the White House is encouraging the formation of large groups of hospitals and doctors that can manage lots of patients, as insurance companies move from simply reimbursing providers for tests and procedures to paying them to keep people healthy. The Obama administration refers to these groups as accountable care organizations, or ACOs.

   It's one of the White House's chief strategies for lowering health-care costs. "We created the concept of the ACO on paper in '08," de la Torre says. "Our business plan is an ACO on steroids" (See Devin Leonard, "Private Equity's Hospitals: A Business Model for the Obamacare Era?," *Business Week*, August 29, 2013).

   Answer the following:
   a. Is there any downside to Torre's "no-frills" hospitals?
   b. Is there a better alternative for making health care more readily accessible?

4. In their essay on global health justice Gostin and Dhai point out that we tend to focus on high-profile, heart-wrenching cases in health care rather than systemic problems. Can you think of examples of such wrenching cases that grab our attention instead of health issues related to survival needs? What steps do you think should be taken to make systemic change on the global level so issues like poverty, access to vaccinations, and medication could be addressed?

5. Gostin and Dhai argue that the root of poverty and health problems links to the power differentials between economic classes—not those of the North versus the South. Poor people in rich countries may be at the same level of disadvantage as their counterparts in poor nations, even if they are living in a wealthier society. Picture yourself as the member of a team of advocates who are undertaking a special kind of ad campaign—to address global health inequities. What are three things you'd do in your campaign to try to turn things around to improve the life expectancy of the poor?

6. Given limited access to health care, should groups form their own health maintenance organizations (HMOs)? And could this be accomplished on an international scale? One possible model is with Native American tribes that negotiated with the state of New Mexico about setting up their own managed care health organization in conjunction with state programs like Medicaid. In 2001, Kaiser put in an HMO for Native Americans in California:

Available to all 103 federally recognized tribes throughout California (approximately 50,000 members), this program provides affordable access to Blue Cross coverage including office visits, prescription benefits, hospitalization and other services.

"As Native Americans become more economically self-sufficient, they have sought to purchase health insurance with their own funds from private health plans," said Assemblywoman Helen Thomson, who sponsored last year's legislation that allows tribes to purchase private health insurance. "I applaud Blue Cross for its effort in reaching out to a population that has historically had difficulty buying health insurance." (See "Blue Cross of California Today Announced a New Health-Care Program Specifically for Native Americans," *Biz Journals*, July 24, 2001).

7. Consider—and construct—several analogies to health care (e.g., the public school system). What sort of analogy would provide the most equitable model for a universal health care system?

8. How can we balance the needs of the aging with the needs of pregnant women, infants, and children? What sorts of steps should be taken to address the medical—and ethical—issues at the beginning and end of life?

9. In her chapter on global aging, Rosemarie Tong looks at the fact that care for the elderly often falls on the children, and this can be morally problematic. Equally problematic is the question of who should care for elderly who have no children to care for them (or whose children refuse to help them). Tong notes that many women and men are childless because they lose their children to disease or war. In addition, childless single men and women are particularly

vulnerable in their old age if they are poor. Can you suggest three or four ideas for addressing this situation?

10. Michael Boylan looks at the issues of public safety and the notion of acceptable risk. Movies like *Outbreak* and *Contagion* present the dilemmas that arise around fast-moving epidemics. One such issue is that, in many cases, there is no readily available supply of vaccines, and those available are in limited supply. This leads to questions about triage.
   Answer the following:
   a. How do we decide, and who decides, which individuals or groups have priority in access to such resources as vaccines, treatment centers, and so on?
   b. What sorts of plan(s) should we put in effect now—before an epidemic or a pandemic strikes?

11. Speaking of acceptable risk and public health, a number of hospital patients were put at risk from contaminated surgical equipment used on a patient with Creutzfeldt-Jakob disease (aka "mad cow" disease). Read about the incident in New Hampshire reported on September 21, 2013:

   Health officials have confirmed that a patient who underwent neurosurgery at a New Hampshire hospital earlier this year had Creutzfeldt-Jakob disease. The death . . . prompted authorities in two states to warn that as many as 13 patients may have been exposed to surgical equipment used during the patient's surgery, thus to the same disease.

   The now-deceased patient had undergone neurosurgery at Catholic Medical Center in Manchester. . . . By the time this diagnosis was suspected, equipment used in the patient's surgery had been used [in] several other operations. This raised the possibility that the equipment might have been contaminated—especially since normal sterilization procedures are not enough to get rid of the disease proteins, known as prions, tied to Creutzfeldt-Jakob disease—thus potentially exposing the other patients to infection.

   Eight other patients at the same Manchester hospital were being monitored for Creutzfeldt-Jakob disease. Massachusetts health authorities noted the next day that five Cape Cod Hospital patients may have been exposed to Creutzfeldt-Jakob disease too because their surgeons this summer later used the same potentially contaminated medical equipment as in the New Hampshire facility (See Greg Botelho, "Case of Creutzfeldt-Jakob Disease Confirmed in New Hampshire," *CNN*, September 21, 2013).
   Answer the following:
   a. To what degree should steps be taken to go beyond normal sterilization procedures in medical settings?
   b. What is an acceptable risk in such cases—though very rare—as here with Creutzfeldt-Jakob disease? Offer some ideas about what should be done to minimize or prevent such incidents as this.

12. Foster Farms, the tenth largest chicken producer in the United States, with $2.3 billion in sales for 2012, is now facing a public relations disaster with an outbreak of salmonella that has sickened hundreds of people. The U.S.

Department of Agriculture (USDA) cited the company for unsanitary plant conditions and a dozen instances of fecal matter on carcasses. David Pierson, Diana Marcum, and Tiffany Hsu report:

Foster Farms is an example of how salmonella has become an increasingly potent threat to consumer safety. "This is not your grandmother's salmonella anymore," said Caroline Smith DeWaal, food safety director for the Center for Science in the Public Interest. "It's a new salmonella, much more potent, and modified with the use of antibiotics on the farm." At least 278 people reportedly have been sickened in 18 states since March [2013] by a strain of Salmonella Heidelberg that has shown signs of resistance to antibiotics.

In addition,

Food safety advocates said that underscores a glaring weakness in the inspection system. They say virulent forms of antibiotic resistant salmonella should be handled like E. coli O157:H7, which triggers an automatic recall. "Producers have been successful at deflecting blame back on to consumers for not cooking poultry properly. It's nonsensical," said Bill Marler, a food safety lawyer who represented dozens of plaintiffs after an E. coli outbreak at Jack in the Box restaurants in the Pacific Northwest in the early 1990s ("Poultry Plants Linked to Outbreaks Won't Be Closed," *Los Angeles Times*, October 10, 2013). http://articles.latimes.com/2013/oct/10/news/chi-no-closing-poultry-plants-linked-to-outbreak-20131010.

Answer the following:

a. What counts as "acceptable risk" when it comes to food-borne diseases, like antibiotic-resistant salmonella and E. coli? Where should we draw the line?

b. There has yet to be a recall of Foster Farm chickens, even though 278 people have been hospitalized. The company insists that cooking at a sufficiently high temperature will destroy the bacteria—but should that be enough to stop a recall? Share your recommendations.

13. In 2005, *Scientific American* looked at preparations for a pandemic (such as influenza). Given the report by W. Wayt Gibbs and Christine Soares below, what sorts of ethical issues arise—and how should they be resolved?

The lethargic, poorly coordinated and undersized response [to Hurricane Katrina in the US] raises concerns about how nations would cope with a much larger and more lethal kind of natural disaster that scientists warn will occur, possibly soon: a pandemic of influenza. . . . As a sense of urgency grows, governments and health experts are working to bolster four substantial lines of defense against a pandemic: surveillance, vaccines, containment measures and medical treatments. . . . Authorities probably have no realistic chance of halting a nascent pandemic unless they can contain it within 30 days. . .

And there will undoubtedly be a line. Total worldwide production of flu vaccine amounts to roughly 300 million doses a year. Most of that is made in Europe; only two plants operate in the U.S. Last winter, when contamination shut down a Chiron facility in Britain, Sanofi Pasteur and MedImmune pulled out all stops on their American lines—and produced 61 million doses. The CDC recommends annual flu immunization for high-risk groups that in the U.S. include some 185 million people (See "Preparing for a Pandemic," *Scientific American*, October 24, 2005).

14. *Scientific American* (2005) pointed out that the need for vaccines would outpace the supplies in the event of an influenza pandemic. In light of the following, what should be the priorities?

Because delays and shortages in producing vaccine against a pandemic are unavoidable, one of the most important functions of national pandemic plans is to push political leaders to decide in advance which groups will be the first to receive vaccine and how the government will enforce its rationing. The U.S. national vaccine advisory committee recommended in July that the first shots to roll off the lines should go to key government leaders, medical caregivers, workers in flu vaccine and drug factories, pregnant women, and those infants, elderly, and ill people who are already in the high-priority group for annual flu shots. That top tier includes about 46 million Americans.

Note also:

Caching large amounts of prepandemic vaccine, though not impossible, is clearly a challenge. Vaccines expire after a few years. At current production rates, a stockpile would never grow to the 228 million doses needed to cover the three highest priority groups, let alone to the roughly 600 million doses that would be needed to vaccinate everyone in the U.S. Other nations face similar limitations (See W. Wayt Gibbs and Christine Soares, "Preparing for a Pandemic," *Scientific American*, October 24, 2005).

15. How much is your medical privacy worth? Would you accept $50 to allow prying eyes into your medical records?
Craig Klugman posted in a blog on *Bioethics.net* on August 23, 2013, that CVS Caremark pharmacies started a program early in 2013 in which "for every 10 prescriptions filled, a customer can receive $5 worth of credits to be used at CVS up to a maximum of $50 per year." That may sound good—but such loyalty means the company acquires information about your health.
Answer the following:
a. Is it worth $50 to retain privacy? Should this be a concern?
b. Who is most vulnerable? What ethical questions do you foresee?

16. Movies like *The Impossible* show how quickly lives can change because a natural disaster (in this case a tsunami). What sorts of preventive measures might be taken to try to make the medical response to environmental catastrophes as fair/just as possible?

17. Sanghamitra Padhy looks at the extent to which environmental issues are also bioethics issues. In the case of the Bhopal gas leak, the source of the problem

was *not* an "Act of God" (that is, a natural disaster) but the company, Union Carbide.

Answer the following:

a. How might corporations take steps to work with medical teams and the medical profession as a whole to set out policies and procedures in the event of environmental disasters?

b. What sort of efforts should we be doing *now* to prepare for the ethical problems that arise in the face of natural disasters such as Bhopal, Chernobyl, Katrina, Fukushima, and Hurricane Sandy?

18. Medical anthropologist Nancy Scheper-Hughes spoke on organ trafficking in a July 30, 2009, radio show *Talk of the Nation* on National Public Radio (NPR). Read her comments, and then answer the questions below.

There's many different routes into buying and selling kidneys. Some are organized by international brokers, as in the case of Izhak Rosenbaum [an organ broker targeted in a sting operation]. He was linked to a very, very large and extensive trafficking network that originates in Israel but is in about 12 countries, with brokers placed, like Izhak, in all of these locations, some, you know, some to hunt for kidney sellers, some to hunt on dialysis units to produce people who will travel and take the risk of breaking laws and doing this on faith. You often have to pay, in advance, large portions of money. . .

I went to Moldova and found out that over 300 men . . . had been recruited by brokers, local kidney hunters, and then passed on to higher-up brokers, trafficked to Turkey, and then some of them even came into New York City. . . . [Also] there was, until I closed it down, a website in China that would sell livers and—even from living people, but mostly from executed prisoners. And selling a half of your liver is not something that any righteous transplant surgeon would take part in, in taking a half of a liver (NPR).

Answer the following:

a. Do you think it is necessarily wrong to trade, purchase, or barter organs such as kidneys that are needed for transplant? Share your thoughts.

b. What might be done to better protect people from being exploited by international organ brokers?

Further Readings on Global Bioethics

Wanda Teays, John-Stewart Gordon, and Alison Dundes Renteln

GLOBAL BIOETHICS OVERVIEW

Andorno, Roberto. 2007. "Global Bioethics at UNESCO: In Defence of the Universal Declaration on Bioethics and Human Rights." *Journal of Medical Ethics* 33:150–4. http://uzh .academia.edu/RobertoAndorno/Papers/444663/Global_Bioethics_at_UNESCO_In_ Defence_of_the_Universal_Declaration_on_Bioethics_and_Human_Rights.

Rennie, Stuart. 2008. "Defining 'Responsiveness' in Global Health Research." *Global Bioethics Blog*. http://globalbioethics.blogspot.com/2008/07/defining-responsiveness-in-global.html.

United Nations. n.d. Convention on the Rights of Persons with Disabilities. http://www .un.org/disabilities/convention/facts.shtml.

United Nations Educational, Scientific and Cultural Organization (UNESCO). n.d. Global Ethics Observatory Database 4: Ethics Related Legislation and Guidelines. http://www .unesco.org/new/en/social-and-human-sciences/themes/global-ethics-observatory/access-geobs/.

———. n.d. International Bioethics Committee (IBC). http://www.unesco.org/new/en/social-and-human-sciences/themes/bioethics/international-bioethics-committee/.

World Health Organization (WHO). n.d. Constitution of the World Health Organization. http://whqlibdoc.who.int/hist/official_records/constitution.pdf.

———. n.d. Definition of Health. http://www.who.int/about/definition/en/print.html

———. n.d. Preamble to the Constitution of the World Health Organization (*World Health Organization: Basic Documents, 26th ed.*). http://www.who.int/governance/eb/who_consti tution_en.pdf.

FURTHER READING: GLOBAL BIOETHICS
AND HUMAN RIGHTS

Airhihenbuwa, Collins O. 1995. *Health and Culture: Beyond the Western Paradigm.* Thousand Oaks: Sage Publications.

Annas, George J. 2005. *American Bioethics Crossing Human Rights and Health Law Boundaries.* New York: Oxford University Press.

———. 2010. *Worst Case Bioethics: Death, Disaster, and Public Health.* New York: Oxford University Press.

Annas, George J., and Michael A. Grodin. 1992. *The Nazi Doctors and the Nuremberg Code: Human Rights in Human Experimentation.* New York: Oxford University Press.

Atighetchi, Dariusch. 2007. *Islamic Bioethics: Problems and Perspectives.* New York: Springer.

Bandman, Elsie L., and Bertram Bandman. 1978. *Bioethics and Human Rights: A Reader for Health Professionals.* Lanham, MD: University Press of America.

Beauchamp, Tom L. 2011. *Standing on Principles: Collected Essays.* New York: Oxford University Press.

Beyleveld, Deryck, and Roger Brownsword. 2002. *Human Dignity in Bioethics and Biolaw.* New York: Oxford University Press.

Biller-Andorno, Nikola, Peter Schaber, and Annette Schulz-Baldes. 2008. *Gibt es eine Universale Bioethik?* Paderborn: Mentis-Verlag.

Boyland, Michael, ed. 2008. *International Public Health Policy and Ethics.* Dordrecht: Springer.

———. 2013. *Environmental Ethics,* 2nd ed. Malden: Wiley-Blackwell.

Brannigan, Michael C., ed. 2004. *Cross-Cultural Biotechnology.* Lanham, MD: Rowman & Littlefield.

Butt, Leslie. 2002. "The Suffering Stranger: Medical Anthropology and International Morality." *Medical Anthropology* 21:1–24; discussion 25–33.

Callahan, Daniel. 1973. "The WHO Definition of 'Health.'" *The Hastings Center Studies* 1 (3): 77–78.

Capron, Alexander Morgan. 2007. "Imagining a New World: Using Internationalism to Overcome the 10/90 Gap in Bioethics [IAB Presidential Address]." *Bioethics* 21 (8): 409–12.

Davis, Lennard J. 2010. *The Disability Studies Reader,* 3rd ed. New York: Routledge.

Easterbrook, Catherine, and Guy Maddern. 2008. "Porcine and Bovine Surgical Products: Jewish, Muslim, and Hindu Perspectives." *Archives of Surgery* 143 (4): 366–70.

Engelhardt, Jr., and Hugo Tristram. 2003. "Introduction: Bioethics as a Global Phenomenon." In *Regional Perspectives in Bioethics,* edited by J. Peppin and M. J. Cerry, xiii–xxii. Lisse: Swets and Zeitlinger Publishers.

———. 2006. *Global Bioethics: The Collapse of Consensus.* Salem, MA: M & M Scrivener Press.

Fan, Rui-Ping, ed. 1999). *Confucian Bioethics (Philosophy and Medicine/Asian Studies in Bioethics and the Philosophy of Medicine).* Dordrecht, The Netherlands: Kluwer.

French, Stanley, Wanda Teays, and Laura Purdy, eds. 1998. *Violence Against Women: Philosophical Perspectives.* Ithaca, NY: Cornell University Press.

Geis, Gilbert, and Gregory C. Brown. 2008. "The Transnational Traffic in Human Body Parts." *Journal of Contemporary Criminal Justice* 24 (3): 212–24.

Gert, Bernard, Charles M. Culver, and K. Danner Clouser. 1997. *Bioethics: A Return to Fundamentals.* New York: Oxford University Press.

Goodman, Ryan, and Mindy Jane Roseman. 2009. *Interrogations, Forced Feedings, and the Role of Health Professionals.* Cambridge, MA: Harvard University Press.

Gordon, John-Stewart. 2008. "Poverty, Human Rights and Justice Distribution." In *International Public Health Policy and Ethics*, edited by M. Boylan. Dordrecht: Springer.

Gordon, John-Stewart, ed. 2010. *Morality and Justice: Reading Boylan's A Just Society.* Boulder: Westview Press.

Gordon, John-Stewart, O. Rauprich, and J. Vollmann. 2011. "Applying the Four-Principle Approach." *Bioethics* 25 (6): 293–300.

Greek, Ray, Annalea Pippus, and Lawrence A. Hansen. 2013. "The Nuremberg Code Subverts Human Health and Safety by Requiring Animal Modeling." *BMC Medical Ethics* 2012, 13:16.

Gruessner, Ranier W. G., and Enrico Benedetti, eds. 2007. *Living Donor Organ Transplantation.* New York: McGraw Hill Medical.

Ingstad, Benedicte, and Susan Reynolds Whyte, eds. 2007. *Disability in Local and Global Worlds.* Berkeley: University of California Press.

Keown, Damien. 2001. *Buddhism and Bioethics.* New York: Palgrave Macmillan.

Lenoir, Noelle. 1999. "Universal Declaration on the Human Genome and Human Rights: The First Legal and Ethical Framework at the Global Level." *Columbia Human Rights Law Review* 30 (1): 537–87.

Levinson, Sanford, ed. 2004. *Torture: A Collection.* Oxford: Oxford University Press.

Mahowald, Mary Briody. 2006. *Bioethics and Women: Across the Life Span.* New York: Oxford University Press.

Mann, Jonathan M., Sofia Gruskin, Michael A. Grodin, and George J. Annas. 1999. *Health and Human Rights: A Reader.* New York: Routledge.

Marks, Jonathan H. 2005. "Doctors of Interrogation." *The Hastings Center Report* 35 (4): 265–70, 295.

Marshall, Patricia. 2008. "'Cultural Competence' and Informed Consent in International Health Research." *Cambridge Quarterly of Healthcare Ethics* 17 (2): 206–15.

Marshall, Patricia, David C. Thomasma, and Jurrit Bergsma. 1994. "Intercultural Reasoning: The Challenge for International Bioethics." *Cambridge Quarterly of Healthcare Ethics* 3 (3): 321–28.

McGrath, P., and E. Phillips. 2008. "Western Notions of Informed Consent and Indigenous Cultures: Australian Findings at the Interface." *Journal of Bioethical Inquiry* 5 (1): 21–31.

Miles, Steven H. 2009. *Oath Betrayed: America's Torture Doctors*, 2nd ed. New York: Random House.

Moreno, Jonathan D. 2000. *Undue Risk: Secret State Experiments on Humans.* London: Routledge.

Nichter, Mark. 2008. *Global Health: Why Cultural Perceptions, Social Representations, and Biopolitics Matter.* Tucson: University of Arizona Press.

Omonzejele, Peter F. 2012. *The Ethics of Medical Research in Africa.* Saarbrücken: Lambert Academic Publishing.

O'Neill, Onora. 2002. *Autonomy and Trust in Bioethics.* Cambridge: Cambridge University Press.

Pellegrino, Edmund D., Robert M. Veatch, and John P. Langan, eds. 1991. *Ethics, Trust, and the Professions: Philosophical and Cultural Aspects.* Washington, DC: Georgetown University Press.

Pornpimon Adams, Waranya Wongwit, Krisana Pengsaa, Srisin Khusmith, Wijitr Fungladda, Warissara Chaiyaphan, Chanthima Limphattharacharoen, Sukanya Prakobtham, and Jaranit Kaewkungwal. 2013. "Ethical Issues in Research Involving Minority Populations: The Process and Outcomes of Protocol Review by the Ethics Committee of the Faculty of Tropical Medicine, Mahidol University, Thailand." *BMC Medical Ethics* 14:33.

Proctor, Robert N. 1989. *Racial Hygiene: Medicine under the Nazis.* Cambridge, MA: Harvard University Press.

Prograis, Lawrence J., and Edmund Pellegrino, eds. 2007. *African American Bioethics: Culture, Race, and Identity.* Washington, DC: Georgetown University Press.

Rachels, J. "Active and Passive Euthanasia" [the classic argument]. http://www2.sunysuffolk .edu/pecorip/scccweb/etexts/deathanddying_text/Active%20and%20Passive%20Euthana sia.pdf.

Radoilska, Lubomira, and Elizabeth Fistein. 2010. "Intellectual Disabilities and Personal Autonomy." http://www.phil.cam.ac.uk/news_events/intellectual_disabilities_autonomy.pdf.

Renteln, Alison Dundes. 1992. "Sex Selection and Reproductive Freedom." *Women's Studies International Forum* 15 (3): 405–42.

———. 2004. *The Cultural Defense.* New York: Oxford University Press.

Roberts, Dorothy E. 1999. *Killing the Black Body: Race, Reproduction, and the Meaning of Liberty.* New York: Vintage Books.

Rodley, Nigel S. 2011. *The Treatment of Prisoners under International Law,* 3rd ed. New York: Oxford University Press.

Rosner, Fred. 1999. "Pig Organs for Transplantation into Humans: A Jewish View." *The Mount Sinai Journal of Medicine* 66 (5 & 6): 314–19.

Sabatello, Maya. 2009. *Children's Bioethics: The International Biopolitical Discourse on Harmful Traditional Practices and the Right of the Child to Cultural Identity.* Boston: Martinus Nijhoff.

Schildmann, Jan, John-Stewart Gordon, and Jochen Vollmann, eds. 2010. *Clinical Ethics Consultation: Theories and Methods, Implementation, Evaluation.* Farnham: Ashgate Publishing.

Singer, Peter A., and A. M. Viens, eds. 2008. *The Cambridge Textbook of Bioethics.* Cambridge: Cambridge University Press.

Tangwa, Godfrey B. 2010. *Elements of African Bioethics in a Western Frame.* Mankon: Langaa Research & Publishing.

Tao Lai Po-Wah, Julia. 2002. *Cross-Cultural Perspectives on the (Im)possibility of Global Bioethics.* Dordrecht: Kluwer Academic Publishers.

Teays, Wanda. 2008. "Torture and Public Health." In *International Public Health Policy and Ethics,* edited by Michael Boylan. Dordrecht: Springer.

———. 2012. *Seeing the Light: Exploring Ethics through Movies.* Malden: Wiley-Blackwell.

———. 2013. "Patently Wrong: The Commercialization of Life Forms." In *Environmental Ethics,* 2nd ed., edited by Michael Boylan. Malden: Wiley-Blackwell.

Teays, Wanda, and Laura Purdy. 2001. *Bioethics, Justice, and Health Care.* Belmont, CA: Wadsworth.

Tong, Rosemarie. 1997. *Feminist Approaches to Bioethics: Theoretical Reflections and Practical Applications.* Boulder, CO: Westview Press.

Tong, Rosemarie, Gwen Anderson, and Aida F. Santos. 2001. *Globalizing Feminist Bioethics: Cross-Cultural Perspectives.* Boulder, CO: Westview Press.

Turner, Bryan, and Zheng Yangwen, eds. 2009. *The Body in Asia.* Oxford: Berghahn Books.

Turner, Leigh. 1997. "Bioethics, Public Health, and Firearm-Related Violence: Missing Links Between Bioethics and Public Health." *Journal of Law, Medicine & Ethics* 25 (1): 42–48.

———. 2012. "News Media Reports of Patient Deaths Following 'Medical Tourism' for Cosmetic Surgery and Bariatric Surgery." *Developing World Bioethics* 12 (1): 21–34.

Warren, Mary Anne. 1985. *Gendercide: The Implications of Sex Selection*. Totowa, New Jersey: Roman and Allanheld.

———. 2000. *Moral Status: Obligations to Persons and Other Living Things*. New York: Oxford University Press.

Wolf, Susan M. 1996. *Feminism & Bioethics: Beyond Reproduction*. New York: Oxford University Press.

Wright, Galen E. B., Pieter G. J. Koornhof, Adebowale A. Adeyemo, and Nicki Tiffin. 2013. "Ethical and Legal Implications of Whole Genome and Whole Exome Sequencing in African Populations." *BMC Medical Ethics* 14 (1): 21.

OATHS AND CODES

American Medical Association. n.d. AMAs Code of Medical Ethics. http://www.ama-assn.org/ama/pub/physician-resources/medical-ethics/code-medical-ethics.page.

American Nurses Association. n.d. Code of Ethics for Nurses. http://www.nursingworld.org/codeofethics.

Jewish Virtual Library. 1947. The Nuremberg Code (August 19, 1947). http://www.jewishvirtuallibrary.org/jsource/Holocaust/Nuremberg_Code.html.

Nuremberg Code, 1947. 1996. *British Medical Journal* 313 (7070): 1448. http://www.cirp.org/library/ethics/nuremberg/.

Tyson, Peter. 2001. "The Hippocratic Oath Today [Classic and modern versions]." PBS.org. http://www.pbs.org/wgbh/nova/body/hippocratic-oath-today.html.

United Nations. 1971. Declaration on the Rights of Mentally Retarded Persons. University of Minnesota.edu. http://www1.umn.edu/humanrts/instree/t1drmrp.htm.

———. 1993. The Standard Rules on the Equalization of Opportunities for Persons with Disabilities. http://www.un.org/esa/socdev/enable/dissre00.htm.

———. n.d. The Special Rapporteur on Disability of the Commission for Social Development. http://www.un.org/esa/socdev/enable/rapporteur.htm.

———. n.d. The Universal Declaration of Human Rights. http://www.un.org/en/documents/udhr/.

———. n.d. World Programme of Action Concerning Disabled Persons. http://www.un.org/disabilities/default.asp?id=23.

United Nations Educational, Scientific and Cultural Organization (UNESCO). n.d. Universal Declaration on Bioethics and Human Rights. http://www.unesco.org/new/en/social-and-human-sciences/themes/bioethics/bioethics-and-human-rights/.

United Nations Human Rights. Office of the High Commissioner for Human Rights. 1975. Declaration on the Rights of Disabled Persons (1975). http://www2.ohchr.org/english/law/res3447.htm.

World Medical Association (WMA). n.d. WMA Declaration of Helsinki—Ethical Principles for Medical Research Involving Human Subjects. http://www.wma.net/en/30publications/10policies/b3/.

World Medical Association (WMA). n.d. WMA International Code of Medical Ethics. http://www.wma.net/en/30publications/10policies/c8/.

POSITION STATEMENTS

American Medical Association. n.d. "Opposing Cooperation of Physicians and Health Professionals in Torture." www.ama-assn.org/meetings/public/annual05/10a05.doc.

Physicians for Human Rights (PHR). n.d. Dual Loyalties in US Immigration Detention. http://physiciansforhumanrights.org/issues/torture/asylum/dual-loyalties-immigration-detention.html.

Physicians for Human Rights (PHR). 2003. Dual Loyalty and Human Rights in Health Professional Practice (Guidelines). http://www.physiciansforhumanrights.org/library/reports/dual-loyalty-and-human-rights-2003.html.

Society of Obstetricians and Gynaecologists of Canada. 2007. Fetal Sex Determination and Disclosure. SOGC Policy Statement. Ottawa (ON): The Society, 2007. http://www.sogc.org/guidelines/documents/192E-PS-April2007.pdf.

Electronic Resources on Global Bioethics

Willow Bunu, Wanda Teays, and Alison Dundes Renteln

GLOBAL BIOETHICS LINKS

Bioethics.net
Website of the *American Journal of Bioethics*
A range of useful resources, including ethics in the news, links, and coming events
  in the field.
http://www.bioethics.net/

British Broadcasting Corporation (BBC) Ethics Guides
Brief guides to various ethical issues (including medical issues such as contraception,
  abortion, and euthanasia). Some include links to recent related news articles or
  television or radio programs.
http://www.bbc.co.uk/ethics/guide/

Center for Bioethics & Human Dignity
The Center provides resources from varying perspectives on issues such as reproductive ethics, organ donation, end of life, stem cell research, disabilities, and cloning.
  The website includes the audio from presentations given at their past conventions.
http://www.cbhd.org/

Ethics Updates
The website includes information on ethical theories and applications such as bioethics, animal rights, environmental ethics, racism, sexism, and world affairs.
http://ethics.sandiego.edu/

GUIDES, DIRECTORIES AND GENERAL REFERENCES

Globethics.net
http://www.globethics.net/web/ge/library/browse-the-journals/by-subjects-ethics

Human Rights Education Associates: Study Guides
This site provides introductions to many common human rights topics. The guides
   present definitions, key rights at stake, human rights instruments, and protection
   and assistance agencies.
http://www.hrea.org/index.php?doc_id=145

Human Rights Education Associates: The Rights of Ethnic and Racial Minorities
A study guide on the rights of ethnic minorities that includes a description of the
   rights to be protected and instruments for protecting those rights, as well as links
   to advocacy organizations.
http://www.hrea.org/index.php?base_id=142

Markkula Center for Applied Ethics
A resource for the analysis of issues in medical ethics, business ethics, government
   ethics, and character education, as well as the process of ethical decision making.
http://www.scu.edu/ethics/

Pew Forum on Religion & Public Life
The forum contains information on various issues of public concern, presented by
   the Pew Research Center, an independent, nonpartisan, public-opinion research
   organization that studies attitudes toward politics, the press, and public policy issues.
http://pewforum.org/
They also study science and bioethics.
http://pewforum.org/Topics/Issues/Science-and-Bioethics/

Phil Papers
A comprehensive directory of online philosophy articles and books by academic
   philosophers. You may set up automatic proxy browsing to connect to campus
   databases using this site.
http://philpapers.org/

Public Agenda for Citizens: Race
This site gives an overview of viewpoints about a variety of issues concerning race-
   based civil rights, as well as charts of relevant data.
http://www.publicagenda.org/citizen/issueguides/race

Stanford Encyclopedia of Philosophy
http://plato.stanford.edu/

University of Minnesota Human Rights Library
The Library houses sixty thousand core human rights documents, including several
hundred human rights treaties and other primary international human rights
instruments, as well as topical guides to various human rights issues. The site also
provides access to more than four thousand links and the ability to search multiple
human rights sites.
http://www1.umn.edu/humanrts/

Women's Health Bibliography at the Center for Bioethics & Human Dignity
http://cbhd.org/womens-health/bibliography

RESOURCES ON CHILDREN'S RIGHTS

American Bar Association Center on Children and the Law
http://www.americanbar.org/groups/child_law.html

Cornell University Law School Legal Information Institute
This site provides a brief overview of children's rights as well as links to American
and international legal statutes concerning children's rights and links to topically
relevant websites.
http://topics.law.cornell.edu/wex/Childrens_rights

Human Rights Watch: Children's Rights
A division of Human Rights Watch, an independent international organization dedicated to defending and protecting human rights, focused on the rights of children.
http://www.hrw.org/topic/childrens-rights

UNICEF: Convention on the Rights of the Child
Part of the United Nations, UNICEF's mission is to advocate for the protection of
children's rights.
http://www.unicef.org/crc/

U.S. Department of Health and Human Services: Administration for Children and
Families
The website for the federal agency that funds state, territory, local, and tribal organizations to provide family assistance, including intervening in child abuse and
human trafficking cases.
http://www.acf.hhs.gov/

Global Bioethics on the Screen

Wanda Teays

GENERAL RESOURCES

Documentary Films on Health (Free), TopDocumentaryFilms.com
http://topdocumentaryfilms.com/category/health/

Frontline Documentary Films
http://www.pbs.org/wgbh/pages/frontline/

NOVA
http://www.pbs.org/wgbh/nova/

Stanford School of Medicine Center for Biomedical Ethics http://medethicsfilms.
stanford.edu

FILMS AND DOCUMENTARIES

Health Care: Global Perspectives

- *Between Two Worlds: The Hmong Shaman in America* (Produced by Taggart Siegel and Dwight Conquergood; released in 1996 by Filmakers Library)
- *Donka: X-Ray of an African Hospital* (Thierry Michel documentary, 1997, Icarus Films)
- *Global Health Documentaries* (on two doctors working in global health care):
- http://www.secondstory.com/project/global-health-documentaries
- *Malaria: Fever Wars* (2006, PBS documentary)

- *Sick around the World* (global look at health care—*Frontline* documentary): http://www.pbs.org/wgbh/pages/frontline/sickaroundtheworld/
- *Sicko* (2007, Dog Eat Dog Films, director and writer Michael Moore)
- *Uninsured in the Mississippi Delta* (poverty/healthcare documentary by Katie Falkenberg): http://www.mediathatmattersfest.org/films/uninsured_in_the_mississippi_delta
- *Untitled Global Health Documentary* (Sundance Institute and the Skoll Foundation, director Kief Davidson): http://www.sundance.org/storiesofchange/film/untitled-global-health-documentary/
- WHO International Media Centre: http://www.who.int/mediacentre/en/

MEDICINE AND MEDICAL ETHICS

- *Alternative Medicine* (PBS documentary): http://www.pbs.org/newshour/health/alt_medicine/index.html
- Feature film: *The Doctor* (1991, from Silver Screen Partners IV and Touchstone Pictures, director Randa Haines)
- *Dr. Stanley Vollant* (Inuit surgeon, documentary, *The Current* with Anna Maria Tremonti): http://www.cbc.ca/thecurrent/episode/2010/12/13/dr-stanley-vollant/*NewsHour with Jim Lehrer* Medical Ethics and Issues Anthology
- (Films for the Humanities Item #37178): http://ffh.films.com/ItemDetails.aspx?TitleId=13860
- *Worlds Apart* (navigating the health care system; directed by Maren Grainger-Monsen and Julia Haslett): http://medethicsfilms.stanford.edu/worldsapart/

ILLNESS AND DISEASE

Doctor-Patient Communication on Serious Illness

- *Grave Words* (documentary on discussing options with patients—e.g., resuscitation; Stanford Center for Biomedical Ethics): http://medethicsfilms.stanford.edu/gravewords/

Alzheimer's Disease

- Feature film: *Away from Her* (2006, Foundry Films, director Sarah Polley)

Parkinson's Disease

- *My Father, My Brother, and Me* (personal story on Parkinson's, *Frontline* documentary by Dave Iverson): http://www.pbs.org/wgbh/pages/frontline/parkinsons/

HIV/AIDS

- *A Closer Walk* (documentary on the global AIDS crisis by Robert Bilheimer): http://www.acloserwalk.org/
- *The Age of AIDS* (*Frontline*): http://www.pbs.org/wgbh/pages/frontline/aids/
- *Endgame: AIDS in Black America* (PBS *Frontline* documentary): http://www.pbs.org/wgbh/pages/frontline/endgame-aids-in-black-america/
- Documentaries on AIDS: *The Lazarus Effect* (2010, Isotope Films, director Lance Bangs); *The Origins of AIDS* (TopDocumentaryFilms.com); *The Other City* (Cabin Films, director Susan Koch); *House of Numbers: Anatomy of an Epidemic* (2009, Knowledge Matters, director Brent Leung); *Angels in America* (2003, Avenue Pictures Productions and HBO Films, director Mike Nichols)

Memory and Personal Identity

- Feature films: *Eternal Sunshine of the Spotless Mind* (2004, Focus Features, director Michel Gondry); *Inception* (2010, Warner Bros., director Christopher Nolan); *All of Me* (1984, Kings Road Entertainment, director Carl Reiner)

Epidemics/Scarce Resources

- Feature films: *Outbreak* (1995, Warner Bros., director Wolfgang Petersen); *Contagion* (2011, Warner Bros., director Steven Soderbergh)

Environmental Issues

- *The Bhopal Disaster* (PBS documentary): http://www.pbs.org/wnet/need-to-know/tag/union-carbide/
- *Flow* (documentary on the water crisis, by Irena Salina): http://www.flowthefilm.com
- *Inside Japan's Nuclear Meltdown* (*Frontline* documentary): http://www.pbs.org/wgbh/pages/frontline/japans-nuclear-meltdown/
- *Seeds of Death* (documentary on genetically modified food, TopDocumentary Films.com): http://topdocumentaryfilms.com/seeds-death/
- *Semper Fi: Always Faithful* (documentary on U.S. water contamination—conspiracy angle, directed by Rachel Libert and Tony Harmon): http://semperfi alwaysfaithful.com
- Documentaries: *Forks over Knives* (2011, Monica Beach Media, director Lee Fulkerson); *Food, Inc.* (2008, Magnolia Pictures, director Robert Kenner); *Darwin's Nightmare* (2004, Mille et Une Productions, director Hubert Sauper)

Organ Transplants

- Feature Films: *Dirty Pretty Things* (2002, BBC Films, director Stephen Frears); *Never Let Me Go* (2010, DNA Films, director Mark Romanek); *21 Grams* (2003, This Is That Productions, director Alejandro González Iñárritu)
- Documentaries: *Transplant: A Gift for Life* (PBS documentary, director Dennis Mahoney); *Organ Donors/Organ Transplants* (BBC documentary—YouTube): http://www.youtube.com/watch?v=hSEkV6Lpkts.
- *Organ Farm* (PBS *Frontline* documentary)]
- *Dying to Live* (documentary by Chuck Boller): http://www.transplantdocu mentary.com/organizations.htm
- *Tales from the Organ Trade* (by Ric Esther Bienstock. Official website: http://www.talesfromtheorgantrade.com)

Transgenic Animals

- Human-Animal Hybrid Embryos (BBC documentary): http://www.bbc.co.uk/ethics/animals/using/hybridembryos_1.shtml
- *Animal Farm* (documentary, the first in a series, has an extended commentary as well on BioethicsBytes, presented by Olivia Judson and Giles Coren): http://www.channel4.com/programmes/animal-farm
- *The Pharmaceutical Farm* (second in the series, presented by Olivia Judson and Giles Coren): http://bioethicsbytes.wordpress.com/2007/06/20/the-"pharmaceutical-farm"-004708---animal-farm-episode-2/
- *Making Creatures That Work for Us* (third in the series, presented by Olivia Judson and Giles Coren): http://bioethicsbytes.wordpress.com/2007/06/20/making-creatures-that-work-for-us-000317-animal-farm-episode-3/

REPRODUCTIVE FREEDOM AND HEALTH

Abortion/Reproductive Health

- *Abortion Clinic* (*Frontline* documentary—may be hard to access due to heavy demand): http://www.pbs.org/wgbh/pages/frontline/twenty/watch/abortion.html
- *Grace under Fire* (documentary on Dr. Grace Kodindo, who works for reproductive health in the Congo, Television Trust for the Environment, directed by Bruno Sorrentino)
- *The Last Abortion Clinic* (*Frontline* documentary on diminishing access to abortion): http://www.pbs.org/wgbh/pages/frontline/clinic/
- Feature films: *4 Months, 3 Weeks and 2 Days* (2007, Mobra Films, director Cristian Mungiu); *Juno* (2007, Fox Searchlight Pictures, director Jason Reitman);

Citizen Ruth (1996, Independent Pictures and Miramax Films, director Alexander Payne); *The Cider House Rules* (1999, FilmColony and Miramax Films, director Lasse Hallström)

Birth/Children

- *Born into Brothels* (2004, Red Light Films and HBO/Cinemax, directors Zana Briski and Ross Kauffman)
- *By the Numbers: Childhood Poverty in the U.S.* (*Frontline* documentary): http:// www.pbs.org/wgbh/pages/frontline/social-issues/poor-kids/by-the-numbers-childhood-poverty-in-the-u-s/
- *Ladies in Waiting* (poor, pregnant women in the Congo, Icarus Films documentary directed by Dieudo Hamadi and Divita Wa Lusala)
- *The Medicated Child* (*Frontline* documentary): http://www.pbs.org/wgbh/pages/ frontline/medicatedchild/
- *Outside Looking In: Transracial Adoption in America* (ITVS documentary produced by Phil Bertelsen and Katy Chevigny)

Older Parents Freezing Eggs

- Older Parents/Freezing Eggs (documentary on *The Current* with Anna Maria Tremonti): http://www.cbc.ca/thecurrent/shift/2010/10/21/older-parentsegg-freezing-oct-2010/

Death, Euthanasia, and Assisted Suicide/Suicide

- Feature films: *The Sea Inside* (2004, Sogepaq, Sociedad General de Cine, director Alejandro Amenábar); *Million Dollar Baby* (2004, Warner Bros., director Clint Eastwood); *The Hours* (2002, Paramount Pictures, director Stephen Daldry); *After the Wedding* (2006, Zentropa Entertainments, director Susanne Bier); *Ikiru* (1952, Toho Company, director Akira Kurosawa)
- *Difficult Decisions: When a Loved One Approaches Death* (2000, Films for the Humanities Item #11016)
- *Facing Death* (*Frontline* documentary): http://www.pbs.org/wgbh/pages/front-line/facing-death/
- *Life and Death: Medical Ethics of the Schiavo Case* (2005, Films for the Humanities Item #53559)
- *The Suicide Plan* (PBS *Frontline* documentary): http://www.pbs.org/wgbh/ pages/frontline/suicide-plan/
- Documentaries: *Calling Dr. Kevorkian: A Date with Dr. Death* (on Jack Kevorkian, 1997); *Facing Death* (*Frontline*); *The Suicide Tourist* (*Frontline*); *H.H. Dalai Lama: Facing Death and Dying Well* (*Frontline*)

Genetics/Genetic Privacy, Stem Cell Research, and Cloning

- Feature films: *Gattaca* (1997, Columbia Pictures, director Andrew Niccol); *The Island* (2005, DreamWorks SKG, director Michael Bay); *Boys from Brazil* (1978, Lew Grade, director Franklin J. Schaffner); *Multiplicity* (1996, Columbia Pictures, director Harold Ramis)
- *Genetic Science: Where Is It Leading Us?* (Films for the Humanities Item #40382) copyright ©2007. http://ffh.films.com/id/16336/Genetic_Science_Where_Is_It_Leading_Us.htm.
- *Weighing the Decision: The Ethics and Science of Stem Cell Research* (2001, Films for the Humanities Item #37367)
- *Who Gets to Know? Genetics and Privacy—A Fred Friendly Seminar*
- (Films for the Humanities Item #30800) *Who's Afraid of Designer Babies? The Ethics of Genetic Screening* (2004, Films for the Humanities Item #36105)

Disabilities

- Feature films: *Regarding Henry* (1991, Paramount, director Mike Nichols); *Planet of Snail* (2011, CreativeEAST, director Yi Seung-jun); *Benda Bilili!* (2010, Screen Runner, director Renaud Barret); *Children of a Lesser God* (1986, Paramount Pictures, director Randa Haines)
- *Sound and Fury* (2000, documentary on deafness, Next Wave Films, director Josh Aronson): http://www.imdb.com/title/tt0240912/
- *Through Deaf Eyes* (documentary by Diane Garey and Lawrence R. Hott): http://www.pbs.org/weta/throughdeafeyes/

Medical Experimentation and Informed Consent

- Feature films: *Miss Evers' Boys* (1997, Anasazi Productions, director Joseph Sargent); *The Constant Gardener* (2005, Focus Features, director Fernando Meirelles); *District 9* (2009, TriStar Pictures, director Neill Blomkamp); *The Bourne Identity* (2002, Universal Pictures, director Doug Liman)
- Documentaries: *In the Shadow of the Reich: Nazi Medicine* (1997, director John Michalczyk); *Deadly Deception* (1993, NOVA); *Code Name: Artichoke* (documentary on CIA scientist Dr. Frank Olson—conspiracy angle): http://topdocumentaryfilms.com/code-name-artichoke/

Racism in Health Care

- Feature film: *John Q* (2002, New Line Cinema, director Nick Cassavetes)
- *Racism Hurts Your Health* (2008, NPR audio, Michel Martin, host): http://www.npr.org/templates/story/story.php?storyId=89678892
- *Racism in America: Small Town 1950s Case Study* (2012, YouTube): http://www.youtube.com/watch?v=OCIYPCYAf7s

- *In the Shadow of the Reich: Nazi Medicine* (1997, director John Michalczyk); *Night and Fog* (1955, Argos Films, director Alain Resnais); *Deadly Deception* (1991, directed by Debra Chasnoff)
- *The Angry Heart: The Impact of Racism on Heart Disease of African Americans* (2001, Fanlight Productions, produced by Jay Fedigan)

Female Circumcision

- *Female Circumcision* (PBS documentary): July 15, 2011. http://video.pbs.org/video/2056789248/.
- BBC documentary: http://www.bbc.com/news/education-26049727.
- *The Right to Femininity: Fighting Female Circumcision in Africa Today* (2010, Multiple Perspectives: Films for the Humanities Item #34539)

Battered Women/Domestic Violence

- Feature films: *Sleeping with the Enemy* (1991, Twentieth Century Fox Film Corporation, director Joseph Ruben); *Enough* (2002, Columbia Pictures, director Michael Apted); *What's Love Got to Do With It?* (1993, Touchstone Pictures, director Brian Gibson); *The Burning Bed* (1984, Tisch/Avnet Productions, director Robert Greenwald)
- *Defending Our Lives* (Award-winning documentary on women who kill their abuser, 1994, Cambridge Documentary Films, directors Margaret Lazarus and Renner Wunderlich)
- *Abused: The Documentary* (Braverman Productions, produced and directed by Chuck Braverman, produced by Marilyn Braverman): http://www.abuseddocumentary.com/index.html
- *Domestic Violence Documentary* (2011): http://www.youtube.com/watch?v=3umi3K64Uqo
- *A Cry for Help: The Tracey Thurman Story* (docudrama, 1989, Dick Clark Productions, director Robert Markowitz)

Torture/Abuse

- Feature films: *Lost Boys of Sudan* (2003, Actual Film, directors Megan Mylan and Jon Shenk); *Last King of Scotland* (2006, Fox Searchlight, director Kevin Macdonald); *Rendition* (2007, Warner Bros., director Gavin Hood); *Hotel Rwanda* (2004, United Artists, director Terry George), *Storm* (2009, Filmproduktion GmbH, director Hans-Christian Schmid)
- Documentaries: *Taxi to the Dark Side* (2007, Discovery Channel, director Alex Gibney); *Ghosts of Abu Ghraib* (2007, HBO Documentary Films, director Rory Kennedy); *Standard Operating Procedure* (2008, Participant Media,

director Errol Morris); *Doctors of the Dark Side* (2011, director Martha Davis); *The Torture Question* (*Frontline*); *Extraordinary Rendition* (*Frontline*)

Incarceration

- Documentaries: *The House I Live In* (2012, Al Jazeera Documentary Channel, director Eugene Jarecki); *My Home, My Prison* (1993, directors Susana Blaustein Muñoz and Erica Marcus); *The Farm: Angola, USA* (1998, Gabriel Films, directors Liz Garbus, Wilbert Rideau, and Jonathan Stack); *Innocent Until Proven Guilty* (1999, director Kirsten Johnson); *Deadline* (2004, Arts Engine, directors Katy Chevigny and Kirsten Johnson)
- *Solitary Confinement* (National Geographic documentary, 2010, director Peter Yost)
- *Solitary Confinement* (PBS video), October 11, 2013, http://www.pbs.org/wnet/religionandethics/2014/02/28/october-11-2013-solitary-confinement/20631/.

Lethal Injection

- *Texas Uses Single-Drug Lethal Injection in Execution* (PBS video): July 19, 2012, http://www.pbs.org/newshour/bb/law-july-dec12-death_07-19/.

Death Penalty

- Feature films: *In Cold Blood* (1967, Columbia Pictures, director Richard Brooks); *Dead Man Walking* (1995, Havoc, director Tim Robbins); *Return to Paradise* (1998, Polygram Filmed Entertainment, director Joseph Ruben)
- *Capital Punishment: Retribution or Justice?* (PBS video), May 11, 2001, http://video.pbs.org/video/2221031994/.
- *Deadline* (documentary on the state of Illinois' death penalty law, 2004, Big Mouth Productions, directors Katy Chevigny and Kirsten Johnson)
- *The Execution* (PBS video), February 1999, http://www.pbs.org/wgbh/pages/frontline/shows/execution/.

Appendix: Human Rights and Disability Rights

Akiko Ito

II. Progressive Development of International Norms and Standards on Disability

1. International Bill of Human Rights

The Universal Declaration of Human Rights (UDHR) (UN 1948),[1] the foundational document of modern human rights law, expresses general human rights principles in the area of civil, political, economic, social, and cultural rights. UDHR emphasizes its applicability to all people, underscoring that "[a]ll human beings are born free and equal in dignity and rights[2] . . . [a]ll are equal before the law, and [all] are entitled without any discrimination to equal protection of the law."[3] Insofar as the UDHR applies to all human beings, it provides an important source of human rights of persons with disabilities. However, it provides no specific guidance regarding disability rights and does not explicitly include disability among the prohibited grounds of discrimination.

The adoption of the UDHR was followed by the drafting of two international treaties that, together with the UDHR, comprise the International Bill of Human Rights, the core of modern international human rights law. In 1996, the United Nations General Assembly opened for signature for the International Covenant on Civil and Political Rights (ICCPR) (UN 1966)[4] and the International Covenant on Economic, Social and Cultural Rights (ICESCR) (UN 1966).[5] Like the UDHR, while the two Covenants provide protections applicable to all people, there is no explicit mention regarding disability. Where disability is addressed in the International Bill of Rights "it is only in connection with social security and preventive health policy,"[6] and not as a comprehensive human rights issue.

These facilitate moving beyond the narrow scheme of state responsibility for the protection of aliens scheme and limited minorities protections[7] and embracing a broader conceptualization of rights protection. The violation of human rights obligations by a state against its own nationals is indeed a matter of international concern. Additional legal measures were required to address human rights abuses experienced throughout the world by individuals belonging to particular social, ethnic, religious, and other groups.

Through the end of the last century, the United Nations adopted a total of seven core human rights conventions, each containing legal obligations that are applicable to persons with disabilities. These include the five listed here:

- The International Convention on the Elimination of All Forms of Racial Discrimination (ICERD) (UN 1965),[8]
- The UN Convention on the Elimination of All Forms of Discrimination Against Women (CEDAW) (UN 1979),[9]
- The Convention against Torture and Other Cruel, Inhuman or Degrading Treatment or Punishment (CAT) (UN 1984),
- The Convention on the Rights of the Child (CRC) (UN 1989),[10]
- The International Convention on the Protection of the Rights of All Migrant Workers and Members of Their Families (ICRMW) (UN 1990).[11]

However, the human rights provisions reflected in the core conventions before the drafting of the Convention on the Rights of Persons with Disabilities (CRPD) did not address the specific barriers facing persons with disabilities. In due course, however, their monitoring bodies, in some instances, sought to clarify the application of the treaties to persons with disabilities or otherwise drew attention to human rights and disabled persons.

2. Declaration on the Rights of Mentally Retarded Persons (1971)

One of the first UN policy instruments to directly focus on the integration of persons with disabilities into society was the 1969 Declaration on Social Progress and Development. It advocates the provision of measures to rehabilitate persons with mental and physical disabilities to facilitate their integration into society.

The integration focus continued with the December 20, 1971, Declaration on the Rights of Mentally Retarded Persons, which states that the persons with intellectual disabilities have to the maximum degree feasible the same rights as other human beings, including those related to proper medical care and education, economic security, guardianship, and protection from exploitation and legal procedures. It stresses that persons with intellectual disabilities should live with their families and participate in the community.

The Declaration represented a significant step in raising awareness about the human rights of persons with intellectual disabilities. However, it has come under heavy criticism by the disability community for its outmoded medical and charity models of disability, which reinforce paternalistic attitudes. The former Special Rapporteur on Disability, Bengt Lindqvist, noted that the Declaration is in many ways outdated by reflecting an approach to disability (the "medical model") "in which persons with disabilities are primarily seen as individuals with medical problems, dependent on social security and welfare and in need of separate services and institutions."[12]

3. Declaration on the Rights of Disabled Persons (1975)

In December 1975, the General Assembly adopted the Declaration on the Rights of Disabled Persons, which states that all persons with disabilities have the same rights as other persons. This culminated the beginning of a new conceptual approach to disability. This expanded the coverage to include all persons with disabilities.[13] It acknowledged that persons with disabilities have the right to respect for human dignity, the same civil and political rights as others,[14] the right to medical treatment, and economic and social security. It set the standard for equal treatment and access to services that help develop the capabilities of persons with disabilities and accelerate their social integration.

These two disability-specific instruments reflect an earlier era. Though serving to raise awareness about disability issues, they were not crafted in the language of modern human rights law—and did little to shape national law and policy and had no monitoring and implementation measures to facilitate national action. Moreover, they did not fully reflect current human rights principles.

4. The World Programme of Action Concerning Disabled Persons (1982)

In 1976, the General Assembly declared 1981 as the International Year for Disabled Persons (IYDP). The International Year[15] and the World Programme of Action adopted in 1982 provided a strong impetus for progress on the rights of persons with disabilities. Among the major outcomes of the Decade of Disabled Persons (1983–1992),[16] the Standard Rules on the Equalization of Opportunities for Persons with Disabilities was adopted by the General Assembly on March 4, 1994.[17]

The World Programme is a global strategy to enhance disability prevention, rehabilitation, and equalization of opportunities—a central theme of the World Programme. It sought to achieve full participation of persons with disabilities in all aspects of social and economic life. An important underlying principle is that issues concerning persons with disabilities should not be treated in isolation, but within the context of community services. The inclusion of the goal of equalization of opportunities represents an important shift toward a rights-based approach. However, the "caring" model, or the World Programme, was still based on so-called medical/charity or personal tragedy models of disability.[18]

In addition, its characterization of terms such as *disability, impairment,* and *handicap* are now outdated. In this approach, *impairment* was defined as any "loss or abnormality of psychological, physiological, or anatomical structure or function," and *disability* was defined as any "restriction or lack (resulting from an impairment) of ability to perform an activity in the manner or within the range considered normal for a human being."[19] Finally, *handicap* was defined as "a disadvantage for a given individual, resulting from an impairment or disability, that limits or prevents the fulfilment of a role that is normal, depending on age, sex, social and cultural factors, for that individual."[20]

5. The Standard Rules on the Equalization of Opportunities for Persons with Disabilities (1993)

In 1993, the General Assembly passed the Standard Rules on the Equalization of Opportunities for Persons with Disabilities. It consists of twenty-two rules aimed at elaborating the message of the World Programme of Action, providing a basis for technical and economic cooperation among States, the United Nations, and other international stakeholders.[21] The purpose of the Standard Rules is "to ensure that girls, boys, women and men with disabilities, as members of their societies, may exercise the same rights and obligations as others."[22] Their core concept is the "equalization of opportunities for persons with disabilities" as "an essential contribution in the general and worldwide effort to mobilize human resources."[23]

The Standard Rules represent an advance in stressing that persons with disabilities may exercise the same rights and obligations as others. The Rules acknowledge that barriers in society prevent the full participation of persons with disabilities and that the population of persons with disabilities is diverse, suggesting that some groups, such as women with disabilities or racial minorities, experience multiple or multidimensional forms of discrimination.[24]

The rules show an expansion into areas not traditionally viewed as human rights concerns. The World Programme of Action's first two goals of prevention and rehabilitation are viewed from the human rights perspective. In the area of prevention, Standard Rule 2 offers several provisions for States to ensure effective medical care to persons with disabilities. In the area of rehabilitation, persons with disabilities and their families have stressed the importance of Community-Based Rehabilitation (CBR) programs to facilitate integration into the community. Standard Rule 3 provides a consumer-based approach to the provision of such services. Thus, even the programs that traditionally focused on changing the person are urged to consider environmental issues in designing programs. The Standard Rules clearly focus on the concept of accessibility in Rule 5, though it is viewed as pertaining to the physical environment and information and communication.

6. Special Rapporteur on Disability

The Standard Rules established a Special Rapporteur on Disability to monitor the implementation of the Rules at the international level. He/she is appointed by and reports to the Commission for Social Development.[25] Bengt Lindqvist (Sweden) was the first Special Rapporteur on Disability from 1994 to 2000. Sheikha Hissa Khalifa bin al-Thani (Qatar) served from 2003 to 2006, and, in 2008, Shuaib Chalklen (South Africa) was appointed as the Special Rapporteur. The absence of a permanent budgetary allocation for servicing the Special Rapporteur is a weakness.

The Special Rapporteur presents findings on the promotion and monitoring of the implementation of the Standard Rules and presents recommendations as requested by the Commission for Social Development. In carrying out his/ her functions, the Special Rapporteur establishes a direct dialogue with member states and with local nongovernmental organizations and experts, seeking their views and comments on any information intended to be included in the reports. This process does not happen on a consistent periodic basis.

7. Other United Nations Disability Policy Mechanisms

Most of the instruments cited thus far refer to General Assembly resolutions. However, within the United Nations system, there exist other policy mechanisms. Two important instruments are the Salamanca Statement and Framework for Action and the International Labour Organization's (ILO) Convention No. C159.

8. Convention on the Rights of Persons with Disabilities

Acting on earlier proposals to address the lack of a legally binding human rights instrument addressing the rights of persons with disabilities, the General Assembly established an ad hoc committee to consider the feasibility of a disability-specific human rights treaty in December 2001.[26] In 2002 it delegated a working group composed of States, nongovernmental organizations, and national human rights institutions to draft a foundational text.[27] On January 16, 2004, the working group issued draft CRPD articles for consideration, and on August 25, 2006, the ad hoc committee adopted the CRPD.[28] It was adopted by the General Assembly on December 13, 2006.[29] It entered into force on May 3, 2008, after a requisite twenty ratifications had been duly deposited with the United Nations.[30]

Article 1 provides that the Convention's explicit purpose is "to promote, protect and ensure the full and equal enjoyment of all human rights and fundamental freedoms by all persons with disabilities, and to promote respect for their inherent dignity."[31] Its Optional Protocol provides mechanisms for individual and group communications and as well as a procedure of inquiry.[32]

Article 1 conceives of disability as including, but not limited to, "long-term physical, mental, intellectual or sensory impairments."[33] The CRPD establishes disability as a social category arising from "interaction with various barriers [that] may hinder their full and effective participation in society on an equal basis with others," rather than as an inherent limitation.[34] In this regard, the Convention adopts a rights-based, social model of disability and marks a major shift away from the traditional way in which human rights conventions and national law and policies around the world typically characterize disability.

Drafters of the CRPD were highly critical of the medical and personal tragedy models of disability that have long been the lens through which the non-disabled majority has viewed persons with disabilities. Its embrace of the social model of disability in the CRPD is a critical shift in approach, intending to impact the reform and development of national-level disability law and policy.

The specific substantive articles of the CRPD provide coverage of the full range and spectrum of life activities of persons with disabilities in Articles 10 to 30. These human rights include the right to life;[35] freedom from torture;[36] freedom from violence and abuse;[37] the right to education;[38] employment;[39] political participation;[40] legal capacity;[41] access to justice;[42] freedom of expression and opinion;[43] privacy;[44] participation in cultural life, sports, and recreation;[45] respect for home and family;[46] personal integrity;[47] liberty of movement and nationality;[48] liberty and security of the person;[49] and adequate standard of living.[50] Other provisions help to clarify human rights within the context of disability and directly link to other CRPD rights.[51] For example, the articles on living independently,[52] personal mobility,[53] and habilitation and rehabilitation[54] are intrinsic to the attainment of historically recognized human rights.

Articles 31 to 40 of the CRPD set forth implementation and monitoring measures,[55] as does the Optional Protocol.[56] The implementation and monitoring mechanisms were established, for the first time. CRPD Article 40 provides for a periodic meeting of State parties to assess implementation and is thus unique for core human rights conventions.[57] The Conferences of States Parties are meant to facilitate the implementation of the Convention by drawing together a wide range of actors, including State parties, relevant UN agencies, organizations of persons with disabilities, nongovernmental organizations, and others to provide a forum for discussion and reflection on how to best operationalize the Convention.[58]

NOTES

1. G.A. Res. 217A (III), U.N. Doc. A/810 at 71 (1948).

2. Universal Declaration of Human Rights, Dec. 10, 1948, art. 1, G.A. Res. 217A (III), U.N. Doc A/810 at 71 (1948) [hereinafter UDHR].

3. *Id.* at art. 7.

4. G.A. Res. 2200A, 21 U.N. GAOR, Supp. No. 16 at 52, U.N. Doc. A/6316 (1966).

5. G.A. Res. 2200A, 21 U.N. GAOR, Supp. No. 16 at 49, U.N. Doc. A/6316 (1966).

6. Theresia Degener, *Disabled Persons and Human Rights: The Legal Framework*, in Human Rights and Disabled Persons, *supra* note 6 at 94.

7. *See generally* Louis B. Sohn, *The New International Law: Protection of the Rights of Individuals Rather Than States*, 32 Am. U.L. Rev. 1, 16–17 (1982).

8. *See* CERD, *supra* note 12.

9. *See* CEDAW, *supra* note 12.

10. *See* CRC, *supra* note 7.

11. *See* ICRMW, *supra* note 12.

12. A/58/181, paragraph 11.

13. 1975 Declaration, *supra* note 25.

14. The 1975 Declaration notes that this provision is limited by paragraph 7 of the Declaration of the Rights of Mentally Retarded People 1971.

15. International Year of Disabled Persons, G.A. Res. 36/77, at 176, U.N. GAOR, 36th Sess., Supp. No. 77, U.N. Doc. A/RES/36/77 (December 8, 1981).

16. Implementation of the World Programme of Action Concerning Disabled Persons, G.A. Res. 37/53, at 186–87, paragraph 11, U.N. GAOR, 37th Sess., Supp. No. 53, U.N. Doc. A/RES/37/53 (December 3, 1982).

17. General Assembly Resolution A/RES/48/96, March 4, 1994, which annexed thereto (resolution 48/96 annex, December 20, 1993), found at: http://www.un.org/disabilities/documents/gadocs/standardrules.pdf.

18. *Id.*

19. *Id.* at paragraph 6.

20. *Id.* at paragraph 7.

21. *See* Standard Rules, *supra* note 2, at Purpose and content, paragraph 14.

22. *Id.* at 15.

23. *Id.*

24. *Id.*

25. See Standard Rules, *supra* note 2 at Monitoring mechanism, paragraph 2.

26. CRPD, *supra* note 1.

27. Ad Hoc Comm. on a Comprehensive and Integral International Convention on the Prot. & Promotion of the Rights & Dignity of Pers. with Disabilities, Report of the Working Group to the Ad Hoc Committee, U.N. Doc. A/AC.265/2004/WG.1 paragraph 1 (January 27, 2004). The working group included twelve nongovernmental organizations ("NGOs"). *See id.* at paragraph 2.

28. The Ad Hoc Committee held eight sessions in total, in addition to the January 2004 Working Group meeting. Documents for all sessions are available online at http://www.un.org/esa/socdev/enable/rights/adhoccom.htm. The sessions ran from 2002 until August 2006, after which the adopted draft Convention was submitted to a technical drafting committee to be reviewed and "cleaned" and made ready for submission to the entire General Assembly. More on each session of the ad hoc committee sessions is available online at http://www.un.org/esa/socdev/enable/rights/adhoccom.htm.

29. *See* General Assembly Adopts Groundbreaking Convention, Optional Protocol on Rights of Persons with Disabilities: Delegations, Civil Society Hail First Human Rights Treaty of Twenty-First Century, GA/105554 (United Nations Department of Public Information December 13, 2006), available online at http://www.un.org/News/Press/docs/2006/ga10554.doc.htm.

30. The CRPD text, along with its drafting history, resolutions, and updated list of States Parties is posted on the United Nations Enable website, available online at http://www.un.org/esa/socdev/enable/rights/convtexte.htm. Readers are encouraged to visit this site to obtain more recent information.

31. CRPD, *supra* note 1, at art. 1. For an overview of the CRPD, see UNDESA, OHCHR, IPU, *From Exclusion to Equality: Realizing the Rights of Persons with Disabilities* (2007).

32. *See* Optional Protocol, *supra* note 1.

33. CRPD, *supra* note 1, at art. 1.

34. *See id.*

35. *See* CRPD, *supra* note 1, at art. 10.

36. *See id.* at art. 15.

37. *See id.* at art. 16.
38. *See id.* at art. 24.
39. *See id.* at art. 27.
40. *See id.* at art. 29.
41. *See id.* at art. 12.
42. *See id.* at art. 13.
43. *See id.* at art. 21.
44. *See id.* at art. 22.
45. *See id.* at art. 30.
46. *See id.* at art. 23.
47. *See id.* at art. 17.
48. *See id.* at art. 18.
49. *See id.* at art. 14.
50. *See id.* at art. 28.
51. A recurrent theme echoed throughout the Convention negotiations was the notion that the draft text did not reflect "new" rights but instead articulated existing human rights within the specific context of disability. This view is summarized by the UN Department of Economic and Social Affairs in its question-and-answer resource on the Convention, which states: "The convention does not create any 'new rights' or 'entitlements.' What the convention does, however, is express existing rights in a manner that addresses the needs and situation of persons with disabilities." Convention on the Rights of Persons with Disabilities: Why a Convention?, available online at http://www.un.org/disabilities/convention/questions.shtml#one.
52. *See* CRPD, *supra* note 1, at art. 19.
53. *See id.* at art. 20.
54. *See id.* at art. 26.
55. *See* CRPD, *supra* note 1, at arts. 31–40.
56. *See* Optional Protocol, *supra* note 2.
57. *See id.* at art 40.
58. *See id.*

Index

Contributors

Robert Baker is the William D. Williams Professor of Philosophy at Union College and the director of Union's Rapaport Ethics across the Curriculum initiative. He is also professor of Bioethics and the founding director of the Union Graduate College-Icahn School of Medicine at Mount Sinai Bioethics Program. He has authored/coauthored and edited/coedited numerous books, articles, and reports, including the *American Medical Ethics Revolution* (1999), *The Cambridge World History of Medical Ethics* (2009), and *Before Bioethics: A History of American Medical Ethics from the Colonial Period to the Bioethics Revolution* (2013).

Tom L. Beauchamp is a professor of Philosophy and senior research scholar at the Kennedy Institute of Ethics. His publications include *Principles of Biomedical Ethics* (6th ed., 2009), *The Human Use of Animals* (2nd ed., 2008), *Philosophical Ethics* (3rd ed., 2001), and *A History and Theory of Informed Consent* (1986). He has edited/coedited numerous anthologies and over 150 scholarly articles, as well as *The Oxford Handbook of Animal Ethics* and *The Oxford Handbook of Business Ethics*.

Michael Boylan is a professor of Philosophy and the department chair of Philosophy, Theology, and Religious Studies at Marymount University. He has published twenty-six books and over one hundred articles in philosophy and ethics, including his recent edited volume, *Environmental Ethics* (2nd ed., 2014). He is also the subject of the anthology *Morality and Justice: Reading Boylan's* A Just Society (2009).

Marlene Brant Castellano is a Mohawk of the Bay of Quinte Band and professor emeritus of Trent University, Ontario. As co-director of research with the Royal Commission on Aboriginal Peoples (RCAP), she helped draft the integrated research plan and the Aboriginal subcommittee's draft of RCAP's Ethical Guidelines for Research. Her teaching and research are bicultural, promoting discourse between Aboriginal peoples and academics and policymakers. She is the recipient of the Order of Ontario and a National Aboriginal Achievement Award, and, in 2005, was named an Officer of the Order of Canada.

Cher Weixia Chen is an assistant professor of International Studies, New Century College, George Mason University. She is the author of *Compliance and Compromise: The Jurisprudence of Gender Pay Equity* (2011). Her research focuses on comparative law and human rights, particularly the rights of marginalized groups, such as women's rights, children's rights, and the rights of indigenous people.

Ames Dhai is the director of the Steve Biko Centre for Bioethics, Witwatersrand University, Johannesburg. She is the editor-in-chief of the *South African Journal of Bioethics & Law* and *Bioethics*, coeditor of *Human Rights and Health Law Principles and Practice*, and author of over eighty journal articles. She is president of the South African Medical Association (SAMA) and recipient of SAMA's 2012 Doctors Certificate Award for patriotism, courage, and contributions made in the struggle for the liberation of the medical profession.

Bernard Gert was the late Stone Professor of Intellectual and Moral Philosophy at Dartmouth College. His works include *The Moral Rules: A New Rational Foundation for Morality* (1973), *Morality and the New Genetics: A Guide for Students and Health Care Providers* (1996), and *Common Morality: Deciding What to Do* (2004). He is the coauthor of *Bioethics: A Return to Fundamentals* (1997) and *Bioethics: A Systematic Approach* (2006).

Heather Gert is a visiting associate professor at the University of North Carolina at Chapel Hill. She specializes in ethics, bioethics, metaphysics, epistemology, and Wittgenstein and has numerous publications in these fields.

John-Stewart Gordon is the W1 Professor in Anthropology and Ethics at the Faculty of Human Sciences and codirector of the Hans Jonas Institute at Cologne University, Germany. He has a BA and MA (University of Konstanz, Germany) and PhD (University of Göttingen, Germany). In 2012 he was appointed permanent visiting professor of philosophy at Vytautas Magnus University in Kaunas, Lithuania. He has numerous publications in the field of practical philosophy.

Lawrence O. Gostin is a professor in Global Health Law at Georgetown University, faculty director of the O'Neill Institute for National and Global Health Law, and director of the WHO Collaborating Center on Public Health Law and Human Rights. He drafted a framework convention on global health, a model public health law for WHO and the CDC and the UK's Mental Health Act, and he has argued before the European Court of Human Rights. He was awarded the Rosemary Delbridge Prize for the person most influencing the UK Parliament and government to act for the welfare of society.

Darragh Hare is a doctoral candidate at the Department of Natural Resources at Cornell University. His research focuses on environmental ethics and governance, and in particular on the relationships between humans, other species, and the environment. He is a Fellow of the Royal Society of Art.

Søren Holm holds a chair in Bioethics at the Centre for Social Ethics and Policy at the School of Law, University of Manchester. He has served as editor of the *Journal of Medical Ethics* and has published extensively in the area of medical ethics and philosophy. He is the coeditor of *The Future of Human Reproduction* (1998).

Ilhan Ilkiliç is an associate professor at the Department of History of Medicine and Ethics at the Istanbul University Faculty of Medicine. He has an MD and PhD and has studied medicine, philosophy, Islamic science, and oriental philology in Istanbul, Bochum, and Tübingen. His publications focus on genetics and ethics, cloning, intercultural bioethics, Islamic biomedical ethics, and ethical issues at the end of life. He is a member of the German Ethics Council.

Akiko Ito is the chief of the Secretariat of the Convention on the Rights of Persons with Disabilities/Global Programme on Disability at the United Nations.

Rita Manning is a professor of Philosophy at San Jose State University, California. She has published widely in ethics, applied ethics, and social justice. Her books include *Speaking from the Heart: A Feminist Perspective on Ethics* (1992), the coedited *Social Justice in a Diverse Society* (1996), and coauthored *A Guide to Practical Ethics: Living and Leading with Integrity* (2008).

Peter F. Omonzejele is a senior lecturer in Bioethics and Health Policy at the Department of Philosophy, University of Benin. He is also an international clinical and research ethics consultant and is the head of the Bioethics Research Unit of the Women's Health and Action Research Centre (WHARC) in Benin City. His research interests are cross-cultural bioethics. He is a member of the editorial board of the *Developing World Bioethics Journal* and the author of *The Ethics of Medical Research in Africa* (2012).

Sanghamitra Padhy is an assistant professor of Law and Society at Ramapo College, New Jersey. Her PhD is from the University of Southern California (Law and Public Policy) and her MPhil in Political Studies is from Jawaharlal Nehru University, New Delhi. Her areas of expertise include water rights, natural resources and public policy, and environmental law and ethics in Asia, especially in India and China.

Vibhuti Patel is a professor and director, Centre for the Study of Social Exclusion and Inclusive Policy and head of the Department of Economics at SNDT Women's University, Mumbai, India. She is a member of the advisory board in the Department of Women's Studies of the National Council of Education, Research and Training (NCERT), Delhi, as well as on the expert committee on the School of Gandhian Thoughts, the board of the School of Extension and Development Studies, and the School of Gender and Development Studies for Indira Gandhi Open University.

Pinit Ratanakul is an associate professor and director of the College of Religious Studies, Mahidol University, Thailand. He has a BA (Chulalongkorn University) and a PhD (Yale University). He is a Buddhist scholar who initiated the study of bioethics in Thailand and Southeast Asia and who promotes the study of Buddhism-science relations and dialogue. His research interests include bioethics, religion and science, religion and culture, and religion and psychology.

Alison Dundes Renteln is a professor of political science at the University of Southern California (USC) where she teaches international human rights law and policy. Her PhD in jurisprudence and social policy is from the University of California, Berkeley, and her JD is from USC. Her publications include *The Cultural Defense* (2004); *Cultural Law* (coauthored with James Nafziger and Robert Paterson, 2010); *International Human Rights: Universalism Versus Relativism* (1990, 2013); and three co-edited volumes, *Folk Law* (1994), *Multicultural Jurisprudence* (2009), and *Cultural Diversity and the Law* (2010).

Maya Sabatello is a postdoctoral Fellow at Columbia University's Center for Research on Ethical, Legal, and Social Implications of Psychiatric, Neurologic, and Behavioral Genetics. Since 2006, she has been teaching at NYU's Center for Global Affairs and Columbia University's Institute for the Study of Human Rights. Her publications are in the areas of international and comparative human rights law, disability, public health, and bioethics. She is the author of *Children's Bioethics* (2009), and she is coeditor of *Human Rights and Disability Advocacy* (2013).

Udo Schüklenk is the Ontario Research Chair in Bioethics and Public Policy at Queen's University, Kingston, Ontario. He is a joint editor-in-chief of *Bioethics*, the journal of the International Association of Bioethics. He coauthored with Russell Blackford *50 Great Myths about Atheism* (2013).

Scott David Stonington is a physician and anthropologist (PhD University of California-San Francisco/University of California-Berkeley; MD UCSF). He is a Clinical Fellow in Internal Medicine at Brigham and Women's Hospital, Boston, and a postdoctoral Fellow in Global Health and Social Medicine at Harvard Medical School. His research is based in Thailand and Boston, Massachusetts. The former addresses the globalization of end-of-life care, bioethics, pain management, and

Buddhism, and the latter (in Boston) focuses on medical epistemology and equitable health care. His forthcoming book is *The Spirit Ambulance: Life, Death and Ethical Tension in Thailand.*

Peter Tagore Tan is an associate professor of Philosophy at Mount St. Mary's College, Los Angeles, and West Coast Program Chair for the Association of Informal Logic and Critical Thinking. He has an MA (Boston College) and a PhD (Fordham University). His research interests lie in the area of health equity, global learning, and diversity. He is currently working on an allegory, *The Ascent of Mont Ventoux: Part II.*

Godfrey B. Tangwa is a professor of Philosophy and chair of the Cameroon Bioethics Initiative (CAMBIN), a nongovernmental organization dedicated to bioethics and research ethics in Cameroon and Africa. He has numerous publications in bioethics, with his academic work anchored in Africa. His conviction is that useful theorizing should arise from empirical data while good practice and policy should be informed by and based on a justifiable, coherent theory. He is a member of several professional associations and of many ethics review committees in Cameroon and abroad.

Wanda Teays is a professor and chair of the Philosophy Department at Mount St. Mary's College, Los Angeles. Her publications are in the areas of philosophy, bioethics, and human rights, including torture and interpersonal violence. She is coeditor of *Bioethics, Justice, & Health Care* (2001) and *Violence against Women: Philosophical Perspectives* (1998). She is the author of *Second Thoughts* (4th ed., 2012) and *Seeing the Light: Ethics through Movies* (2013).

Rosemarie Tong is the Distinguished Professor of Health Care Ethics in the Department of Philosophy and former director of the Center for Professional and Applied Ethics at UNC Charlotte. She is internationally known for her work in bioethics and feminist philosophy and has authored or edited thirteen books and over one hundred articles on feminist theory, reproductive and genetic technology, biomedical research, global bioethics, aging, and health care reform.

Cecilia Wee is an associate professor of philosophy at the National University of Singapore. Her research interests are in early modern philosophy, with an emphasis on Descartes, as well as classical Confucianism and environmental ethics. In addition to her many articles she is the author of *Material Falsity and Error in Descartes's Meditations* (2006).

CPSIA information can be obtained at www.ICGtesting.com
Printed in the USA
BVOW04*0657040414

349583BV00004B/9/P